Vascular, Oxidative and Inflammatory Dysregulation in Neurodegenerative Diseases: Current Status and Future Therapeutic Perspectives

Vascular, Oxidative and Inflammatory Dysregulation in Neurodegenerative Diseases: Current Status and Future Therapeutic Perspectives

Editor

Nicoletta Marchesi

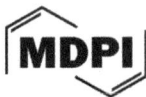

Basel • Beijing • Wuhan • Barcelona • Belgrade • Novi Sad • Cluj • Manchester

Editor
Nicoletta Marchesi
Department of Drug Sciences
University of Pavia
Pavia
Italy

Editorial Office
MDPI
St. Alban-Anlage 66
4052 Basel, Switzerland

This is a reprint of articles from the Special Issue published online in the open access journal *International Journal of Molecular Sciences* (ISSN 1422-0067) (available at: www.mdpi.com/journal/ijms/special_issues/9FJAOU6W54).

For citation purposes, cite each article independently as indicated on the article page online and as indicated below:

Lastname, A.A.; Lastname, B.B. Article Title. *Journal Name* **Year**, *Volume Number*, Page Range.

ISBN 978-3-7258-1434-3 (Hbk)
ISBN 978-3-7258-1433-6 (PDF)
doi.org/10.3390/books978-3-7258-1433-6

© 2024 by the authors. Articles in this book are Open Access and distributed under the Creative Commons Attribution (CC BY) license. The book as a whole is distributed by MDPI under the terms and conditions of the Creative Commons Attribution-NonCommercial-NoDerivs (CC BY-NC-ND) license.

Contents

About the Editor vii

Preface ix

Yizhou Hu, Feng Zhang, Milos Ikonomovic and Tuo Yang
The Role of NRF2 in Cerebrovascular Protection: Implications for Vascular Cognitive Impairment and Dementia (VCID)
Reprinted from: *Int. J. Mol. Sci.* **2024**, *25*, 3833, doi:10.3390/ijms25073833 1

Angela Dziedzic, Karina Maciak, Elżbieta Dorota Miller, Michał Starosta and Joanna Saluk
Targeting Vascular Impairment, Neuroinflammation, and Oxidative Stress Dynamics with Whole-Body Cryotherapy in Multiple Sclerosis Treatment
Reprinted from: *Int. J. Mol. Sci.* **2024**, *25*, 3858, doi:10.3390/ijms25073858 23

Daria Gendosz de Carrillo, Olga Kocikowska, Małgorzata Rak, Aleksandra Krzan, Sebastian Student and Halina Jedrzejowska-Szypułka et al.
The Relevance of Reperfusion Stroke Therapy for miR-9-3p and miR-9-5p Expression in Acute Stroke—A Preliminary Study
Reprinted from: *Int. J. Mol. Sci.* **2024**, *25*, 2766, doi:10.3390/ijms25052766 41

Eveljn Scarian, Camilla Viola, Francesca Dragoni, Rosalinda Di Gerlando, Bartolo Rizzo and Luca Diamanti et al.
New Insights into Oxidative Stress and Inflammatory Response in Neurodegenerative Diseases
Reprinted from: *Int. J. Mol. Sci.* **2024**, *25*, 2698, doi:10.3390/ijms25052698 67

Yuewei Chen, Peiwen Lu, Shengju Wu, Jie Yang, Wanwan Liu and Zhijun Zhang et al.
CD163-Mediated Small-Vessel Injury in Alzheimer's Disease: An Exploration from Neuroimaging to Transcriptomics
Reprinted from: *Int. J. Mol. Sci.* **2024**, *25*, 2293, doi:10.3390/ijms25042293 89

Nicoletta Marchesi, Pasquale Linciano, Lucrezia Irene Maria Campagnoli, Foroogh Fahmideh, Daniela Rossi and Giosuè Costa et al.
Short- and Long-Term Regulation of HuD: A Molecular Switch Mediated by Folic Acid?
Reprinted from: *Int. J. Mol. Sci.* **2023**, *24*, 12201, doi:10.3390/ijms241512201 109

Giovanni Napoli, Martina Rubin, Gianni Cutillo, Paride Schito, Tommaso Russo and Angelo Quattrini et al.
Tako-Tsubo Syndrome in Amyotrophic Lateral Sclerosis: Single-Center Case Series and Brief Literature Review
Reprinted from: *Int. J. Mol. Sci.* **2023**, *24*, 12096, doi:10.3390/ijms241512096 122

Caterina Claudia Lepre, Marina Russo, Maria Consiglia Trotta, Francesco Petrillo, Fabiana Anna D'Agostino and Gennaro Gaudino et al.
Inhibition of Galectins and the P2X7 Purinergic Receptor as a Therapeutic Approach in the Neurovascular Inflammation of Diabetic Retinopathy
Reprinted from: *Int. J. Mol. Sci.* **2023**, *24*, 9721, doi:10.3390/ijms24119721 130

Katarzyna Pawletko, Halina Jedrzejowska-Szypułka, Katarzyna Bogus, Alessia Pascale, Foroogh Fahmideh and Nicoletta Marchesi et al.
After Ischemic Stroke, Minocycline Promotes a Protective Response in Neurons via the RNA-Binding Protein HuR, with a Positive Impact on Motor Performance
Reprinted from: *Int. J. Mol. Sci.* **2023**, *24*, 9446, doi:10.3390/ijms24119446 150

Mirco Masi, Fabrizio Biundo, André Fiou, Marco Racchi, Alessia Pascale and Erica Buoso
The Labyrinthine Landscape of APP Processing: State of the Art and Possible Novel Soluble APP-Related Molecular Players in Traumatic Brain Injury and Neurodegeneration
Reprinted from: *Int. J. Mol. Sci.* **2023**, *24*, 6639, doi:10.3390/ijms24076639 . . . . **173**

About the Editor

Nicoletta Marchesi

In 2008, Dr. Marchesi obtained a degree in Biology, University of Pavia, Italy. In 2010, Nicoletta was awarded cum laude in Experimental and Applied Biology, University of Pavia, Italy. From 2010 to 2013, Nicoletta completed the Ph.D. with IUSS fellowship at the Department of Drug Science, Cellular and Molecular Neuropharmacology Group with supervision from Professor Govoni Stefano, University of Pavia, Italy. From August 2013 to October 2013, Nicoletta completed an FBML fellowship in Ophthalmology Unit Research with supervision from Professor Kaarniranta Kai, University of Eastern Finland, Kuopio. From October 2015 to June 2017, Nicoletta was a research assistant at NeuHeart Srl. From 2017 to 2023, Nicoletta completed the post-doc at the Department of Drug Science, Cellular and Molecular Neuropharmacology Group with supervision from Professors Govoni Stefano and Pascale Alessia, University of Pavia. From July 2023 to present, Nicoletta is involved in RTDa.

Her research interests are the study and characterization of proteins able to bind specific mRNA, particularly ELAV proteins. This includes studying a particular ELAV, HuR, which is involved in the post-transcriptional regulation of key proteins involved in the AMD (in Finland), diabetic retinopathy, and autophagy. She is also interested in the molecular and cellular changes following the silencing of a protein ELAV neuronal, HuD, in neuroblastoma cells. Regarding HuD, she studies its involvement in neurodegenerative disorders and its correlation with BDNF and GAP-43. During SpinOff, she analysed the concentrations of NGF in human serum samples derived from patients with heart failure, conducted a novel in vitro experiment with IVTech Bioreactors, and utilized an in vitro model to test new molecules (drug discovery). She also investigated the role of microbiota and dietary supplements in different fields: glaucoma, pain, and neurodegenerative disorders. From 2021, she has been a member of RedyNeuheart s.r.l., a biotech start-up focused on new molecules and new drug targets for known molecules in pai. She is interested in the discovery of new mechanism-based targets for integrators for nociplastic pain.

Preface

Dear Colleagues,

A new report from the World Health Organization (WHO) shows that neurological disorders affect up to one billion people worldwide. Neurological disorders are medically defined as disorders that affect the brain as well as the nerves found throughout the human body and the spinal cord. Structural, biochemical, or electrical abnormalities in the brain, spinal cord, or other nerves can result in a range of symptoms. Some of the most common are epilepsy, Alzheimer's and other dementias, stroke, migraine, multiple sclerosis, Parkinson's disease, Amyotrophic lateral sclerosis, polyneuropathies, neurological infections, brain tumours, traumatic conditions of the nervous system such as head injuries, and disorders caused by malnutrition or by an imbalance in metabolism such as diabetes (i.e., diabetic retinopathy).

In this Special Issue for *IJMS*, we will focus on new discoveries and treatments of neurological disorders. New therapies in this area must be aimed at improving the quality of life, symptoms, and treatment of the disease itself.

Thanks to all the scientists and colleagues who decided and chose this Special Issue.

Nicoletta Marchesi
Editor

The Role of NRF2 in Cerebrovascular Protection: Implications for Vascular Cognitive Impairment and Dementia (VCID)

Yizhou Hu [1,2,3], Feng Zhang [1,2], Milos Ikonomovic [1,4,5] and Tuo Yang [1,2,6,*]

1. Department of Neurology, University of Pittsburgh, Pittsburgh, PA 15216, USA; huy5@upmc.edu (Y.H.); zhanfx2@upmc.edu (F.Z.); ikonomovicmd@upmc.edu (M.I.)
2. Pittsburgh Institute of Brain Disorders and Recovery, University of Pittsburgh, Pittsburgh, PA 15216, USA
3. Department of Internal Medicine, University of Pittsburgh Medical Center (UPMC) McKeesport, McKeesport, PA 15132, USA
4. Department of Psychiatry, University of Pittsburgh, Pittsburgh, PA 15216, USA
5. Geriatric Research Education and Clinical Center, VA Pittsburgh Healthcare System, Pittsburgh, PA 15240, USA
6. Department of Internal Medicine, University of Pittsburgh Medical Center (UPMC), Pittsburgh, PA 15216, USA
* Correspondence: yangt@upmc.edu

Abstract: Vascular cognitive impairment and dementia (VCID) represents a broad spectrum of cognitive decline secondary to cerebral vascular aging and injury. It is the second most common type of dementia, and the prevalence continues to increase. Nuclear factor erythroid 2-related factor 2 (NRF2) is enriched in the cerebral vasculature and has diverse roles in metabolic balance, mitochondrial stabilization, redox balance, and anti-inflammation. In this review, we first briefly introduce cerebrovascular aging in VCID and the NRF2 pathway. We then extensively discuss the effects of NRF2 activation in cerebrovascular components such as endothelial cells, vascular smooth muscle cells, pericytes, and perivascular macrophages. Finally, we summarize the clinical potential of NRF2 activators in VCID.

Keywords: aging; blood–brain barrier; oxidative stress; neuroinflammation; perivascular macrophage; lymphatic system

1. Introduction

Vascular cognitive impairment and dementia (VCID), an age-related neurodegenerative disorder, is the second most common cause of dementia after Alzheimer's disease with no available treatment yet [1]. VCID accounts for approximately 20% of dementia cases in the developed world such as North America and Europe, with an even higher percentage in the developing world and Asia [2–4]. The prevalence of VCID rises rapidly with increasing age. It is estimated that 1.6% of individuals over 65 years old are suffering from VCID, and the figure increases up to 5.2% among those over 90 years old [2]. In an epidemiological study, the disability-adjusted life year (DALY), a parameter that measures the number of years lost due to illness, disability, or early death, has been estimated as 316 per 100,000 person-years for vascular dementia, and the years of life lived with disability as 85 per 100,000 [5]. It has been estimated that VCID patients have the highest annual cost of care among dementia patients [6]. Hypoperfusion due to vascular dysfunction is the key pathophysiology of VCID [7]. In fact, vascular pathology is fairly common in all types of dementia, and is present in up to 75% of dementia patients upon autopsy [8].

Nuclear factor erythroid 2-related factor 2 (NRF2) plays a crucial protective role in oxidative stress and inflammation [9]. NRF2/Kelch-like ECH-associated protein 1 (Keap1)–antioxidant response element (ARE) signaling is potentially the most important regulation in redox homeostasis [10–12]. NRF2 has robust potential for attenuating oxidative and hemodynamic stress in cardiovascular diseases [13]. In this regard, NRF2 is essential for protecting microvasculature, especially when under oxidative stress [14].

In this review article, we first briefly introduce the concept of cerebrovascular aging in VCID and the NRF2 pathway. We then more extensively address the effects of NRF2 in cerebrovascular components such as endothelial cells (ECs), vascular smooth muscle cells (VSMCs), pericytes, and perivascular macrophages (PVMs). Finally, we summarize the clinical potentials of the currently available NRF2 activators in VCID.

2. An Overview of Vascular Aging in VCID and the NRF2 Pathway

2.1. Cerebrovascular Aging in VCID

The term VCID needs clarification due to the inconsistent and often interchangeable use of the terms vascular dementia (VaD), vascular cognitive impairment (VCI), and vascular cognitive impairment and dementia (VCID), which has been addressed in detail by John et al. [1]. VCI is a recently coined term referring to cognitive impairment caused predominantly by cerebrovascular diseases. It includes a wide spectrum of diseases ranging from mild cognitive impairment to VaD [15]. VaD refers to a broader variant of VCI where disruption to daily activities is present. In the present review, we use the term VCID, which encompasses the full range of disease severity.

Several risk factors have been identified for VCID, with aging and vascular disease considered the most important. Female sex, hypertension, stroke, and brain atrophy on structural magnetic resonance imaging (MRI) also play a role [2,16–19]. Deterioration of vascular function at different levels of the cerebral vasculature, especially structural components of the blood–brain barrier (BBB) (Figure 1), can occur in normal aging and is associated with dementia [20]. Although accounting for only 2% of body mass, the brain consumes 20% of oxygen and 25% of glucose [21]. Due to the limited ability of the brain to store energy, a constant and sufficient blood supply is essential for the brain to carry out complex and highly energy-consuming tasks [22]. The exchange of nutrients and metabolic waste products occurs predominantly at the capillary level of the brain vasculature [21]. Mounting evidence suggests that aging-related dysfunction of brain microvasculature contributes to neurodegeneration [23–26].

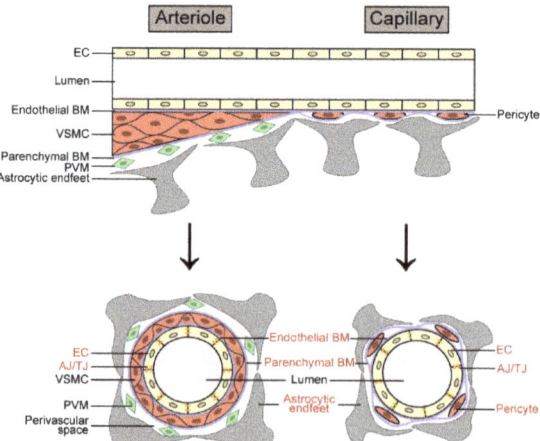

Figure 1. Schematic image showing cell types and structure of the arteriole and capillary/venule levels of the cerebral vasculature. In the lower panel, structural components of the blood–brain barrier are labeled in red. Abbreviations: AJ—adherens junction; BM—basement membrane; EC—endothelial cell; TJ—tight junction; PVM—perivascular macrophage; VSMC—vascular smooth muscle cell.

VCI can be caused by the "entire spectrum of vascular brain pathology" including infarcts, hemorrhages, and diffuse hypoperfusion [27]. The pathobiology of VCID is highly complex, and most commonly involves brain infarcts and white matter (WM) injury [28,29]. Cerebral infarction due to large vessel atherosclerosis and arteriolosclerosis with microbleeds both contribute to the development of VCID [1], with direct tissue injury playing a major role. At autopsy, up to 80% of patients with dementia demonstrate evidence of vascular pathology [30]. Macrovascular infarcts are historically recognized as the major pathophysiology of VCID and are associated with a higher risk of dementia [31]. On the other hand, microvascular infarcts are more common in VCID patients [27,32]; they are present in 20–40% of individuals aged 80 years or older [33] and in nearly half (48.0%) of dementia patients at autopsy [34]. The reasons why microvascular infarcts can cause cognitive impairment are not fully understood, but may involve inappropriate immune response and impairments in waste protein removal [35–37] and cerebral hypoperfusion [38]. According to Costantino et al., there are multiple mechanisms that can explain the pathophysiology of cognitive impairment in diseases such as VCID, including WM infarction, BBB breakdown, oxidative stress, inflammation, trophic uncoupling, demyelination and remyelination, neurovascular coupling dysfunction, and disposal of unwanted proteins. The current review focuses on several of these mechanisms to address how NRF2 can play a role in fighting against VCID.

In addition to gray matter injury, WM injury can negatively affect the cognitive function of the brain, as the latter is critical for fidelity and precision of information transfer [39]. Compared to gray matter, WM is more vulnerable to ischemia insult because of its physiologically lower perfusion and grey matter steal [40]. WM lesions are very common in VCID, and their presentation on MRI scans in the form of WM hyperintensities is regarded as the hallmark of small vessel diseases [41–43].

Aging is inevitable and irreversible [44]. As an organ mostly composed of postmitotic cells such as neurons and oligodendrocytes, the brain is especially vulnerable to DNA damage which increases and accumulates with advanced aging [44,45]. The association between neuroinflammation and neurodegeneration has been consistently reported. Chronic inflammation, primarily in response to DNA damage, produces excessive reactive oxygen species (ROS) and accelerates the process of age-related neurodegenerative diseases and aging itself [44,46,47]. On top of that, mitochondrial dysfunction is one of the antagonistic responses to DNA damage. Although initially compensatory, the overwhelming ROS production beyond the mitochondrial compensatory capacity eventually increases NF-κB signaling and causes chronic inflammation, which leads to further damage and tissue degeneration [44,48]. Indeed, in a recent VCID study imperatorin was found to reduce mitochondrial membrane potential and thereby ameliorate cobalt chloride-mediated primary hippocampal neuronal damage dependent on the NRF2 signaling pathway [49].

2.2. An Overview of the NRF2 Pathway and Its Implications in VCID

NRF2 plays an essential role in the regulation of redox hemostasis and protection of endothelial cells, potentially by targeting ARE-regulated antioxidants through a variety of downstream players such as heme oxygenase-1 (HO-1) and NAD(P)H quinone dehydrogenase 1 [10,50]. Keap1 is the major regulator controlling the activation of NRF2/ARE (Figure 2). Details on the NRF2/Keap1 pathway and its regulation have been thoroughly reviewed by us and other groups elsewhere [51–54]. In brief, in non-stress conditions, NRF2 is sequestered by the Cul3-Keap1 complex in the cytosol and subjected to proteasomal degradation. NRF2 can be released in response to oxidative stress and subsequently translocated to the nucleus, serving as a transcription factor for downstream antioxidant genes [55,56]. The deactivation of NRf2 is regulated by negative feedback, where NRF2 accumulation induces the expression of the Rbx1-Cul3-Keap1 complex, leading to rapid elimination and deactivation of NRF2 [57]. It is worth mentioning that activation of NRF2/HO-1 also leads to downregulation of proinflammatory cytokines and ameliorates systemic inflammation [58]. The interplay between NRF2 and nuclear factor (NF)-κB tunes the equilibrium of oxidation and inflammation [59,60]. NRF2 regulates inflammation through downregulation of proinflammatory gene expression such as interleukin (IL)-1β and IL-6 and upregulation of anti-inflammatory factors such as HO-1.

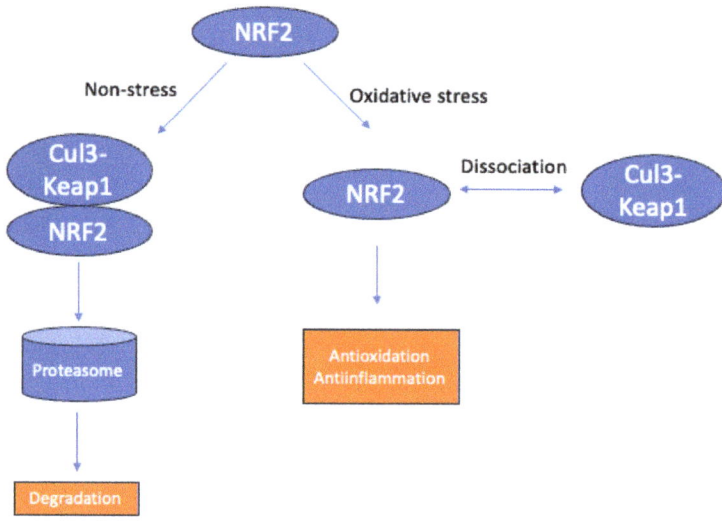

Figure 2. Simplified schematic image of the NRF2/Keap1 pathway.

NRF2 activity is positively related to species longevity, and NRF2 dysfunction plays an essential role in aging [61]. Indeed, multiple age-related transcriptomic changes, such as proteinopathy, have been observed in NRF2-knockout mice [47]. Accumulating evidence suggests that NRF2 expression and activity decrease in an age-dependent manner [62–64]. Similar results were reported in rat and Rhesus monkey aorta organoid cultures [65,66]. In rat livers, NRF2 expression has been confirmed to decrease in an age-dependent manner [62], while the opposite has been observed in the brain, liver, and lungs of young mice [67]. Although NRF2 expression may increase or decrease with age, studies have consistently reported declining efficiency of NRF2 signaling with aging, which is related to decreased antioxidant response [68]. A possible explanation for this is that an age-dependent increase in NRF2 protein levels serves as an internal compensatory mechanism in early aging, while later on a decline in NRF2 expression ensues. In fact, given the multifaceted involvement of the NRF2/KEAP1 pathway in aging physiology and disease pathology, this pathway is currently an emerging hot topic in many fields, including but not limited to metabolic disorders, degenerative disorders, inflammatory disorders, and cancerous disorders [69–72]. Therefore, it is reasonable to propose that activating NRF2 may be a potential approach to managing age-related and vascular-oriented neurodegenerative disorders such as VCID.

Aging is in a close relationship with vascular dysfunction in both primates and rodents [65,66]. Chronic inflammation has been observed in normal aging, leading to damage and microvascular barrier dysfunction, which might in turn accelerate brain aging [73], forming a vicious cycle. Because NRF2 plays a role in BBB preservation [59] and mitigates inflammation through complex interactions with nuclear factor (NF)-κB signaling, NRF2 may be a promising target for vascular protection in VCID [59]. In addition, the aging process can potentially be slowed down by NAD-dependent enzymes such as SIRT1 that serve to protect the endothelium from oxidative stress [74]. In light of the complex interconnection between NRF2 and SIRT1, it is highly likely that targeting NRF2 might also mitigate vascular aging indirectly through regulating SIRT1 signaling [75–77]. The following review of NRF2 functions in different cell types in the brain vasculature is intended to provide a better understanding of its protective role in VCID (Figure 3).

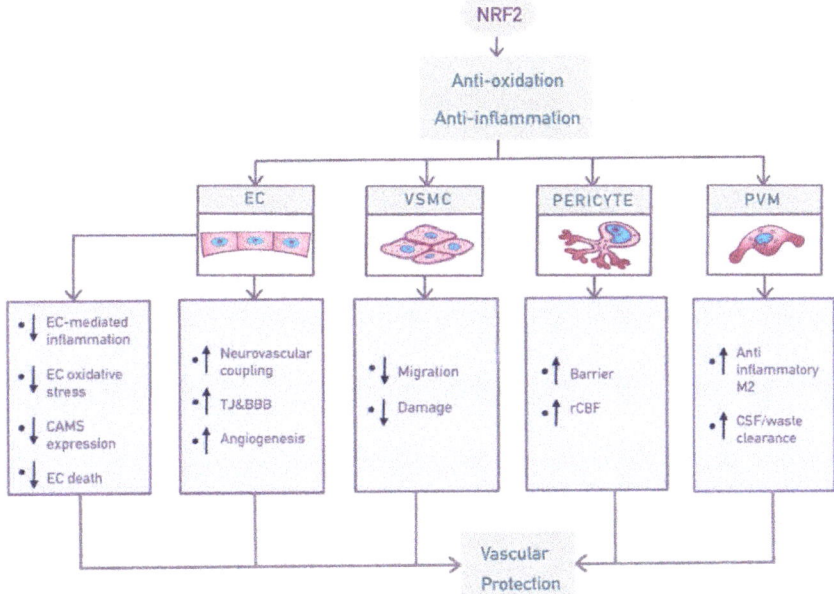

Figure 3. Schematic image showing NRF2 effects in different cell types of the cerebral vasculature in VCID. BBB, blood–brain barrier; CAM, cell adhesion molecule; CSF, cerebrospinal fluid; EC, endothelial cell; PVM, perivascular macrophage; rCBF, regional cerebral blood flow; TJ, tight junction; VSMC, vascular smooth muscle cell. ↑: increase/upregulate. ↓: decrease/downregulate.

3. Effects of NRF2 in Vasculature Components

3.1. Endothelial Cells (ECs)

ECs line the lumen of blood vessels and play multiple roles in permeability, inflammation, thrombosis, and regulation of blood flow [78]. In particular, cerebrovascular ECs line the border between the central nervous system (CNS) and the periphery, playing important roles in BBB function and neuroinflammation [79]. One of the earliest manifestations of vascular aging is impaired endothelial-dependent vasodilation function [80]. ECs regulate blood flow by releasing vasodilators such as nitric oxide (NO), and dysfunction of this process plays a major role in the pathophysiology of VCID.

3.1.1. Role of ECs in Inflammation and Oxidative Stress

Inflammation and oxidative stress are important in the pathophysiology of VCID, where aging alone leads to low-grade inflammation [59]. The inflammatory cascade starts with proinflammatory cytokines such as tumor necrosis factor (TNF)-α and IL-1β [60], which subsequently increase ROS production (serving as a major source of oxidative stress [10]) and represent the hallmark of vascular aging [20,59]. ECs play a pivotal role in the inflammatory processes. ECs per se can be activated by proinflammatory molecules such as TNF-α and IL-1, and respond by producing NO and prostaglandin I_2 which increase the leakiness of venules [81]. ECs can also respond to chronic inflammation with angiogenesis [82–84]. In addition, leukocyte and macromolecule extravasation during inflammation penetrates ECs either intracellularly or transcellularly through EC junction proteins [85]

ROS are produced through complex enzyme-mediated processes during aging and cerebral hypoperfusion, and mitochondria are considered their major source [86–90]. Alteration of mitochondrial metabolism causes excessive generation of ROS due to interruption of the electron transport chain [91]. Recent studies have demonstrated that NRF2-Keap1 senses the ROS produced by mitochondria, and it has been suggested that NRF2 plays a role in regulating mitochondrial ROS [92]. Indeed, upregulation of HO-1, a downstream effector of NRF2, has been found to prevent H_2O_2-mediated cytotoxicity [50].

NFR2 is related to decreased EC inflammation as well. For example, overexpression of NRF2 through adenoviral transduction significantly decreased expression levels of proinflammatory cytokines, including TNF-α and vascular cell adhesion molecule-1 (VCAM-1), and remarkably increased the expression of antioxidant proteins such as HO-1 and glutathione in aortic EC cultures [93]. NRF2 improved brain EC permeability by reducing inflammation in an in vitro model [94]. As a downstream effector of NRF2, targeted expression of HO-1 demonstrated atheroprotective effects in low-density lipoprotein-receptor knockout mice [95].

3.1.2. Cell Adhesion Molecules (CAMs)

During chronic hypoperfusion and VCID, CAMs are upregulated on EC surfaces to facilitate white blood cell extravasation [96–98]. Proinflammatory cytokines such as TNF-α and IL-1β induce upregulation of CAMs such as intracellular cell adhesion molecule-1 (ICAM-1) and VCAM-1 on ECs [99,100]. Therefore, CAMs are important molecules for leukocyte recruitment, which generates oxidative stress and inflammation.

NRF2 may play a protective role in decreasing CAM expression induced by TNF-α [101]. In a mouse model of brain ischemia, NRF2 was found to confer protection by suppressing CAM upregulation in brain EC [102]. In traumatic brain injury (TBI), NRF2 knockdown was found to activate NF-κB and induce proinflammatory cytokines secretion, and resulted in overexpression of CAMs such as ICAL-1 [103]. In human umbilical vein ECs, hydroxyanthranilic acid was found to upregulate NRF2 translocation and subsequently induce HO-1 expression in association with reduced VCAM-1 expression [104]. In cancer studies, NRF2 was found to downregulate the expression of E-cadherin [105]. These findings demonstrate the universal and crucial role that NRF2 plays in regulating CAMs and CAM-induced inflammation.

3.1.3. Neurovascular Coupling (NVC)

Blood flow control is regulated by different cells in different blood vessels. In large arteries, lumen diameter control is endothelial-dependent [106,107]. In small arteries and arterioles, vascular smooth muscle cells control the lumen diameter [108]. The term NVC describes the phenomenon that increasing neural activity leads to increasing local blood supply [109]. EC-dependent NO synthesis and release serve as the predominant modulator of local cerebral blood flow (CBF) for normal NVC functioning [110].

NO synthase (NOS) is critical for matching regional CBF with neural activities, as NOS inhibitors can reduce NVC response by 30% in humans [111]. In addition, endothelial NOS (eNOS) activity is essential for EC proliferation, pericyte recruitment, and angiogenesis after ischemia injury in vivo [112,113]. Aging is related to decreased levels of NO and antioxidant enzymes, and impaired vasodilation is a typical manifestation of aging [20,114–117]. In addition, chronic brain hypoperfusion is associated with EC dysfunction leading to NVC failure, which is also responsible for WM lesions [97,98]. Impaired NVC is a key pathobiology in neurodegenerations such as VCID [38,118–120]. Therefore, maintenance and restoration of normal EC functioning is critical for NVC and VCID management.

EC dysfunction and chronic hypoperfusion are closely associated with oxidative stress, and are modulated by the balance between ROS and NO [10]. ROS inhibits the activity of eNOS, decreasing the level of NO and eventually compromising EC-mediated vasodilation [121]. As we previously described, NRF2 plays a vital role in facilitating NVC by modulating eNOS and tetrahydrobiopterin [59].

It is worth noting that vasodilation is one of the primary pathobiological events during tissue inflammation, and NO is the primary vasorelaxant [83,122]. NO directly facilitates acute inflammation by vasodilation, increasing endothelial permeability and angiogenesis [83]; therefore, it is recognized as a marker of acute inflammation. Proper control of NO levels to allow appropriate vasodilation without compromising its integrity is critical for maintaining normal NVC function.

3.1.4. Junction Protein and BBB

BBB breakdown has been observed in numerous neurodegenerative diseases, including VCID, and may contribute to early stages of cognitive dysfunction [123,124]. The breakdown of BBB leads to neurotoxic chemicals entering the brain and tissue inflammation arising from leukocyte extravasation into the brain parenchyma [125–127]. Junction proteins such as the adherens junction (AJ) and tight junction (TJ) are critical for BBB function and participate in regulating the paracellular permeability for the diffusion of water, ions, and small molecules [59,128,129]. The production of TJ proteins relies on normal mitochondrial and NVU function, both of which are vulnerable to oxidative stress [130–133]. Indeed, decreased expression of claudin-5 protein, the most enriched TJ protein, is observed in ECs with NRF2-knockdown [134,135].

Chronic inflammation and atherosclerosis, which typically accompany VCID, cause excessive blood coagulation, which leads to EC damage and BBB disruption [136]. Subsequent release of cytokines, including vascular endothelial growth factor (VEGF), can further disrupt cerebral vasculature, forming a vicious cycle [137,138]. Chronic cerebral hypoperfusion is directly related to TJ loss, as the release of proinflammatory cytokines such as TNF-α can upregulate the apoptosis signaling–regulating kinase 1 (ASK1), leading to angiotensin II-related EC apoptosis and degeneration of TJ proteins such as claudin and occludin [139,140]. This process could contribute to VCI, as it has been shown that inhibiting ASK1 activation can alleviate memory loss in VaD mice [141].

NRF2 is important for BBB integrity. In vitro models have demonstrated BBB disruption in NRF2 knockout samples, along with reduced expression of junction proteins such as occludin and claudin-5 [134,142]. Through promoter analysis, NRF2 seems to be able to directly target the claudin-5 gene and contribute to stable BBB integrity [134]. Interestingly, obese mice lacking NRF2 have a higher degree of BBB disruption along with a significant increase in blood protein leakage, which is associated with a higher level of oxidative stress [14]. Sulforaphane (Sfn), a potent NRF2 activator, has demonstrated a protective effect against claudin-5 loss through an NRF2-dependent pathway in VCID mice [134,143]. Sfn has proven effective in protecting BBB in stroke and TBI models [144]. Importantly, such a protective effect of Sfn is lacking in NRF2 knockdown mice, supporting a pivotal role of NRF2 in the protection of the BBB [143,145]. Mechanistically, NRF2 directly acts on the promoters of the claudin-5 and VE-cadherin genes, as evidenced by promoter analysis and promoter activity studies [134,144].

Interestingly, in a study with a VCID rat model, oral administration of *Artemisia annua Linné*, a plant harboring antioxidant properties, helped to maintain BBB integrity by increasing platelet-derived growth factor (PDGF) receptor β and platelet-endothelial CAM-1 levels associated with NRF2/Keap1 pathway [145], although CAMs are generally believed to be inflammatory markers and may lead to BBB breakdown.

3.1.5. Cell Death and Angiogenesis

NRF2 dysfunction results in increased ROS-mediated EC apoptosis [65,66,146]. Aging-associated NRF2 dysfunction causes significant endothelial apoptosis and vascular rarefaction [65,147–151]. Without a properly functioning NRF2, ECs lose their protection against physiological ROS production, becoming more vulnerable to pro-apoptotic factors such as H_2O_2 or high glucose, as observed in an obesity mouse model [152].

Mitochondrial protection is another important mechanism in NRF2 antiapoptotic function. NRF2 takes part in mitophagy by upregulating PINK1 or p62 expression. NRF2 also plays a role in mitochondrial biogenesis, which compensates for the natural loss of mitochondria, by modulating the expression of related mitochondrial genes [153]. As the upstream gene of NRF2, PI3K/Akt plays an important role during oxidative stress by upregulating NRF-2/HO-1 expression. On the other hand, extracellular regulated kinase (ERK) works directly on the dissociation of NRF2 and Keap1 by phosphorylation of NRF2, which promotes the transcription of NRF2 and thereby upregulates HO-1 expression. PI3/Akt and ERK work together to tune the expression of NRF2. Hypoxia activates PI3K/AKT, while HIF-1α is regulated by ERK1/2. In a lung tissue injury model induced by cerebral ischemia/reperfusion in rats, PI3K and ERK levels were significantly higher compared to the sham group and trended consistently with NRF2/HO-1 [154]. In another study using a rat ischemia/reperfusion model, brain endothelial cells responded to oxidative stress with increased NRF2/HO-1 levels through ERK and Akt phosphorylation [155].

Angiogenesis is an important rescue pathway under the circumstances of hypoperfusion. Evidence suggests that angiogenesis occurs at the same time as neurogenesis and synaptogenesis after ischemic brain injury [156,157]. In angiogenesis, angiogenic growth factors such as VEGF and insulin-like growth factor activate NRF2 at the level of both expression and transcription, the latter of which is likely achieved by activating Akt1 [158,159]. NRF2, on the other hand, promotes angiogenesis by regulating the serine/threonine domain of growth factor receptor [160]. ROS act as a double-edged sword for endothelial angiogenesis [161]. At the physiological level, ROS are essential, and may have a beneficial effect during the tissue repair process by regulating angiogenesis [162]. Acting as signaling molecules, ROS take part in angiogenesis and maintain newly formed blood vessels [163–165]. Mechanistically, ROS upregulate angiogenic factors such as VEGF and promote the response of these factors by upregulating their receptors [166–168]. On the other hand, pathological levels of ROS may exceed the antioxidant capacity and result in cell death. Moreover, excessive ROS levels are involved in pathological angiogenesis such as in cancer and atherosclerosis [169].

Studies in different models have consistently proved that NRF2 promotes angiogenesis in many organs. For example, knockdown of NRF2 or overexpression of Keap1 impaired angiogenic processes in human coronary artery EC cultures, with abnormal EC adhesion, migration, and microtubule formation [152]. In cardiac microvascular ECs, NRF2 knockdown was associated with reduced VEGF expression level [170]. In the developing retina, NRF2 deficiency reduced angiogenic sprouting and vascular density [171]. In a rodent model of myocardial infarction, resveratrol, an NRF2 activator, promoted angiogenesis [172–174]. In VCID models, resveratrol has shown the ability to improve NVC responses by restoring EC function and subsequently improving cognitive function in aging mice [175]. Mechanistically, NRF is critical to preserving mitochondrial structural and functional integrity in ECs [176,177], in particular endothelial progenitor cells [178].

In light of the complicated and dual-directional role of ROS in regulating angiogenesis, the extent to which ROS should be eliminated by NRF2 activity is an important issue to consider. Unfortunately, the vast majority of studies have not addressed this concern. In addition, the time window for manipulating angiogenesis might be a critical issue. For example, in the retinopathy of a prematurity model where retinal vessel obliteration was present due to hyperoxia-mediated oxidative stress, Nrf2 was found to be critical for preserving the retinal vessels in P9 mice, but not in those after P12 [179].

3.2. Vascular Smooth Muscle Cell (VSMC)

Impaired CBF contributes to cognitive dysfunction, as decreased baseline CBF has been shown to correlate with the severity of cognitive impairment [180]. Atherosclerosis and arteriosclerosis both contribute to the development of VCID [1]; however, dementia caused solely by vascular pathology is rare, and results mostly from large vessel disease, while small vessel disease accounts for most milder forms of VCID [1].

Contractile VSMC phenotype, as its name suggests, controls blood vessel diameters by relaxation and contraction [181]. The local renin–angiotensin (Ang) system (RAS) is critical in vasoconstriction, while NO plays a pivotal role in vasodilation [182,183]. RAS changes contribute to neurodegenerative diseases such as Parkinson's disease, while Ang II can promote inflammation by producing ROS [184,185]. Synthetic VSMC phenotype, on the contrary, has lower contractile phenotype-related protein expression but is active in the synthesis of proinflammatory factors and matrix proteins as well as in proteins associated with migration and proliferation [181]. Synthetic VSMCs such as H_2O_2 proliferate after ischemic arterial injury mediated by ROS [186], which in turn narrows the lumen, leading to reduced CBF. Additionally, they secrete inflammatory factors such as IL-6, indirectly disrupting BBB integrity [187]. Indeed, oral administration of an ROS scavenger reduced proinflammatory cytokines in synthetic VSMCs in a traumatic carotid injury model [55].

Limited evidence is present on the role of NRF2 in VSMCs in VCID. Ang II could induce abnormal proliferation of VSMCs through NADPH-oxidase-mediated ROS production and inflammation, which has been proven to exacerbate pre-existing vascular damage and accelerate atherosclerosis [188]. NRF2 demonstrates antiproliferative effects and is capable of suppressing VSMC migration through the NOX4/ROS/NRF2 pathway. NRF2 depletion, on the other hand, enhanced ROS-dependent VSMC migration upon PDGF stimulation [189,190]. Another research studying the relationship between NRF2 and abdominal aortic aneurysm (AAA) showed similar results; increased NFR2 degradation by Keap1 overexpression resulted in tremendous VSMC-mediated inflammatory factor expression, which subsequently disrupted the aortic structure and led to AAA formation [191,192].

3.3. Pericytes—Oxidative Stress and Microvascular Barrier Dysfunction

Pericytes are closely associated with microvasculature, in line with their distribution in small vessels such as arterioles, capillaries, and venules [193]. Pericytes play an essential role in maintaining BBB integrity and in regulating vascular permeability, angiogenesis, capillary diameters, and blood flow, as well as in the removal of toxic metabolites [194,195].

3.3.1. Barrier Function

The location and contractile nature of pericytes suggests their function in regulating microvascular permeability. Increased vascular permeability in the setting of inflammation mostly occurs at the level of venules, the majority of which are surrounded by pericytes. In an in vitro lung pericyte/EC co-culture study, pericytes were proven to serve as an additional barrier compared to EC alone [73]. Permeability of water and a range of different molecular weight tracers were significantly increased in pericyte-deficient mice [194,196,197], suggesting that pericytes may serve as a means of salvage to prevent a higher degree of leakage when EC dysfunction occurs [73]. Several potential mechanisms have been proposed. First, pericytes participate in BBB maintenance, which is highly dependent on redox balance. In a mouse model of hypoglycemia-mediated cognitive dysfunction, both pericyte loss and BBB leakage were restored by Mito-TEMPO, a mitochondria-targeted antioxidant shown to reduce ROS in pericyte cultures [198]. Indeed, in a mouse traumatic brain injury model, TNFα-related oxidative stress and inflammation were responsible for pericyte loss, BBB damage, and vasogenic edema [199]. Second, pericytes interact with ECs to regulate BBB permeability by regulating BBB-specific gene expression on ECs, such as Glut1 and transferrin receptor [194,200]. Last but not least, pericytes promote astrocyte endfeet attachment and normal polarization, thereby maintaining the normal functioning of the BBB [194]. Given the robust antioxidant and anti-inflammatory effect of NRF2, it is plausible that pericytes could be protective of the BBB in VCID, although more direct evidence is required.

3.3.2. Contractile Function/Cerebral Blood Flow

Whether the contractile function of pericytes plays an important role in CBF is controversial. Though studies in the cortex and retina have proved the contractility of pericytes, it is questionable whether and to what extent this contraction impacts the rCBF [201,202]. It has been reported that, unlike VSMCs, pericytes are unable to contract in response to multiple stimuli, which may be due to their lack of smooth muscle actin [203]. In contrast, other studies have suggested that, as compared to VSMC-dominant penetrating arterioles, the majority of CBF upregulation after neuronal activation takes place at the pericyte-dominant capillary level, supporting a crucial role of pericytes in CBF regulation [204–206].

Small vessel disease (SVD) is the most common cause of VCID, and it plays a significant role in stroke and Alzheimer's disease (AD) [207–209]. CBF decrease and amyloid β (Aβ) changes are present in both AD and VCID. In AD, Aβ deposition generates excessive ROS and triggers the release of vasoconstrictive peptides such as endothelin-1, altering pericyte tone and causing vasoconstriction [210,211]. Therefore, it is reasonable to hypothesize that NRF2 may rescue pericyte dysfunction and increase CBF in both AD and VCID.

3.4. Perivascular Macrophage

Brain-proximal arterioles and venules are surrounded by perivascular space, which hosts perivascular macrophages (PVMs) [212–215]. PVMs are specialized myeloid cells that play an active role in the maintenance of BBB integrity and lymphatic drainage under physiologic conditions. Increased PVM numbers are observed in diseases associated with infection, vascular impairment, and amyloid deposition [215].

3.4.1. Inflammation/Oxidative Stress

As the resident macrophages in the CNS, PVMs are an important source of ROS [216]. For example, in spontaneous hypertensive mice, damage to the BBB resulted in Ang II accessing the perivascular space, leading to activation of PVMs which produce excessive ROS and resulting in cognitive impairment [216]. On the other hand, BBB breakdown facilitates penetration of fibrinogen into brain tissue, which turns to fibrin and activates microglia, causing inflammation [217]. Several experimental studies have examined the relationship between fibrin and perivascular macrophages. In a rabbit retina model, perivascular macrophages accumulated around fibrin in the setting of IL-1-induced inflammation [218]. Fibrin in the brain tissue was associated with Aβ deposits and loss of pericytes [217]. NRF2 has great potential to break these pathological cascades by eliminating ROS and rescuing cognitive function in VCID.

Two traditional categories of activated macrophages, M1 (pro-inflammatory) and M2 (anti-inflammatory), have been identified [219], though this concept has been increasingly questioned in the field. Our group has demonstrated the presence of PVM subtypes by examining their specific markers [215]. Importantly, NRF2 plays a role in phenotype shifting in macrophages and microglia. For example, human umbilical cord mesenchymal stem cell-derived extracellular vesicles were found to inhibit M1 differentiation of microglia and thereby decrease inflammation levels in a VCID rat model through the PI3K/AKT/NRF2 pathway [220]. In mice modeling Parkinson's disease, NRF2 KO was associated with significantly increased proinflammatory M1 cytokine levels and decreased anti-inflammatory M2 cytokine levels [221]. In a stroke model, activated microglia converted to pro-inflammatory M1 and anti-inflammatory M2, acting as double-edged sword. Therefore, it could be important to promote differentiation towards the anti-inflammatory state in patients with stroke [222]. NRF2 can likely facilitate the formation of M2 an anti-inflammatory phenotype in PVMs, which would benefit cognitive function in VCID.

3.4.2. Clearance of Interstitial Fluid (ISF) or Metabolic Waste (e.g., Aβ)

Lymphatic drainage is somewhat unique in the CNS because the brain parenchyma lacks lymphatic vasculature. Details on brain lymphatic pathways have been thoroughly reviewed elsewhere [223]. Importantly, perivascular space serves as an important route for the removal of waste products such as Aβ [224]. In transgenic AD mice, an impaired lymphatic system enhanced Aβ deposition [224]. PVMs contribute to lymphatic clearance in two major pathways: the glymphatic pathway and the intramural perivascular pathway [215].

Interestingly, PVMs appear to be a double-edged sword in the pathogenesis of aging-related proteinopathies such as diseases characterized by the pathological accumulation of Aβ, α-synuclein, and p-Tau [225]. Aβ has been reported to impact neurovascular coupling and contribute to impaired cognition [226]. Perivascular space is a major site for both disposal and accumulation of Aβ [37,227–230]. Residing in the perivascular space, PVMs are, on the one hand, involved in Aβ clearance through phagocytosis; this lessens Aβ deposition in the brain tissue as well as in the blood vessels in the setting of cerebral amyloid angiopathy [231]. On the other hand, PVMs release large amounts of ROS in response to excessive Aβ [232]; in this way, selective removal of PVMs using clodronate liposomes was able to reduce ROS production, preserve BBB integrity, and protect cognitive function in AD mice and spontaneous hypertension mice [232,233].

NRF2 has been proven to influence Aβ levels in the brain. For example, NRF2 deficiency was associated with upregulated Aβ precursor protein (APP) gene expression in obese mice [14]. When crossed with transgenic AD mice with APP or Tau mutations, NRF2 KO led to increased Aβ and p-Tau, resulting in early-onset cognitive dysfunction [47]. Hexahydrocurcumin was found to decrease Aβ and p-Tau production, which are associated with increased NRF2 activity, and to improve memory function in a VCID rat model [234]. In addition, transcriptomic analysis of NRF2-KO mouse brains revealed pathways replicating those in human aging and AD brains. Persistent activation of proinflammatory microglia and expression of proinflammatory cytokines induced by Aβ play a vital role in cellular senescence and the progression of neurodegenerative diseases. At the same time, the SIRT1/NRF2 pathway is partially blocked and NRF2 translocation is diminished by Aβ stimulation, which was reversed by aspirin in a mouse model [232].

4. Future Perspectives on NRF2 in VCID

Though preclinical studies support the potential value of NRF2 in VCID prevention and/or management, clinical trials are still lacking at this time. It should be noted that NRF2 dysfunction occurs with aging, which can impair expected responses upon NRF2 activation [59,235]. This is especially important in VCID, where cerebrovascular aging appears to play a central pathogenetic role. Another point to consider is that BBB permeability may or may not be crucial for drug efficacy, given that the vasculature, rather than the brain parenchyma, could be the major site of drug action in VCID, which greatly expands the candidate pool for clinical trial design. In addition, VCID comorbidities such as hypercapnia may impose an additional layer of complexity on NRF2 expression [236], which is commonly the case in the real world given the demographic characteristics of the VCID population.

Studies have identified that NRF2 plays a protective role against newly identified forms of cell death, such as ferroptosis and pyroptosis. Ferroptosis is characterized by iron accumulation and lipid peroxidation [10,11]. In a VCID rat model, gastrodin has been proven to inhibit ferroptosis and improve memory impairment through the NRF2/Keap1–glutathione peroxidase 4 pathway [11]. Pyroptosis is a form of inflammatory programmed cell death mediated by the NLRP3 inflammasome. Activation of ChemR23, a G-protein-coupled receptor, was observed to inhibit pyroptosis and improve cognitive function via the PI3K/AKT/NRF2 pathway in a chronic cerebral hypoperfusion rat model [12]. These could be novel mechanisms for future NRF2-VCID research.

NRF2 activators have been extensively studied in preclinical settings; however, which compounds to proceed with in VCID clinical trials is hard to determine. Five candidate compounds (curcumin, trichostatin-a, panobinostat, parthenolide, and entinostat) have been identified for AD treatment based on structural similarities, NRF2-diseasome, targeted pathways, and modes [237]. A selected list of NRF2 activators that are currently being trialed in CNS diseases is listed in Table 1. Because no NRF2 activators are currently being trialed in VCID studies, patient selection, drug dose, delivery modalities, timing of administration, and administration protocol need to be developed and optimized for the best therapeutic effects while avoiding potential side effects.

Table 1. NRF2 activators that are being trialed in CNS diseases.

Compounds	Trial ID	Disease	Comments	References
Dimethyl fumarate	NCT02634307	Multiple sclerosis	• FDA approved, currently in phase III trial. • Good tolerance. • Improvements from baseline in clinical and radiological efficacy outcomes, including significantly reduced annualized relapse rates.	[77]
Omaveloxone	NCT02255435	Friedreich ataxia	• Significantly improved neurological function with good tolerance. • Mild adverse effects. • High accumulation in the brain with significant and stable upregulation of NRF2 downstream genes in monkeys and humans.	[238,239]
Sfn	NCT02561481	Autism spectrum disorder	• Only small non-significant changes were found in the primary outcome measures (Ohio Autism Clinical Impressions Scale). • Safety and tolerance were confirmed. • Significant changes in glutathione redox status, mitochondrial respiration, inflammatory markers, and heat shock proteins.	[240]
SFX-01 (Evgen Pharma)	NCT02614742, NCT01948362, NCT02055716	SAH	• Currently in phase II trial. • No serious adverse events were reported in healthy volunteers per phase I trials.	[241]

In conclusion, NRF2 is a promising target for the management of VCID in light of its robust protective effects in the cerebral vasculature and its multimodal anti-aging potency. In-depth preclinical and clinical trials are needed for better VCID outcomes.

Author Contributions: Conceptualization, Y.H. and T.Y.; writing—original draft preparation, Y.H. and T.Y.; writing—review and editing, F.Z. and M.I.; visualization, Y.H. and T.Y.; supervision, F.Z., M.I. and T.Y.; funding acquisition, M.I. All authors have read and agreed to the published version of the manuscript.

Funding: This research was funded by National Institutes of Health (NS103810) and start-up funds from the Pittsburgh Institute of Brain Disorders and Recovery and the Department of Neurology of the University of Pittsburgh. The article processing charge was funded by National Institutes of Health (NS103810).

Acknowledgments: We thank Pat Strickler for her administrative support.

Conflicts of Interest: The authors declare no conflict of interest.

References

1. O'Brien, J.T.; Thomas, A. Vascular dementia. *Lancet* **2015**, *386*, 1698–1706. [CrossRef]
2. Lobo, A.; Launer, L.J.; Fratiglioni, L.; Andersen, K.; Di Carlo, A.; Breteler, M.M.; Copeland, J.R.; Dartigues, J.F.; Jagger, C.; Martinez-Lage, J.; et al. Prevalence of dementia and major subtypes in Europe: A collaborative study of population-based cohorts. Neurologic Diseases in the Elderly Research Group. *Neurology* **2000**, *54*, S4–S9.
3. Rizzi, L.; Rosset, I.; Roriz-Cruz, M. Global Epidemiology of Dementia: Alzheimer's and Vascular Types. *BioMed. Res. Int.* **2014**, *2014*, 908915. [CrossRef] [PubMed]
4. Kalaria, R.N.; Maestre, G.E.; Arizaga, R.; Friedland, R.P.; Galasko, D.; Hall, K.; Luchsinger, J.A.; Ogunniyi, A.; Perry, E.K.; Potocnik, F.; et al. Alzheimer's disease and vascular dementia in developing countries: Prevalence, management, and risk factors. *Lancet Neurol.* **2008**, *7*, 812–826. [CrossRef]
5. Moon, W.; Han, J.W.; Bae, J.B.; Suh, S.W.; Kim, T.H.; Kwak, K.P.; Kim, B.J.; Kim, S.G.; Kim, J.L.; Moon, S.W.; et al. Disease Burdens of Alzheimer's Disease, Vascular Dementia, and Mild Cognitive Impairment. *J. Am. Med. Dir. Assoc.* **2021**, *22*, 2093–2099.e3. [CrossRef] [PubMed]
6. Hill, J.; Fillit, H.; Shah, S.N.; del Valle, M.C.; Futterman, R. Patterns of healthcare utilization and costs for vascular dementia in a community-dwelling population. *J. Alzheimer's Dis.* **2005**, *8*, 43–50. [CrossRef]

7. Canobbio, I.; Abubaker, A.A.; Visconte, C.; Torti, M.; Pula, G. Role of amyloid peptides in vascular dysfunction and platelet dysregulation in Alzheimer's disease. *Front. Cell Neurosci.* **2015**, *9*, 65. [CrossRef]
8. Neuropathology Group; Medical Research Council Cognitive Function and Aging Study. Pathological correlates of late-onset dementia in a multicentre, community-based population in England and Wales. Neuropathology Group of the Medical Research Council Cognitive Function and Ageing Study (MRC CFAS). *Lancet* **2001**, *357*, 169–175. [CrossRef] [PubMed]
9. He, F.; Ru, X.; Wen, T. NRF2, a Transcription Factor for Stress Response and Beyond. *Int. J. Mol. Sci.* **2020**, *21*, 4777. [CrossRef]
10. Chen, B.; Lu, Y.; Chen, Y.; Cheng, J. The role of Nrf2 in oxidative stress-induced endothelial injuries. *J. Endocrinol.* **2015**, *225*, R83–R99. [CrossRef]
11. Li, Y.; Zhang, E.; Yang, H.; Chen, Y.; Tao, L.; Xu, Y.; Chen, T.; Shen, X. Gastrodin Ameliorates Cognitive Dysfunction in Vascular Dementia Rats by Suppressing Ferroptosis via the Regulation of the Nrf2/Keap1-GPx4 Signaling Pathway. *Molecules* **2022**, *27*, 6311. [CrossRef] [PubMed]
12. Zhang, Y.; Zhang, J.; Zhao, Y.; Zhang, Y.; Liu, L.; Xu, X.; Wang, X.; Fu, J. ChemR23 activation attenuates cognitive impairment in chronic cerebral hypoperfusion by inhibiting NLRP3 inflammasome-induced neuronal pyroptosis. *Cell Death Dis.* **2023**, *14*, 721. [CrossRef] [PubMed]
13. Vashi, R.; Patel, B.M. NRF2 in Cardiovascular Diseases: A Ray of Hope! *J. Cardiovasc. Transl. Res.* **2021**, *14*, 573–586. [CrossRef] [PubMed]
14. Tarantini, S.; Valcarcel-Ares, M.N.; Yabluchanskiy, A.; Tucsek, Z.; Hertelendy, P.; Kiss, T.; Gautam, T.; A Zhang, X.; E Sonntag, W.; de Cabo, R.; et al. Nrf2 Deficiency Exacerbates Obesity-Induced Oxidative Stress, Neurovascular Dysfunction, Blood–Brain Barrier Disruption, Neuroinflammation, Amyloidogenic Gene Expression, and Cognitive Decline in Mice, Mimicking the Aging Phenotype. *J. Gerontol. Ser. A* **2018**, *73*, 853–863. [CrossRef]
15. Rundek, T.; Tolea, M.; Ariko, T.; Fagerli, E.A.; Camargo, C.J. Vascular Cognitive Impairment (VCI). *Neurotherapeutics* **2022**, *19*, 68–88. [CrossRef] [PubMed]
16. Pendlebury, S.T.; Rothwell, P.M. Prevalence, incidence, and factors associated with pre-stroke and post-stroke dementia: A systematic review and meta-analysis. *Lancet Neurol.* **2009**, *8*, 1006–1018. [CrossRef] [PubMed]
17. Power, M.C.; Mormino, E.; Soldan, A.; James, B.D.; Yu, L.; Armstrong, N.M.; Bangen, K.J.; Delano-Wood, L.; Lamar, M.; Lim, Y.Y.; et al. Combined neuropathological pathways account for age-related risk of dementia. *Ann. Neurol.* **2018**, *84*, 10–22. [CrossRef] [PubMed]
18. Pendlebury, S.T.; Rothwell, P.M. Incidence and prevalence of dementia associated with transient ischaemic attack and stroke: Analysis of the population-based Oxford Vascular Study. *Lancet Neurol.* **2019**, *18*, 248–258. [CrossRef]
19. Wiesmann, M.; Kiliaan, A.J.; Claassen, J.A. Vascular aspects of cognitive impairment and dementia. *J. Cereb. Blood Flow Metab.* **2013**, *33*, 1696–1706. [CrossRef]
20. El Assar, M.; Angulo, J.; Rodríguez-Mañas, L. Oxidative stress and vascular inflammation in aging. *Free. Radic. Biol. Med.* **2013**, *65*, 380–401. [CrossRef]
21. Sharma, S.; Brown, C.E. Microvascular basis of cognitive impairment in type 1 diabetes. *Pharmacol. Ther.* **2022**, *229*, 107929. [CrossRef] [PubMed]
22. Choi, I.; Seaquist, E.R.; Gruetter, R. Effect of hypoglycemia on brain glycogen metabolism in vivo. *J. Neurosci. Res.* **2003**, *72*, 25–32. [CrossRef] [PubMed]
23. Zhang, S.; Murphy, T.H. Imaging the impact of cortical microcirculation on synaptic structure and sensory-evoked hemodynamic responses in vivo. *PLoS Biol.* **2007**, *5*, e119. [CrossRef] [PubMed]
24. Iadecola, C.; Gottesman, R.F. Neurovascular and Cognitive Dysfunction in Hypertension. *Circ. Res.* **2019**, *124*, 1025–1044. [CrossRef] [PubMed]
25. Yamazaki, Y.; Baker, D.J.; Tachibana, M.; Liu, C.-C.; Van Deursen, J.M.; Brott, T.G.; Bu, G.; Kanekiyo, T. Vascular Cell Senescence Contributes to Blood–Brain Barrier Breakdown. *Stroke* **2016**, *47*, 1068–1077. [CrossRef] [PubMed]
26. Wilhelm, I.; Nyúl-Tóth, Á.; Kozma, M.; Farkas, A.E.; Krizbai, I.A. Role of pattern recognition receptors of the neurovascular unit in inflamm-aging. *Am. J. Physiol. Heart Circ. Physiol.* **2017**, *313*, H1000–H1012. [CrossRef] [PubMed]
27. van der Flier, W.M.; Skoog, I.; Schneider, J.A.; Pantoni, L.; Mok, V.; Chen, C.L.; Scheltens, P. Vascular cognitive impairment. *Nat. Rev. Dis. Primers* **2018**, *4*, 18003. [CrossRef] [PubMed]
28. Gorelick, P.B.; Scuteri, A.; Black, S.E.; DeCarli, C.; Greenberg, S.M.; Iadecola, C.; Launer, L.J.; Laurent, S.; Lopez, O.L.; Nyenhuis, D.; et al. Vascular contributions to cognitive impairment and dementia: A statement for healthcare professionals from the american heart association/american stroke association. *Stroke* **2011**, *42*, 2672–2713. [CrossRef] [PubMed]
29. Román, G.C.; Tatemichi, T.K.; Erkinjuntti, T.; Cummings, J.L.; Masdeu, J.C.; Garcia, J.H.; Amaducci, L.; Orgogozo, J.-M.; Brun, A.; Hofman, A.; et al. Vascular dementia: Diagnostic criteria for research studies. Report of the NINDS-AIREN International Workshop. *Neurology* **1993**, *43*, 250–260. [CrossRef] [PubMed]
30. Smith, E.E. Clinical presentations and epidemiology of vascular dementia. *Clin. Sci.* **2017**, *131*, 1059–1068. [CrossRef] [PubMed]
31. Schneider, J.; Wilson, R.; Cochran, E.; Bienias, J.; Arnold, S.; Evans, D.; Bennett, D. Relation of cerebral infarctions to dementia and cognitive function in older persons. *Neurology* **2003**, *60*, 1082–1088. [CrossRef] [PubMed]
32. Arvanitakis, Z.; Leurgans, S.E.; Barnes, L.L.; Bennett, D.A.; Schneider, J.A. Microinfarct pathology, dementia, and cognitive systems. *Stroke* **2011**, *42*, 722–727. [CrossRef] [PubMed]

33. Brundel, M.; de Bresser, J.; van Dillen, J.J.; Kappelle, L.J.; Biessels, G.J. Cerebral microinfarcts: A systematic review of neuropathological studies. *J. Cereb. Blood Flow Metab.* **2012**, *32*, 425–436. [CrossRef] [PubMed]
34. White, L. Brain lesions at autopsy in older japanese-american men as related to cognitive impairment and dementia in the final years of life: A summary report from the honolulu-asia aging study. *J. Alzheimer's Dis.* **2009**, *18*, 713–725. [CrossRef] [PubMed]
35. Doyle, K.P.; Quach, L.N.; Solé, M.; Axtell, R.C.; Nguyen, T.-V.V.; Soler-Llavina, G.J.; Jurado, S.; Han, J.; Steinman, L.; Longo, F.M.; et al. B-lymphocyte-mediated delayed cognitive impairment following stroke. *J. Neurosci.* **2015**, *35*, 2133–2145. [CrossRef] [PubMed]
36. Jin, W.-N.; Shi, S.X.-Y.; Li, Z.; Li, M.; Wood, K.; Gonzales, R.J.; Liu, Q. Depletion of microglia exacerbates postischemic inflammation and brain injury. *J. Cereb. Blood Flow Metab.* **2017**, *37*, 2224–2236. [CrossRef] [PubMed]
37. Carare, R.O.; Hawkes, C.A.; Jeffrey, M.; Kalaria, R.N.; Weller, R.O. Review: Cerebral amyloid angiopathy, prion angiopathy, CADASIL and the spectrum of protein elimination failure angiopathies (PEFA) in neurodegenerative disease with a focus on therapy. *Neuropathol. Appl. Neurobiol.* **2013**, *39*, 593–611. [CrossRef] [PubMed]
38. Iadecola, C. The pathobiology of vascular dementia. *Neuron* **2013**, *80*, 844–866. [CrossRef] [PubMed]
39. Nave, K.-A. Myelination and support of axonal integrity by glia. *Nature* **2010**, *468*, 244–252. [CrossRef]
40. Mandell, D.M.; Han, J.S.; Poublanc, J.; Crawley, A.P.; Kassner, A.; Fisher, J.A.; Mikulis, D.J. Selective reduction of blood flow to white matter during hypercapnia corresponds with leukoaraiosis. *Stroke* **2008**, *39*, 1993–1998. [CrossRef]
41. Barber, R.; Scheltens, P.; Gholkar, A.; Ballard, C.; McKeith, I.; Ince, P.; Perry, R.; O'Brien, J. White matter lesions on magnetic resonance imaging in dementia with Lewy bodies, Alzheimer's disease, vascular dementia, and normal aging. *J. Neurol. Neurosurg. Psychiatry* **1999**, *67*, 66–72. [CrossRef] [PubMed]
42. Kynast, J.; Lampe, L.; Luck, T.; Frisch, S.; Arelin, K.; Hoffmann, K.-T.; Loeffler, M.; Riedel-Heller, S.G.; Villringer, A.; Schroeter, M.L. White matter hyperintensities associated with small vessel disease impair social cognition beside attention and memory. *J. Cereb. Blood Flow Metab.* **2018**, *38*, 996–1009. [CrossRef] [PubMed]
43. Lampe, L.; Kharabian-Masouleh, S.; Kynast, J.; Arelin, K.; Steele, C.J.; Löffler, M.; Witte, A.V.; Schroeter, M.L.; Villringer, A.; Bazin, P.-L. Lesion location matters: The relationships between white matter hyperintensities on cognition in the healthy elderly. *J. Cereb. Blood Flow Metab.* **2019**, *39*, 36–43. [CrossRef] [PubMed]
44. Hou, Y.; Dan, X.; Babbar, M.; Wei, Y.; Hasselbalch, S.G.; Croteau, D.L.; Bohr, V.A. Ageing as a risk factor for neurodegenerative disease. *Nat. Rev. Neurol.* **2019**, *15*, 565–581. [CrossRef] [PubMed]
45. Madabhushi, R.; Pan, L.; Tsai, L.-H. DNA Damage and Its Links to Neurodegeneration. *Neuron* **2014**, *83*, 266–282. [CrossRef] [PubMed]
46. Shang, D.; Sun, D.; Shi, C.; Xu, J.; Shen, M.; Hu, X.; Liu, H.; Tu, Z. Activation of epidermal growth factor receptor signaling mediates cellular senescence induced by certain pro-inflammatory cytokines. *Aging Cell* **2020**, *19*, e13145. [CrossRef] [PubMed]
47. Rojo, A.I.; Pajares, M.; Rada, P.; Nuñez, A.; Nevado-Holgado, A.J.; Killik, R.; Van Leuven, F.; Ribe, E.; Lovestone, S.; Yamamoto, M.; et al. NRF2 deficiency replicates transcriptomic changes in Alzheimer's patients and worsens APP and TAU pathology. *Redox Biol.* **2017**, *13*, 444–451. [CrossRef] [PubMed]
48. Johri, A.; Beal, M.F. Mitochondrial Dysfunction in Neurodegenerative Diseases. *J. Pharmacol. Exp. Ther.* **2012**, *342*, 619–630. [CrossRef]
49. Liao, X.; Zhang, Z.; Ming, M.; Zhong, S.; Chen, J.; Huang, Y. Imperatorin exerts antioxidant effects in vascular dementia via the Nrf2 signaling pathway. *Sci. Rep.* **2023**, *13*, 1–14. [CrossRef]
50. Chen, J.-S.; Huang, P.-H.; Wang, C.-H.; Lin, F.-Y.; Tsai, H.-Y.; Wu, T.-C.; Lin, S.-J.; Chen, J.-W. Nrf-2 mediated heme oxygenase-1 expression, an antioxidant-independent mechanism, contributes to anti-atherogenesis and vascular protective effects of Ginkgo biloba extract. *Atherosclerosis* **2011**, *214*, 301–309. [CrossRef]
51. Zhang, M.; An, C.; Gao, Y.; Leak, R.K.; Chen, J.; Zhang, F. Emerging roles of Nrf2 and phase II antioxidant enzymes in neuroprotection. *Prog. Neurobiol.* **2013**, *100*, 30–47. [CrossRef]
52. Fadoul, G.; Ikonomovic, M.; Zhang, F.; Yang, T. The cell-specific roles of Nrf2 in acute and chronic phases of ischemic stroke. *CNS Neurosci. Ther.* **2023**, *30*, e14462. [CrossRef] [PubMed]
53. Tejo, F.V.; A Quintanilla, R. Contribution of the Nrf2 Pathway on Oxidative Damage and Mitochondrial Failure in Parkinson and Alzheimer's Disease. *Antioxidants* **2021**, *10*, 1069. [CrossRef] [PubMed]
54. De Freitas Silva, M.; Pruccoli, L.; Morroni, F.; Sita, G.; Seghetti, F.; Viegas, C., Jr.; Tarozzi, A. The Keap1/Nrf2-ARE Pathway as a Pharmacological Target for Chalcones. *Molecules* **2018**, *23*, 1803. [CrossRef]
55. Pi, Y.; Zhang, L.-L.; Li, B.-H.; Guo, L.; Cao, X.-J.; Gao, C.-Y.; Li, J.-C. Inhibition of reactive oxygen species generation attenuates TLR4-mediated proinflammatory and proliferative phenotype of vascular smooth muscle cells. *Mod. Pathol.* **2013**, *93*, 880–887. [CrossRef] [PubMed]
56. Niture, S.K.; Khatri, R.; Jaiswal, A.K. Regulation of Nrf2-an update. *Free Radic. Biol. Med.* **2014**, *66*, 36–44. [CrossRef] [PubMed]
57. Kaspar, J.W.; Jaiswal, A.K. An Autoregulatory Loop between Nrf2 and Cul3-Rbx1 Controls Their Cellular Abundance. *J. Biol. Chem.* **2010**, *285*, 21349–21358. [CrossRef] [PubMed]
58. Chi, X.; Yao, W.; Xia, H.; Jin, Y.; Li, X.; Cai, J.; Hei, Z. Elevation of HO-1 Expression Mitigates Intestinal Ischemia-Reperfusion Injury and Restores Tight Junction Function in a Rat Liver Transplantation Model. *Oxidative Med. Cell. Longev.* **2015**, *2015*, 1–12. [CrossRef]

59. Yang, T.; Zhang, F. Targeting Transcription Factor Nrf2 (Nuclear Factor Erythroid 2-Related Factor 2) for the Intervention of Vascular Cognitive Impairment and Dementia. *Arter. Thromb. Vasc. Biol.* **2021**, *41*, 97–116. [CrossRef]
60. Saha, S.; Buttari, B.; Panieri, E.; Profumo, E.; Saso, L. An Overview of Nrf2 Signaling Pathway and Its Role in Inflammation. *Molecules* **2020**, *25*, 5474. [CrossRef]
61. Yu, C.; Xiao, J.-H. The Keap1-Nrf2 System: A Mediator between Oxidative Stress and Aging. *Oxidative Med. Cell. Longev.* **2021**, *2021*, 6635460. [CrossRef] [PubMed]
62. Shih, P.-H.; Yen, G.-C. Differential expressions of antioxidant status in aging rats: The role of transcriptional factor Nrf2 and MAPK signaling pathway. *Biogerontology* **2007**, *8*, 71–80. [CrossRef] [PubMed]
63. Kapeta, S.; Chondrogianni, N.; Gonos, E.S. Nuclear Erythroid Factor 2-mediated Proteasome Activation Delays Senescence in Human Fibroblasts. *J. Biol. Chem.* **2010**, *285*, 8171–8184. [CrossRef] [PubMed]
64. Suh, J.H.; Shenvi, S.V.; Dixon, B.M.; Liu, H.; Jaiswal, A.K.; Liu, R.-M.; Hagen, T.M. Decline in transcriptional activity of Nrf2 causes age-related loss of glutathione synthesis, which is reversible with lipoic acid. *Proc. Natl. Acad. Sci. USA* **2004**, *101*, 3381–3386. [CrossRef] [PubMed]
65. Ungvari, Z.; Bailey-Downs, L.; Sosnowska, D.; Gautam, T.; Koncz, P.; Losonczy, G.; Ballabh, P.; de Cabo, R.; Sonntag, W.E.; Csiszar, A.; et al. Vascular oxidative stress in aging: A homeostatic failure due to dysregulation of NRF2-mediated antioxidant response. *Am. J. Physiol. Circ. Physiol.* **2011**, *301*, H363–H372. [CrossRef] [PubMed]
66. Ungvari, Z.; Bailey-Downs, L.; Gautam, T.; Sosnowska, D.; Wang, M.; Monticone, R.E.; Telljohann, R.; Pinto, J.T.; de Cabo, R.; Sonntag, W.E.; et al. Age-associated vascular oxidative stress, Nrf2 dysfunction, and NF-κB activation in the nonhuman primate *Macaca mulatta*. *J. Gerontol. A Biol. Sci. Med. Sci.* **2011**, *66*, 866–875. [CrossRef] [PubMed]
67. Zhang, H.; Liu, H.; Davies, K.J.; Sioutas, C.; Finch, C.E.; Morgan, T.E.; Forman, H.J. Nrf2-regulated phase II enzymes are induced by chronic ambient nanoparticle exposure in young mice with age-related impairments. *Free. Radic. Biol. Med.* **2012**, *52*, 2038–2046. [CrossRef] [PubMed]
68. Zhang, H.; Davies, K.J.; Forman, H.J. Oxidative stress response and Nrf2 signaling in aging. *Free. Radic. Biol. Med.* **2015**, *88*, 314–336. [CrossRef]
69. Tossetta, G.; Fantone, S.; Piani, F.; Crescimanno, C.; Ciavattini, A.; Giannubilo, S.R.; Marzioni, D. Modulation of NRF2/KEAP1 Signaling in Preeclampsia. *Cells* **2023**, *12*, 1545. [CrossRef]
70. Xia, L.; Ma, W.; Afrashteh, A.; Sajadi, M.A.; Fakheri, H.; Valilo, M. The nuclear factor erythroid 2-related factor 2/p53 axis in breast cancer. *Biochem. Med.* **2023**, *33*, 030504.
71. Tossetta, G.; Fantone, S.; Marzioni, D.; Mazzucchelli, R. Cellular Modulators of the NRF2/KEAP1 Signaling Pathway in Prostate Cancer. *Front. Biosci.* **2023**, *28*, 143. [CrossRef] [PubMed]
72. Fasipe, B.; Laher, I. Nrf2 modulates the benefits of evening exercise in type 2 diabetes. *Sports Med. Health Sci.* **2023**, *5*, 251–258. [CrossRef] [PubMed]
73. He, P.; Talukder, M.A.H.; Gao, F. Oxidative Stress and Microvessel Barrier Dysfunction. *Front. Physiol.* **2020**, *11*, 472. [CrossRef] [PubMed]
74. Campagna, R.; Mateuszuk, Ł.; Wojnar-Lason, K.; Kaczara, P.; Tworzydło, A.; Kij, A.; Bujok, R.; Mlynarski, J.; Wang, Y.; Sartini, D.; et al. Nicotinamide N-methyltransferase in endothelium protects against oxidant stress-induced endothelial injury. *Biochim. Biophys. Acta* **2021**, *1868*, 119082. [CrossRef] [PubMed]
75. Andrés, C.M.C.; de la Lastra, J.M.P.; Juan, C.A.; Plou, F.J.; Pérez-Lebeña, E. Antioxidant Metabolism Pathways in Vitamins, Polyphenols, and Selenium: Parallels and Divergences. *Int. J. Mol. Sci.* **2024**, *25*, 2600. [CrossRef] [PubMed]
76. Scuto, M.; Modafferi, S.; Rampulla, F.; Zimbone, V.; Tomasello, M.; Spano', S.; Ontario, M.; Palmeri, A.; Salinaro, A.T.; Siracusa, R.; et al. Redox modulation of stress resilience by Crocus sativus L. for potential neuroprotective and anti-neuroinflammatory applications in brain disorders: From molecular basis to therapy. *Mech. Ageing Dev.* **2022**, *205*, 111686. [CrossRef] [PubMed]
77. Di Nicolantonio, J.J.; McCarty, M.F.; Assanga, S.I.; Lujan, L.L.; O'Keefe, J.H. Ferulic acid and berberine, via Sirt1 and AMPK, may act as cell cleansing promoters of healthy longevity. *Open Hear.* **2022**, *9*, e001801. [CrossRef] [PubMed]
78. Schwartz, B.G.; Economides, C.; Mayeda, G.S.; Burstein, S.; A Kloner, R. The endothelial cell in health and disease: Its function, dysfunction, measurement and therapy. *Int. J. Impot. Res.* **2009**, *22*, 77–90. [CrossRef] [PubMed]
79. Ludewig, P.; Winneberger, J.; Magnus, T. The cerebral endothelial cell as a key regulator of inflammatory processes in sterile inflammation. *J. Neuroimmunol.* **2019**, *326*, 38–44. [CrossRef]
80. Seals, D.R.; Moreau, K.L.; Gates, P.E.; Eskurza, I. Modulatory influences on ageing of the vasculature in healthy humans. *Exp. Gerontol.* **2006**, *41*, 501–507. [CrossRef]
81. Teixeira, M.; Williams, T.; Hellewell, P. Role of prostaglandins and nitric oxide in acute inflammatory reactions in guinea-pig skin. *Br. J. Pharmacol.* **1993**, *110*, 1515–1521. [CrossRef] [PubMed]
82. Reglero-Real, N.; Colom, B.; Bodkin, J.V.; Nourshargh, S. Endothelial Cell Junctional Adhesion Molecules: Role and Regulation of Expression in Inflammation. *Arter. Thromb. Vasc. Biol.* **2016**, *36*, 2048–2057. [CrossRef] [PubMed]
83. Pober, J.S.; Sessa, W.C. Evolving functions of endothelial cells in inflammation. *Nat. Rev. Immunol.* **2007**, *7*, 803–815. [CrossRef] [PubMed]
84. Pober, J.S.; Cotran, R.S. The role of endothelial cells in inflammation. *Transplantation* **1990**, *50*, 537–544. [CrossRef] [PubMed]
85. Hellenthal, K.E.M.; Brabenec, L.; Wagner, N.-M. Regulation and Dysregulation of Endothelial Permeability during Systemic Inflammation. *Cells* **2022**, *11*, 1935. [CrossRef] [PubMed]

86. Van der Loo, B.; Schildknecht, S.; Zee, R.; Bachschmid, M.M. Signalling processes in endothelial ageing in relation to chronic oxidative stress and their potential therapeutic implications in humans. *Exp. Physiol.* **2009**, *94*, 305–310. [CrossRef] [PubMed]
87. Ungvari, Z.; Sonntag, W.E.; Csiszar, A. Mitochondria and aging in the vascular system. *J. Mol. Med.* **2010**, *88*, 1021–1027. [CrossRef] [PubMed]
88. Esteras, N.; Dinkova-Kostova, A.T.; Abramov, A.Y. Nrf2 activation in the treatment of neurodegenerative diseases: A focus on its role in mitochondrial bioenergetics and function. *Biol. Chem.* **2016**, *397*, 383–400. [CrossRef] [PubMed]
89. Moreira, P.I.; Carvalho, C.; Zhu, X.; Smith, M.A.; Perry, G. Mitochondrial dysfunction is a trigger of Alzheimer's disease pathophysiology. *Biochim. Biophys. Acta* **2010**, *1802*, 2–10. [CrossRef]
90. Varghese, M.; Zhao, W.; Wang, J.; Cheng, A.; Qian, X.; Chaudhry, A.; Ho, L.; Pasinetti, G. Mitochondrial bioenergetics is defective in presymptomatic Tg2576 AD Mice. *Transl. Neurosci.* **2011**, *2*, 1–5. [CrossRef]
91. Hurd, T.R.; Prime, T.A.; Harbour, M.E.; Lilley, K.S.; Murphy, M.P. Detection of reactive oxygen species-sensitive thiol proteins by redox difference gel electrophoresis: Implications for mitochondrial redox signaling. *J. Biol. Chem.* **2007**, *282*, 22040–22051. [CrossRef] [PubMed]
92. Lo, S.-C.; Hannink, M. PGAM5 tethers a ternary complex containing Keap1 and Nrf2 to mitochondria. *Exp. Cell Res.* **2008**, *314*, 1789–1803. [CrossRef] [PubMed]
93. Chen, X.L.; Dodd, G.; Thomas, S.; Zhang, X.; Wasserman, M.A.; Rovin, B.H.; Kunsch, C. Activation of Nrf2/ARE pathway protects endothelial cells from oxidant injury and inhibits inflammatory gene expression. *Am. J. Physiol. Heart Circ. Physiol.* **2006**, *290*, H1862–H1870. [CrossRef] [PubMed]
94. Wang, Q.; Iketani, S.; Li, Z.; Liu, L.; Guo, Y.; Huang, Y.; Bowen, A.D.; Liu, M.; Wang, M.; Yu, J.; et al. Alarming antibody evasion properties of rising SARS-CoV-2 BQ and XBB subvariants. *Cell.* **2023**, *186*, 279–286.e8. [CrossRef] [PubMed]
95. Ishikawa, K.; Sugawara, D.; Wang, X.-P.; Suzuki, K.; Itabe, H.; Maruyama, Y.; Lusis, A.J. Heme Oxygenase-1 Inhibits Atherosclerotic Lesion Formation in LDL-Receptor Knockout Mice. *Circ. Res.* **2001**, *88*, 506–512. [CrossRef] [PubMed]
96. Candelario-Jalil, E.; Dijkhuizen, R.M.; Magnus, T. Neuroinflammation, Stroke, Blood-Brain Barrier Dysfunction, and Imaging Modalities. *Stroke* **2022**, *53*, 1473–1486. [CrossRef] [PubMed]
97. Kitamura, A.; Manso, Y.; Duncombe, J.; Searcy, J.; Koudelka, J.; Binnie, M.; Webster, S.; Lennen, R.; Jansen, M.; Marshall, I.; et al. Long-term cilostazol treatment reduces gliovascular damage and memory impairment in a mouse model of chronic cerebral hypoperfusion. *Sci. Rep.* **2017**, *7*, 4299. [CrossRef] [PubMed]
98. Huang, Y.; Zhang, W.; Lin, L.; Feng, J.; Chen, F.; Wei, W.; Zhao, X.; Guo, W.; Li, J.; Yin, W.; et al. Is endothelial dysfunction of cerebral small vessel responsible for white matter lesions after chronic cerebral hypoperfusion in rats? *J. Neurol. Sci.* **2010**, *299*, 72–80. [CrossRef]
99. Shah, P.K. Inflammation, neointimal hyperplasia, and restenosis: As the leukocytes roll, the arteries thicken. *Circulation* **2003**, *107*, 2175–2177. [CrossRef]
100. Schiffrin, E.L. Canadian Institutes of Health Research Multidisciplinary Research Group on Hypertension. Beyond blood pressure: The endothelium and atherosclerosis progression. *Am. J. Hypertens* **2002**, *15* (Suppl. S5), 115S–122S. [CrossRef]
101. Kim, J.-H.; Choi, Y.K.; Lee, K.-S.; Cho, D.-H.; Baek, Y.-Y.; Lee, D.-K.; Ha, K.-S.; Choe, J.; Won, M.-H.; Jeoung, D.; et al. Functional dissection of Nrf2-dependent phase II genes in vascular inflammation and endotoxic injury using Keap1 siRNA. *Free. Radic. Biol. Med.* **2012**, *53*, 629–640. [CrossRef] [PubMed]
102. Weng, W.-T.; Kuo, P.-C.; Scofield, B.A.; Paraiso, H.C.; Brown, D.A.; Yu, I.-C.; Yen, J.-H. 4-Ethylguaiacol Modulates Neuroinflammation and Promotes Heme Oxygenase-1 Expression to Ameliorate Brain Injury in Ischemic Stroke. *Front. Immunol.* **2022**, *13*, 887000. [CrossRef] [PubMed]
103. Jin, W.; Wang, H.; Yan, W.; Xu, L.; Wang, X.; Zhao, X.; Yang, X.; Chen, G.; Ji, Y. Disruption of Nrf2 enhances upregulation of nuclear factor-kappaB activity, proinflammatory cytokines, and intercellular adhesion molecule-1 in the brain after traumatic brain injury. *Mediat. Inflamm.* **2008**, *2008*, 725174. [CrossRef] [PubMed]
104. Pae, H.-O.; Oh, G.-S.; Lee, B.-S.; Rim, J.-S.; Kim, Y.-M.; Chung, H.-T. 3-Hydroxyanthranilic acid, one of l-tryptophan metabolites, inhibits monocyte chemoattractant protein-1 secretion and vascular cell adhesion molecule-1 expression via heme oxygenase-1 induction in human umbilical vein endothelial cells. *Atherosclerosis* **2006**, *187*, 274–284. [CrossRef] [PubMed]
105. Arfmann-Knubel, S.; Struck, B.; Genrich, G.; Helm, O.; Sipos, B.; Sebens, S.; Schäfer, H. The Crosstalk between Nrf2 and TGF-beta1 in the Epithelial-Mesenchymal Transition of Pancreatic Duct Epithelial Cells. *PLoS ONE* **2015**, *10*, e0132978. [CrossRef] [PubMed]
106. Glagov, S.; Weisenberg, E.; Zarins, C.K.; Stankunavicius, R.; Kolettis, G.J. Compensatory Enlargement of Human Atherosclerotic Coronary Arteries. *New Engl. J. Med.* **1987**, *316*, 1371–1375. [CrossRef] [PubMed]
107. Langille, B.L.; A Reidy, M.; Kline, R.L. Injury and repair of endothelium at sites of flow disturbances near abdominal aortic coarctations in rabbits. *Arter. Off. J. Am. Hear. Assoc. Inc.* **1986**, *6*, 146–154. [CrossRef] [PubMed]
108. Kauffenstein, G.; Tamareille, S.; Prunier, F.; Roy, C.; Ayer, A.; Toutain, B.; Billaud, M.; Isakson, B.E.; Grimaud, L.; Loufrani, L.; et al. Central Role of P2Y$_6$ UDP Receptor in Arteriolar Myogenic Tone. *Arter. Thromb. Vasc. Biol.* **2016**, *36*, 1598–1606. [CrossRef] [PubMed]
109. Drew, P.J. Neurovascular coupling: Motive unknown. *Trends Neurosci.* **2022**, *45*, 809–819. [CrossRef]
110. Hosford, P.S.; Gourine, A.V. What is the key mediator of the neurovascular coupling response? *Neurosci. Biobehav. Rev.* **2019**, *96*, 174–181. [CrossRef]

111. Hoiland, R.L.; Caldwell, H.G.; Howe, C.A.; Nowak-Flück, D.; Stacey, B.S.; Bailey, D.M.; Paton, J.F.R.; Green, D.J.; Sekhon, M.S.; Macleod, D.B.; et al. Nitric oxide is fundamental to neurovascular coupling in humans. *J. Physiol.* **2020**, *598*, 4927–4939. [CrossRef] [PubMed]
112. Murohara, T.; Asahara, T.; Silver, M.; Bauters, C.; Masuda, H.; Kalka, C.; Kearney, M.; Chen, D.; Symes, J.F.; Fishman, M.C.; et al. Nitric oxide synthase modulates angiogenesis in response to tissue ischemia. *J. Clin. Investig.* **1998**, *101*, 2567–2578. [CrossRef] [PubMed]
113. Ha, J.M.; Jin, S.Y.; Lee, H.S.; Shin, H.K.; Lee, D.H.; Song, S.H.; Kim, C.D.; Bae, S.S. Regulation of retinal angiogenesis by endothelial nitric oxide synthase signaling pathway. *Korean J. Physiol. Pharmacol.* **2016**, *20*, 533–538. [CrossRef] [PubMed]
114. Park, S.Y.; Ives, S.J.; Gifford, J.R.; Andtbacka, R.H.; Hyngstrom, J.R.; Reese, V.; Layec, G.; Bharath, L.P.; Symons, J.D.; Richardson, R.S. Impact of age on the vasodilatory function of human skeletal muscle feed arteries. *Am. J. Physiol. Heart Circ. Physiol.* **2016**, *310*, H217–H225. [CrossRef] [PubMed]
115. Csiszar, A.; Labinskyy, N.; Orosz, Z.; Xiangmin, Z.; Buffenstein, R.; Ungvari, Z. Vascular aging in the longest-living rodent, the naked mole rat. *Am. J. Physiol. Circ. Physiol.* **2007**, *293*, H919–H927. [CrossRef] [PubMed]
116. Warabi, E.; Takabe, W.; Minami, T.; Inoue, K.; Itoh, K.; Yamamoto, M.; Ishii, T.; Kodama, T.; Noguchi, N. Shear stress stabilizes NF-E2-related factor 2 and induces antioxidant genes in endothelial cells: Role of reactive oxygen/nitrogen species. *Free. Radic. Biol. Med.* **2007**, *42*, 260–269. [CrossRef] [PubMed]
117. Xue, M.; Qian, Q.; Adaikalakoteswari, A.; Rabbani, N.; Babaei-Jadidi, R.; Thornalley, P.J. Activation of NF-E2–Related Factor-2 Reverses Biochemical Dysfunction of Endothelial Cells Induced by Hyperglycemia Linked to Vascular Disease. *Diabetes* **2008**, *57*, 2809–2817. [CrossRef] [PubMed]
118. Chen, B.R.; Kozberg, M.G.; Bouchard, M.B.; Shaik, M.A.; Hillman, E.M. A Critical role for the vascular endothelium in functional neurovascular coupling in the brain. *J. Am. Hear. Assoc.* **2014**, *3*, e000787. [CrossRef]
119. Girouard, H.; Iadecola, C. Neurovascular coupling in the normal brain and in hypertension, stroke, and Alzheimer disease. *J. Appl. Physiol.* **2006**, *100*, 328–335. [CrossRef]
120. Hamilton, N.B.; Attwell, D.; Hall, C.N. Pericyte-mediated regulation of capillary diameter: A component of neurovascular coupling in health and disease. *Front. Neuroenergetics* **2010**, *2*, 1453. [CrossRef]
121. Donato, A.J.; Morgan, R.G.; Walker, A.E.; Lesniewski, L.A. Cellular and molecular biology of aging endothelial cells. *J. Mol. Cell. Cardiol.* **2015**, *89*, 122–135. [CrossRef] [PubMed]
122. Schairer, D.O.; Chouake, J.S.; Nosanchuk, J.D.; Friedman, A.J. The potential of nitric oxide releasing therapies as antimicrobial agents. *Virulence* **2012**, *3*, 271–279. [CrossRef] [PubMed]
123. Sweeney, M.D.; Sagare, A.P.; Zlokovic, B.V. Blood–brain barrier breakdown in Alzheimer disease and other neurodegenerative disorders. *Nat. Rev. Neurol.* **2018**, *14*, 133–150. [CrossRef] [PubMed]
124. Erhardt, E.B.; Pesko, J.C.; Prestopnik, J.; Thompson, J.; Caprihan, A.; A Rosenberg, G. Biomarkers identify the Binswanger type of vascular cognitive impairment. *J. Cereb. Blood Flow Metab.* **2019**, *39*, 1602–1612. [CrossRef] [PubMed]
125. Piers, T.M.; East, E.; Villegas-Llerena, C.; Sevastou, I.G.; Matarin, M.; Hardy, J.; Pocock, J.M. Soluble Fibrinogen Triggers Non-cell Autonomous ER Stress-Mediated Microglial-Induced Neurotoxicity. *Front. Cell. Neurosci.* **2018**, *12*, 404. [CrossRef] [PubMed]
126. Ryu, J.K.; McLarnon, J.G. A leaky blood-brain barrier, fibrinogen infiltration and microglial reactivity in inflamed Alzheimer's disease brain. *J. Cell Mol. Med.* **2009**, *13*, 2911–2925. [CrossRef] [PubMed]
127. Miners, J.S.; Schulz, I.; Love, S. Differing associations between Abeta accumulation, hypoperfusion, blood-brain barrier dysfunction and loss of PDGFRB pericyte marker in the precuneus and parietal white matter in Alzheimer's disease. *J. Cereb. Blood Flow Metab.* **2018**, *38*, 103–115. [CrossRef] [PubMed]
128. Obermeier, B.; Daneman, R.; Ransohoff, R.M. Development, maintenance and disruption of the blood-brain barrier. *Nat. Med.* **2013**, *19*, 1584–1596. [CrossRef]
129. Cong, Y.; Wang, X.; Wang, S.; Qiao, G.; Li, Y.; Cao, J.; Jiang, W.; Cui, Y. Tim-3 promotes tube formation and decreases tight junction formation in vascular endothelial cells. *Biosci. Rep.* **2020**, *40*, BSR20202130. [CrossRef]
130. Parodi-Rullán, R.; Sone, J.Y.; Fossati, S. Endothelial Mitochondrial Dysfunction in Cerebral Amyloid Angiopathy and Alzheimer's Disease. *J. Alzheimer's Dis.* **2019**, *72*, 1019–1039. [CrossRef]
131. Rao, A.; Balachandran, B. Role of Oxidative Stress and Antioxidants in Neurodegenerative Diseases. *Nutr. Neurosci.* **2002**, *5*, 291–309. [CrossRef] [PubMed]
132. Goes, A.; Wouters, D.; Pol, S.M.A.; Huizinga, R.; Ronken, E.; Adamson, P.; Greenwood, J.; Dijkstra, C.D.; Vries, H.E. Reactive oxygen species enhance the migration of monocytes across the blood-brain barrier in vitro. *FASEB J.* **2001**, *15*, 1852–1854. [CrossRef] [PubMed]
133. Witt, K.A.; Mark, K.S.; Hom, S.; Davis, T.P. Effects of hypoxia-reoxygenation on rat blood-brain barrier permeability and tight junctional protein expression. *Am. J. Physiol. Circ. Physiol.* **2003**, *285*, H2820–H2831. [CrossRef] [PubMed]
134. Mao, L.; Yang, T.; Li, X.; Lei, X.; Sun, Y.; Zhao, Y.; Zhang, W.; Gao, Y.; Sun, B.; Zhang, F. Protective effects of sulforaphane in experimental vascular cognitive impairment: Contribution of the Nrf2 pathway. *J. Cereb. Blood Flow Metab.* **2019**, *39*, 352–366. [CrossRef] [PubMed]
135. Greene, C.; Hanley, N.; Campbell, M. Claudin-5: Gatekeeper of neurological function. *Fluids Barriers CNS* **2019**, *16*, 3. [CrossRef] [PubMed]

136. Wang, X.-X.; Zhang, B.; Xia, R.; Jia, Q.-Y. Inflammation, apoptosis and autophagy as critical players in vascular dementia. *Eur. Rev. Med. Pharmacol. Sci.* **2020**, *24*, 9601–9614. [CrossRef] [PubMed]
137. Shaik-Dasthagirisaheb, Y.; Varvara, G.; Murmura, G.; Saggini, A.; Potalivo, G.; Caraffa, A.; Antinolfi, P.; Tetè, S.; Tripodi, D.; Conti, F.; et al. Vascular endothelial growth factor (VEGF), mast cells and inflammation. *Int. J. Immunopathol. Pharmacol.* **2013**, *26*, 327–335. [CrossRef] [PubMed]
138. Wallin, A.; Kapaki, E.; Boban, M.; Engelborghs, S.; Hermann, D.M.; Huisa, B.; Jonsson, M.; Kramberger, M.G.; Lossi, L.; Malojcic, B.; et al. Biochemical markers in vascular cognitive impairment associated with subcortical small vessel disease—A consensus report. *BMC Neurol.* **2017**, *17*, 1–12. [CrossRef] [PubMed]
139. Ichijo, H.; Nishida, E.; Irie, K.; ten Dijke, P.; Saitoh, M.; Moriguchi, T.; Takagi, M.; Matsumoto, K.; Miyazono, K.; Gotoh, Y. Induction of Apoptosis by ASK1, a Mammalian MAPKKK That Activates SAPK/JNK and p38 Signaling Pathways. *Science* **1997**, *275*, 90–94. [CrossRef]
140. Yamamoto, E.; Kataoka, K.; Shintaku, H.; Yamashita, T.; Tokutomi, Y.; Dong, Y.F.; Matsuba, S.; Ichijo, H.; Ogawa, H.; Kim-Mitsuyama, S. Novel mechanism and role of angiotensin II induced vascular endothelial injury in hypertensive diastolic heart failure. *Arter. Thromb. Vasc. Biol.* **2007**, *27*, 2569–2575. [CrossRef]
141. Toyama, K.; Koibuchi, N.; Uekawa, K.; Hasegawa, Y.; Kataoka, K.; Katayama, T.; Sueta, D.; Ma, M.J.; Nakagawa, T.; Yasuda, O.; et al. Apoptosis signal-regulating kinase 1 is a novel target molecule for cognitive impairment induced by chronic cerebral hypoperfusion. *Arter. Thromb. Vasc. Biol.* **2014**, *34*, 616–625. [CrossRef] [PubMed]
142. Sajja, R.K.; Green, K.N.; Cucullo, L. Altered Nrf2 Signaling Mediates Hypoglycemia-Induced Blood–Brain Barrier Endothelial Dysfunction In Vitro. *PLoS ONE* **2015**, *10*, e0122358. [CrossRef] [PubMed]
143. Zhao, J.; Moore, A.N.; Redell, J.B.; Dash, P.K. Enhancing Expression of Nrf2-Driven Genes Protects the Blood–Brain Barrier after Brain Injury. *J. Neurosci.* **2007**, *27*, 10240–10248. [CrossRef] [PubMed]
144. Alfieri, A.; Srivastava, S.; Siow, R.C.; Cash, D.; Modo, M.; Duchen, M.R.; Fraser, P.A.; Williams, S.C.; Mann, G.E. Sulforaphane preconditioning of the Nrf2/HO-1 defense pathway protects the cerebral vasculature against blood-brain barrier disruption and neurological deficits in stroke. *Free Radic. Biol. Med.* **2013**, *65*, 1012–1022. [CrossRef] [PubMed]
145. Kim, S.-Y.; Kim, Y.-J.; Cho, S.-Y.; Lee, H.-G.; Kwon, S.; Park, S.-U.; Jung, W.-S.; Moon, S.-K.; Park, J.-M.; Cho, K.-H.; et al. Efficacy of Artemisia annua Linné in improving cognitive impairment in a chronic cerebral hypoperfusion-induced vascular dementia animal model. *Phytomedicine* **2023**, *112*, 154683. [CrossRef] [PubMed]
146. Ungvari, Z.; Kaley, G.; De Cabo, R.; Sonntag, W.E.; Csiszar, A. Mechanisms of vascular aging: New perspectives. *J. Gerontol. Ser. A Boil. Sci. Med. Sci.* **2010**, *65*, 1028–1041. [CrossRef] [PubMed]
147. Csiszar, A.; Labinskyy, N.; Smith, K.; Rivera, A.; Orosz, Z.; Ungvari, Z. Vasculoprotective effects of anti-tumor necrosis factor-α treatment in aging. *Am. J. Pathol.* **2007**, *170*, 388–398. [CrossRef] [PubMed]
148. Csiszar, A.; Ungvari, Z.; Koller, A.; Edwards, J.G.; Kaley, G.; Tarantini, S.; Kirkpatrick, A.C.; Prodan, C.I.; Gautam, T.; Sosnowska, D.; et al. Proinflammatory phenotype of coronary arteries promotes endothelial apoptosis in aging. *Physiol. Genom.* **2004**, *17*, 21–30. [CrossRef] [PubMed]
149. Anversa, P.; Li, P.; Sonnenblick, E.H.; Olivetti, G. Effects of aging on quantitative structural properties of coronary vasculature and microvasculature in rats. *Am. J. Physiol. Circ. Physiol.* **1994**, *267*, H1062–H1073. [CrossRef]
150. Riddle, D.R.; Sonntag, W.E.; Lichtenwalner, R.J. Microvascular plasticity in aging. *Ageing Res. Rev.* **2003**, *2*, 149–168. [CrossRef]
151. Sonntag, W.E.; Lynch, C.D.; Cooney, P.T.; Hutchins, P.M. Decreases in cerebral microvasculature with age are associated with the decline in growth hormone and insulin-like growth factor 1. *Endocrinology* **1997**, *138*, 3515–3520. [CrossRef] [PubMed]
152. Valcarcel-Ares, M.N.; Gautam, T.; Warrington, J.P.; Bailey-Downs, L.; Sosnowska, D.; de Cabo, R.; Losonczy, G.; Sonntag, W.E.; Ungvari, Z.; Csiszar, A. Disruption of Nrf2 signaling impairs angiogenic capacity of endothelial cells: Implications for microvascular aging. *J. Gerontol. Ser. A* **2012**, *67*, 821–829. [CrossRef] [PubMed]
153. Chen, G.-H.; Song, C.-C.; Pantopoulos, K.; Wei, X.-L.; Zheng, H.; Luo, Z. Mitochondrial oxidative stress mediated Fe-induced ferroptosis via the NRF2-ARE pathway. *Free. Radic. Biol. Med.* **2022**, *180*, 95–107. [CrossRef] [PubMed]
154. Fan, J.; Lane, W.; Lawrence, M.; Mixon, T. Adjunctive use of Angio-Seal closure device following transcatheter aortic valve implantation via percutaneous transfemoral approach with incomplete hemostasis after modified Perclose ProGlide preclosure technique. *Bayl. Univ. Med. Cent. Proc.* **2019**, *32*, 34–36. [CrossRef] [PubMed]
155. Lonati, E.; Carrozzini, T.; Bruni, I.; Mena, P.; Botto, L.; Cazzaniga, E.; Del Rio, D.; Labra, M.; Palestini, P.; Bulbarelli, A. Coffee-Derived Phenolic Compounds Activate Nrf2 Antioxidant Pathway in I/R Injury In Vitro Model: A Nutritional Approach Preventing Age Related-Damages. *Molecules* **2022**, *27*, 1049. [CrossRef] [PubMed]
156. Beck, H.; Plate, K.H. Angiogenesis after cerebral ischemia. *Acta Neuropathol.* **2009**, *117*, 481–496. [CrossRef] [PubMed]
157. Yang, J.-P.; Liu, H.-J.; Liu, X.-F. VEGF promotes angiogenesis and functional recovery in stroke rats. *J. Investig. Surg.* **2010**, *23*, 149–155. [CrossRef]
158. Bailey-Downs, L.C.; Mitschelen, M.; Sosnowska, D.; Toth, P.; Pinto, J.T.; Ballabh, P.; Valcarcel-Ares, M.N.; Farley, J.; Koller, A.; Henthorn, J.C.; et al. Liver-Specific Knockdown of IGF-1 Decreases Vascular Oxidative Stress Resistance by Impairing the Nrf2-Dependent Antioxidant Response: A Novel Model of Vascular Aging. *J. Gerontol. Ser. A* **2012**, *67*, 313–329. [CrossRef]
159. Papaiahgari, S.; Zhang, Q.; Kleeberger, S.R.; Cho, H.-Y.; Reddy, S.P. Hyperoxia stimulates an Nrf2-ARE transcriptional response via ROS-EGFR-PI3K-Akt/ERK MAP kinase signaling in pulmonary epithelial cells. *Antioxid. Redox Signal* **2006**, *8*, 43–52. [CrossRef]

160. A Beyer, T.; Xu, W.; Teupser, D.; Keller, U.A.D.; Bugnon, P.; Hildt, E.; Thiery, J.; Kan, Y.W.; Werner, S. Impaired liver regeneration in Nrf2 knockout mice: Role of ROS-mediated insulin/IGF-1 resistance. *EMBO J.* **2008**, *27*, 212–223. [CrossRef]
161. Panieri, E.; Santoro, M.M. ROS signaling and redox biology in endothelial cells. *Experientia* **2015**, *72*, 3281–3303. [CrossRef] [PubMed]
162. Yang, J. The role of reactive oxygen species in angiogenesis and preventing tissue injury after brain ischemia. *Microvasc. Res.* **2019**, *123*, 62–67. [CrossRef] [PubMed]
163. Kim, Y.-W.; Byzova, T.V. Oxidative stress in angiogenesis and vascular disease. *Blood* **2014**, *123*, 625–631. [CrossRef] [PubMed]
164. Zhao, W.; Zhao, T.; Chen, Y.; A Ahokas, R.; Sun, Y. Reactive oxygen species promote angiogenesis in the infarcted rat heart. *Int. J. Exp. Pathol.* **2009**, *90*, 621–629. [CrossRef] [PubMed]
165. García-Quintans, N.; Sánchez-Ramos, C.; Tierrez, A.; Olmo, Y.; Luque, A.; Arza, E.; Alfranca, A.; Redondo, J.M.; Monsalve, M. Control of endothelial function and angiogenesis by PGC-1α relies on ROS control of vascular stability. *Free. Radic. Biol. Med.* **2014**, *75*, S5. [CrossRef] [PubMed]
166. Jiang, F.; Zhang, Y.; Dusting, G.J. NADPH Oxidase-Mediated Redox Signaling: Roles in Cellular Stress Response, Stress Tolerance, and Tissue Repair. *Pharmacol. Rev.* **2011**, *63*, 218–242. [CrossRef] [PubMed]
167. Calvani, M.; Comito, G.; Giannoni, E.; Chiarugi, P. Time-dependent stabilization of hypoxia inducible factor-1α by different intracellular sources of reactive oxygen species. *PLoS ONE* **2012**, *7*, e38388. [CrossRef] [PubMed]
168. Rosenstein, J.M.; Krum, J.M.; Ruhrberg, C. VEGF in the nervous system. *Organogenesis* **2010**, *6*, 107–114. [CrossRef] [PubMed]
169. Fukai, T.; Ushio-Fukai, M. Cross-Talk between NADPH Oxidase and Mitochondria: Role in ROS Signaling and Angiogenesis. *Cells* **2020**, *9*, 1849. [CrossRef] [PubMed]
170. Kuang, L.; Feng, J.; He, G.; Jing, T. Knockdown of Nrf2 inhibits the angiogenesis of rat cardiac micro-vascular endothelial cells under hypoxic conditions. *Int. J. Biol. Sci.* **2013**, *9*, 656–665. [CrossRef]
171. Wei, Y.; Gong, J.; Thimmulappa, R.K.; Kosmider, B.; Biswal, S.; Duh, E.J. Nrf2 acts cell-autonomously in endothelium to regulate tip cell formation and vascular branching. *Proc. Natl. Acad. Sci. USA* **2013**, *110*, E3910–E3918. [CrossRef] [PubMed]
172. Fukuda, S.; Kaga, S.; Zhan, L.; Bagchi, D.; Das, D.K.; Bertelli, A.; Maulik, N. Resveratrol ameliorates myocardial damage by inducing vascular endothelial growth factor-angiogenesis and tyrosine kinase receptor Flk-1. *Cell Biochem. Biophys.* **2006**, *44*, 043–050. [CrossRef] [PubMed]
173. Csiszar, A.; Labinskyy, N.; Podlutsky, A.; Kaminski, P.M.; Wolin, M.S.; Zhang, C.; Mukhopadhyay, P.; Pacher, P.; Hu, F.; de Cabo, R.; et al. Vasoprotective effects of resveratrol and SIRT1: Attenuation of cigarette smoke-induced oxidative stress and proinflammatory phenotypic alterations. *Am. J. Physiol. Heart Circ. Physiol.* **2008**, *294*, H2721–H2735. [CrossRef] [PubMed]
174. Pearson, K.J.; Baur, J.A.; Lewis, K.N.; Peshkin, L.; Price, N.L.; Labinskyy, N.; Swindell, W.R.; Kamara, D.; Minor, R.K.; Perez, E.; et al. Resveratrol delays age-related deterioration and mimics transcriptional aspects of dietary restriction without extending life span. *Cell Metab.* **2008**, *8*, 157–168. [CrossRef] [PubMed]
175. Oomen, C.A. Resveratrol preserves cerebrovascular density and cognitive function in aging mice. *Front. Aging Neurosci.* **2009**, *1*, 4. [CrossRef] [PubMed]
176. Ungvari, Z.; Bagi, Z.; Feher, A.; Recchia, F.A.; Sonntag, W.E.; Pearson, K.; de Cabo, R.; Csiszar, A. Resveratrol confers endothelial protection via activation of the antioxidant transcription factor Nrf2. *Am. J. Physiol. Heart Circ. Physiol.* **2010**, *299*, H18–H24. [CrossRef]
177. Ungvari, Z.; Bailey-Downs, L.; Gautam, T.; Jimenez, R.; Losonczy, G.; Zhang, C.; Ballabh, P.; Recchia, F.A.; Wilkerson, D.C.; Sonntag, W.E.; et al. Adaptive induction of NF-E2-related factor-2-driven antioxidant genes in endothelial cells in response to hyperglycemia. *Am. J. Physiol. Circ. Physiol.* **2011**, *300*, H1133–H1140. [CrossRef] [PubMed]
178. Dai, X.; Wang, K.; Fan, J.; Liu, H.; Fan, X.; Lin, Q.; Chen, Y.; Chen, H.; Li, Y.; Liu, H.; et al. Nrf2 transcriptional upregulation of IDH2 to tune mitochondrial dynamics and rescue angiogenic function of diabetic EPCs. *Redox Biol.* **2022**, *56*, 102449. [CrossRef] [PubMed]
179. Uno, K.; Prow, T.W.; Bhutto, I.A.; Yerrapureddy, A.; McLeod, D.S.; Yamamoto, M.; Reddy, S.P.; Lutty, G.A. Role of Nrf2 in retinal vascular development and the vaso-obliterative phase of oxygen-induced retinopathy. *Exp. Eye Res.* **2010**, *90*, 493–500. [CrossRef]
180. Bracko, O.; Njiru, B.N.; Swallow, M.; Ali, M.; Haft-Javaherian, M.; Schaffer, C.B. Increasing cerebral blood flow improves cognition into late stages in Alzheimer's disease mice. *J. Cereb. Blood Flow Metab.* **2020**, *40*, 1441–1452. [CrossRef]
181. Hayes, G.; Pinto, J.; Sparks, S.N.; Wang, C.; Suri, S.; Bulte, D.P. Vascular smooth muscle cell dysfunction in neurodegeneration. *Front. Neurosci.* **2022**, *16*, 1010164. [CrossRef] [PubMed]
182. Griendling, K.K.; Ushio-Fukai, M.; Lassègue, B.; Alexander, R.W. Angiotensin II signaling in vascular smooth muscle. *Hypertension* **1997**, *29*, 366–370. [CrossRef] [PubMed]
183. Zhao, Y.; Vanhoutte, P.M.; Leung, S.W. Vascular nitric oxide: Beyond eNOS. *J. Pharmacol. Sci.* **2015**, *129*, 83–94. [CrossRef] [PubMed]
184. Parga, J.A.; Rodriguez-Perez, A.I.; Garcia-Garrote, M.; Rodriguez-Pallares, J.; Labandeira-Garcia, J.L. Angiotensin II induces oxidative stress and upregulates neuroprotective signaling from the NRF2 and KLF9 pathway in dopaminergic cells. *Free. Radic. Biol. Med.* **2018**, *129*, 394–406. [CrossRef] [PubMed]
185. Rodriguez-Pallares, J.; Rey, P.; Parga, J.; Muñoz, A.; Guerra, M.; Labandeira-Garcia, J. Brain angiotensin enhances dopaminergic cell death via microglial activation and NADPH-derived ROS. *Neurobiol. Dis.* **2008**, *31*, 58–73. [CrossRef] [PubMed]

186. Rao, G.N.; Berk, B.C. Active oxygen species stimulate vascular smooth muscle cell growth and proto-oncogene expression. *Circ. Res.* **1992**, *70*, 593–599. [CrossRef]
187. Meng, H.; Fan, L.; Zhang, C.-J.; Zhu, L.; Liu, P.; Chen, J.; Bao, X.; Pu, Z.; Zhu, M.-S.; Xu, Y. Synthetic VSMCs induce BBB disruption mediated by MYPT1 in ischemic stroke. *iScience* **2021**, *24*, 103047. [CrossRef]
188. Zhang, M.; Xu, Y.; Qiu, Z.; Jiang, L. Sulforaphane Attenuates Angiotensin II-Induced Vascular Smooth Muscle Cell Migration via Suppression of NOX4/ROS/Nrf2 Signaling. *Int. J. Biol. Sci.* **2019**, *15*, 148–157. [CrossRef] [PubMed]
189. Ashino, T.; Yamamoto, M.; Numazawa, S. Nrf2/Keap1 system regulates vascular smooth muscle cell apoptosis for vascular homeostasis: Role in neointimal formation after vascular injury. *Sci. Rep.* **2016**, *6*, 26291. [CrossRef]
190. Ashino, T.; Yamamoto, M.; Yoshida, T.; Numazawa, S. Redox-sensitive transcription factor Nrf2 regulates vascular smooth muscle cell migration and neointimal hyperplasia. *Arter. Thromb. Vasc. Biol.* **2013**, *33*, 760–768. [CrossRef]
191. Song, H.; Xu, T.; Feng, X.; Lai, Y.; Yang, Y.; Zheng, H.; He, X.; Wei, G.; Liao, W.; Liao, Y.; et al. Itaconate prevents abdominal aortic aneurysm formation through inhibiting inflammation via activation of Nrf2. *EBioMedicine* **2020**, *57*, 102832. [CrossRef] [PubMed]
192. Kopacz, A.; Werner, E.; Grochot-Przęczek, A.; Klóska, D.; Hajduk, K.; Neumayer, C.; Józkowicz, A.; Piechota-Polanczyk, A. Simvastatin Attenuates Abdominal Aortic Aneurysm Formation Favoured by Lack of Nrf2 Transcriptional Activity. *Oxidative Med. Cell. Longev.* **2020**, *2020*, 6340190. [CrossRef] [PubMed]
193. Rucker, H.K.; Wynder, H.J.; Thomas, W. Cellular mechanisms of CNS pericytes. *Brain Res. Bull.* **2000**, *51*, 363–369. [CrossRef] [PubMed]
194. Armulik, A.; Genove, G.; Betsholtz, C. Pericytes: Developmental, physiological, and pathological perspectives, problems, and promises. *Dev. Cell* **2011**, *21*, 193–215. [CrossRef] [PubMed]
195. A Winkler, E.; Bell, R.D.; Zlokovic, B.V. Central nervous system pericytes in health and disease. *Nat. Neurosci.* **2011**, *14*, 1398–1405. [CrossRef] [PubMed]
196. Armulik, A.; Genové, G.; Mäe, M.; Nisancioglu, M.H.; Wallgard, E.; Niaudet, C.; He, L.; Norlin, J.; Lindblom, P.; Strittmatter, K.; et al. Pericytes regulate the blood-brain barrier. *Nature* **2010**, *468*, 557–561. [CrossRef] [PubMed]
197. Daneman, R.; Zhou, L.; Kebede, A.A.; Barres, B.A. Pericytes are required for blood–brain barrier integrity during embryogenesis. *Nature* **2010**, *468*, 562–566. [CrossRef]
198. Lin, L.; Chen, Z.; Huang, C.; Wu, Y.; Huang, L.; Wang, L.; Ke, S.; Liu, L. Mito-TEMPO, a Mitochondria-Targeted Antioxidant, Improves Cognitive Dysfunction due to Hypoglycemia: An Association with Reduced Pericyte Loss and Blood-Brain Barrier Leakage. *Mol. Neurobiol.* **2023**, *60*, 672–686. [CrossRef] [PubMed]
199. Zheng, S.; Wang, C.; Lin, L.; Mu, S.; Liu, H.; Hu, X.; Chen, X.; Wang, S. TNF-α Impairs Pericyte-Mediated Cerebral Microcirculation via the NF-κB/iNOS Axis after Experimental Traumatic Brain Injury. *J. Neurotrauma.* **2023**, *40*, 349–364. [CrossRef]
200. Dente, C.J.; Steffes, C.P.; Speyer, C.; Tyburski, J.G. Pericytes Augment the Capillary Barrier in in Vitro Cocultures. *J. Surg. Res.* **2001**, *97*, 85–91. [CrossRef]
201. Fernández-Klett, F.; Offenhauser, N.; Dirnagl, U.; Priller, J.; Lindauer, U. Pericytes in capillaries are contractile in vivo, but arterioles mediate functional hyperemia in the mouse brain. *Proc. Natl. Acad. Sci. USA* **2010**, *107*, 22290–22295. [CrossRef] [PubMed]
202. Kornfield, T.E.; Newman, E.A. Regulation of Blood Flow in the Retinal Trilaminar Vascular Network. *J. Neurosci.* **2014**, *34*, 11504–11513. [CrossRef] [PubMed]
203. Hill, R.A.; Tong, L.; Yuan, P.; Murikinati, S.; Gupta, S.; Grutzendler, J. Regional Blood Flow in the Normal and Ischemic Brain Is Controlled by Arteriolar Smooth Muscle Cell Contractility and Not by Capillary Pericytes. *Neuron* **2015**, *87*, 95–110. [CrossRef] [PubMed]
204. Hall, C.N.; Reynell, C.; Gesslein, B.; Hamilton, N.B.; Mishra, A.; Sutherland, B.A.; O'Farrell, F.M.; Buchan, A.M.; Lauritzen, M.; Attwell, D. Capillary pericytes regulate cerebral blood flow in health and disease. *Nature* **2014**, *508*, 55–60. [CrossRef] [PubMed]
205. Chaigneau, E.; Oheim, M.; Audinat, E.; Charpak, S. Two-photon imaging of capillary blood flow in olfactory bulb glomeruli. *Proc. Natl. Acad. Sci. USA* **2003**, *100*, 13081–13086. [CrossRef] [PubMed]
206. Peppiatt, C.M.; Howarth, C.; Mobbs, P.; Attwell, D. Bidirectional control of CNS capillary diameter by pericytes. *Nature* **2006**, *443*, 700–704. [CrossRef] [PubMed]
207. Debette, S.; Schilling, S.; Duperron, M.-G.; Larsson, S.C.; Markus, H. Clinical Significance of Magnetic Resonance Imaging Markers of Vascular Brain Injury: A Systematic Review and Meta-analysis. *JAMA Neurol.* **2019**, *76*, 81–94. [CrossRef] [PubMed]
208. Kapasi, A.; DeCarli, C.; Schneider, J.A. Impact of multiple pathologies on the threshold for clinically overt dementia. *Acta Neuropathol.* **2017**, *134*, 171–186. [CrossRef] [PubMed]
209. Bos, D.; Wolters, F.J.; Darweesh, S.K.; Vernooij, M.W.; de Wolf, F.; Ikram, M.A.; Hofman, A. Cerebral small vessel disease and the risk of dementia: A systematic review and meta-analysis of population-based evidence. *Alzheimer's Dement* **2018**, *14*, 1482–1492. [CrossRef]
210. Nortley, R.; Korte, N.; Izquierdo, P.; Hirunpattarasilp, C.; Mishra, A.; Jaunmuktane, Z.; Kyrargyri, V.; Pfeiffer, T.; Khennouf, L.; Madry, C.; et al. Amyloid beta oligomers constrict human capillaries in Alzheimer's disease via signaling to pericytes. *Science* **2019**, *365*, eaav9518. [CrossRef]
211. Nielsen, R.B.; Egefjord, L.; Angleys, H.; Mouridsen, K.; Gejl, M.; Møller, A.; Brock, B.; Brændgaard, H.; Gottrup, H.; Rungby, J.; et al. Capillary dysfunction is associated with symptom severity and neurodegeneration in Alzheimer's disease. *Alzheimer's Dement* **2017**, *13*, 1143–1153. [CrossRef] [PubMed]

212. Bonkowski, D.; Katyshev, V.; Balabanov, R.D.; Borisov, A.; Dore-Duffy, P. The CNS microvascular pericyte: Pericyte-astrocyte crosstalk in the regulation of tissue survival. *Fluids Barriers CNS* **2011**, *8*, 8. [CrossRef] [PubMed]
213. Bosetti, F.; Galis, Z.S.; Bynoe, M.S.; Charette, M.; Cipolla, M.J.; del Zoppo, G.J.; Gould, D.; Hatsukami, T.S.; Jones, T.L.Z.; Koenig, J.I.; et al. "Small Blood Vessels: Big Health Problems?": Scientific Recommendations of the National Institutes of Health Workshop. *J. Am. Hear. Assoc.* **2016**, *5*, e004389. [CrossRef] [PubMed]
214. Brown, L.S.; Foster, C.G.; Courtney, J.-M.; King, N.E.; Howells, D.W.; Sutherland, B.A. Pericytes and Neurovascular Function in the Healthy and Diseased Brain. *Front. Cell. Neurosci.* **2019**, *13*, 282. [CrossRef] [PubMed]
215. Yang, T.; Guo, R.; Zhang, F. Brain perivascular macrophages: Recent advances and implications in health and diseases. *CNS Neurosci. Ther.* **2019**, *25*, 1318–1328. [CrossRef] [PubMed]
216. Faraco, G.; Sugiyama, Y.; Lane, D.; Garcia-Bonilla, L.; Chang, H.; Santisteban, M.M.; Racchumi, G.; Murphy, M.; Van Rooijen, N.; Anrather, J.; et al. Perivascular macrophages mediate the neurovascular and cognitive dysfunction associated with hypertension. *J. Clin. Investig.* **2016**, *126*, 4674–4689. [CrossRef] [PubMed]
217. Petersen, M.A.; Ryu, J.K.; Akassoglou, K. Fibrinogen in neurological diseases: Mechanisms, imaging and therapeutics. *Nat. Rev. Neurosci.* **2018**, *19*, 283–301. [CrossRef] [PubMed]
218. Cuff, C.A.; Berman, J.W.; Brosnan, C.F. The ordered array of perivascular macrophages is disrupted by IL-1-induced inflammation in the rabbit retina. *Glia* **1996**, *17*, 307–316. [CrossRef]
219. Yunna, C.; Mengru, H.; Lei, W.; Weidong, C. Macrophage M1/M2 polarization. *Eur. J. Pharmacol.* **2020**, *877*, 173090. [CrossRef]
220. Wang, P.; Yi, T.; Mao, S.; Li, M. Neuroprotective mechanism of human umbilical cord mesenchymal stem cell-derived extracellular vesicles improving the phenotype polarization of microglia via the PI3K/AKT/Nrf2 pathway in vascular dementia. *Synapse* **2023**, *77*, e22268. [CrossRef]
221. Rojo, A.I.; Innamorato, N.G.; Martín-Moreno, A.M.; De Ceballos, M.L.; Yamamoto, M.; Cuadrado, A. Nrf2 regulates microglial dynamics and neuroinflammation in experimental Parkinson's disease. *Glia* **2010**, *58*, 588–598. [CrossRef] [PubMed]
222. Wang, J.; Xing, H.; Wan, L.; Jiang, X.; Wang, C.; Wu, Y. Treatment targets for M2 microglia polarization in ischemic stroke. *Biomed. Pharmacother.* **2018**, *105*, 518–525. [CrossRef] [PubMed]
223. Sun, B.-L.; Wang, L.-H.; Yang, T.; Sun, J.-Y.; Mao, L.-L.; Yang, M.-F.; Yuan, H.; Colvin, R.A.; Yang, X.-Y. Lymphatic drainage system of the brain: A novel target for intervention of neurological diseases. *Prog. Neurobiol.* **2018**, *163–164*, 118–143. [CrossRef] [PubMed]
224. Da Mesquita, S.; Louveau, A.; Vaccari, A.; Smirnov, I.; Cornelison, R.C.; Kingsmore, K.M.; Contarino, C.; Onengut-Gumuscu, S.; Farber, E.; Raper, D.; et al. Functional aspects of meningeal lymphatics in ageing and Alzheimer's disease. *Nature* **2018**, *560*, 185–191. [CrossRef] [PubMed]
225. Elobeid, A.; Libard, S.; Leino, M.; Popova, S.N.; Alafuzoff, I. Altered Proteins in the Aging Brain. *J. Neuropathol. Exp. Neurol.* **2016**, *75*, 316–325. [CrossRef] [PubMed]
226. Han, B.H.; Zhou, M.L.; Abousaleh, F.; Brendza, R.P.; Dietrich, H.H.; Koenigsknecht-Talboo, J.; Cirrito, J.R.; Milner, E.; Holtzman, D.M.; Zipfel, G.J. Cerebrovascular dysfunction in amyloid precursor protein transgenic mice: Contribution of soluble and insoluble amyloid-beta peptide, partial restoration via gamma-secretase inhibition. *J. Neurosci.* **2008**, *28*, 13542–13550. [CrossRef] [PubMed]
227. Iliff, J.J.; Lee, H.; Yu, M.; Feng, T.; Logan, J.; Nedergaard, M.; Benveniste, H. Brain-wide pathway for waste clearance captured by contrast-enhanced MRI. *J. Clin. Investig.* **2013**, *123*, 1299–1309. [CrossRef] [PubMed]
228. Laman, J.D.; Weller, R.O. Drainage of Cells and Soluble Antigen from the CNS to Regional Lymph Nodes. *J. Neuroimmune Pharmacol.* **2013**, *8*, 840–856. [CrossRef] [PubMed]
229. Ramirez, J.; Berezuk, C.; McNeely, A.A.; Gao, F.; McLaurin, J.; Black, S.E. Imaging the Perivascular Space as a Potential Biomarker of Neurovascular and Neurodegenerative Diseases. *Cell. Mol. Neurobiol.* **2016**, *36*, 289–299. [CrossRef]
230. Weller, R.O.; Subash, M.; Preston, S.D.; Mazanti, I.; Carare, R.O. Perivascular drainage of amyloid-beta peptides from the brain and its failure in cerebral amyloid angiopathy and Alzheimer's disease. *Brain Pathol.* **2008**, *18*, 253–266. [CrossRef]
231. Hawkes, C.A. and J. McLaurin, Selective targeting of perivascular macrophages for clearance of beta-amyloid in cerebral amyloid angiopathy. *Proc. Natl. Acad. Sci. USA* **2009**, *106*, 1261–1266. [CrossRef] [PubMed]
232. Park, L.; Uekawa, K.; Garcia-Bonilla, L.; Koizumi, K.; Murphy, M.; Pistik, R.; Younkin, L.; Younkin, S.; Zhou, P.; Carlson, G.; et al. Brain Perivascular Macrophages Initiate the Neurovascular Dysfunction of Alzheimer Abeta Peptides. *Circ. Res.* **2017**, *121*, 258–269. [CrossRef] [PubMed]
233. Santisteban, M.M.; Ahn, S.J.; Lane, D.; Faraco, G.; Garcia-Bonilla, L.; Racchumi, G.; Poon, C.; Schaeffer, S.; Segarra, S.G.; Körbelin, J.; et al. Endothelium-Macrophage Crosstalk Mediates Blood-Brain Barrier Dysfunction in Hypertension. *Hypertension* **2020**, *76*, 795–807. [CrossRef] [PubMed]
234. Jearjaroen, P.; Thangwong, P.; Tocharus, C.; Lungkaphin, A.; Chaichompoo, W.; Srijun, J.; Suksamrarn, A.; Tocharus, J. Hexahydrocurcumin Attenuates Neuronal Injury and Modulates Synaptic Plasticity in Chronic Cerebral Hypoperfusion in Rats. *Mol. Neurobiol.* **2023**, *2023*, 1–14. [CrossRef] [PubMed]
235. Leonardo, C.C.; Mendes, M.; Ahmad, A.S.; Doré, S. Efficacy of prophylactic flavan-3-ol in permanent focal ischemia in 12-mo-old mice. *Am. J. Physiol. Circ. Physiol.* **2015**, *308*, H583–H591. [CrossRef] [PubMed]
236. Otulakowski, G.; Engelberts, D.; Arima, H.; Hirate, H.; Bayir, H.; Post, M.; Kavanagh, B.P. α-Tocopherol transfer protein mediates protective hypercapnia in murine ventilator-induced lung injury. *Thorax* **2017**, *72*, 538–549. [CrossRef] [PubMed]

237. Bourdakou, M.M.; Fernandez-Gines, R.; Cuadrado, A.; Spyrou, G.M. Drug repurposing on Alzheimer's disease through modulation of NRF2 neighborhood. *Redox Biol.* **2023**, *67*, 102881. [CrossRef] [PubMed]
238. A Reisman, S.; Gahir, S.S.; I Lee, C.-Y.; Proksch, J.W.; Sakamoto, M.; Ward, K.W. Pharmacokinetics and pharmacodynamics of the novel Nrf2 activator omaveloxolone in primates. *Drug Des. Dev. Ther.* **2019**, *13*, 1259–1270. [CrossRef] [PubMed]
239. Lynch, D.R.; Farmer, J.; Hauser, L.; Blair, I.A.; Wang, Q.Q.; Mesaros, C.; Snyder, N.; Boesch, S.; Chin, M.; Delatycki, M.B.; et al. Safety, pharmacodynamics, and potential benefit of omaveloxolone in Friedreich ataxia. *Ann. Clin. Transl. Neurol.* **2019**, *6*, 15–26. [CrossRef]
240. Zimmerman, A.W.; Singh, K.; Connors, S.L.; Liu, H.; Panjwani, A.A.; Lee, L.C.; Diggins, E.; Foley, A.; Melnyk, S.; Singh, I.N.; et al. Randomized controlled trial of sulforaphane and metabolite discovery in children with Autism Spectrum Disorder. *Mol. Autism.* **2021**, *12*, 38. [CrossRef]
241. Zolnourian, A.H.; Franklin, S.; Galea, I.; Bulters, D.O. Study protocol for SFX-01 after subarachnoid haemorrhage (SAS): A multicentre randomised double-blinded, placebo controlled trial. *BMJ Open* **2020**, *10*, e028514. [CrossRef] [PubMed]

Disclaimer/Publisher's Note: The statements, opinions and data contained in all publications are solely those of the individual author(s) and contributor(s) and not of MDPI and/or the editor(s). MDPI and/or the editor(s) disclaim responsibility for any injury to people or property resulting from any ideas, methods, instructions or products referred to in the content.

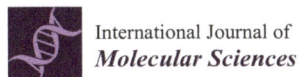 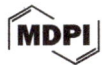

Review

Targeting Vascular Impairment, Neuroinflammation, and Oxidative Stress Dynamics with Whole-Body Cryotherapy in Multiple Sclerosis Treatment

Angela Dziedzic [1], Karina Maciak [1], Elżbieta Dorota Miller [2], Michał Starosta [2] and Joanna Saluk [1,*]

1. Department of General Biochemistry, Faculty of Biology and Environmental Protection, University of Lodz, Pomorska 141/143, 90-236 Lodz, Poland; angela.dziedzic@biol.uni.lodz.pl (A.D.); karina.maciak@edu.uni.lodz.pl (K.M.)
2. Department of Neurological Rehabilitation, Medical University of Lodz, Milionowa 14, 93-113 Lodz, Poland; elzbieta.dorota.miller@umed.lodz.pl (E.D.M.); michal.starosta@umed.lodz.pl (M.S.)
* Correspondence: joanna.saluk@biol.uni.lodz.pl

Abstract: Multiple sclerosis (MS), traditionally perceived as a neurodegenerative disease, exhibits significant vascular alternations, including blood–brain barrier (BBB) disruption, which may predispose patients to increased cardiovascular risks. This vascular dysfunction is intricately linked with the infiltration of immune cells into the central nervous system (CNS), which plays a significant role in perpetuating neuroinflammation. Additionally, oxidative stress serves not only as a byproduct of inflammatory processes but also as an active contributor to neural damage. The synthesis of these multifaceted aspects highlights the importance of understanding their cumulative impact on MS progression. This review reveals that the triad of vascular damage, chronic inflammation, and oxidative imbalance may be considered interdependent processes that exacerbate each other, underscoring the need for holistic and multi-targeted therapeutic approaches in MS management. There is a necessity for reevaluating MS treatment strategies to encompass these overlapping pathologies, offering insights for future research and potential therapeutic interventions. Whole-body cryotherapy (WBCT) emerges as one of the potential avenues for holistic MS management approaches which may alleviate the triad of MS progression factors in multiple ways.

Keywords: multiple sclerosis; neurodegeneration; neuroinflammation; vascular impairment; oxidative stress; whole-body cryotherapy

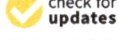

1. Introduction

Clinicians face significant challenges in understanding and treating conditions characterized by a complex, multifactorial, and elusive pathogenesis. A prime example may be multiple sclerosis (MS), an autoimmune and demyelinating disorder that affects the central nervous system (CNS) and is characterized by inflammation, loss of myelin sheaths, and ultimately neurodegeneration [1,2].

The MS pathogenesis is not clearly defined due to its highly varied and heterogeneous clinical and imaging manifestations [3]. Based on immanent features and symptom progression, two main clinical courses may be distinguished. The initially diagnosed relapsing–remitting stage (RR) is the most common form of MS characterized by periods of exacerbation (an acute inflammation relapsing) and followed episode resolutions (remission). The exacerbation usually occurs 1–2 times a year, for several days (from 24 h to one week), and then spontaneously reduces until it disappears, in the initial phase of the disease, but episodes worsen as it progresses [4]. The manifestation of RRMS symptoms during flare periods is the result of autoimmune inflammation in the CNS. Autoreactive immune cells, primarily T cells, are activated and cross the blood–brain barrier (BBB), leading to the destruction of myelin sheaths surrounding nerve fibers. However, inflammation is

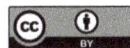

transient and remyelination occurs, and although it is not durable, neurological symptoms resolve completely in the initial phase of the disease [5]. Typically, as the disease develops, after an average of approximately 15 years since the first symptoms occur, approximately three-fourths of patients with RRMS advance into the secondary progressive stage (SP), which is marked by the progression of neurodegenerative phenomena leading to disability [4]. So, in the progressive subtype, during disease duration, the neurodegeneration processes are more prominent features than inflammation and gradually increase, leading to progressive deterioration of the patient's disability. In addition to RRMS and SPMS, there is also primary progressive multiple sclerosis (PPMS), which is the rarest type of MS (observed only in approximately 10% of diagnosed individuals). The typical progression of symptoms seen in PPMS makes it appear similar to SPMS; however, in PPMS, the progressive disability begins at the very onset of the disease [6]. In progressive MS subtypes, over time, long-standing established astroglia activation, secretion of pro-inflammatory cytokines, chemokines, and free radicals cause persistent lesions in the gray and white matter of the brain and spinal cord. Demyelination and neurodegeneration in the CNS are associated with profound astroglia reactions, forming a dense glial scar in long-standing established inflammatory lesions. Focal demyelinated plaques diffuse and create large confluent demyelinated lesions. This includes deprivation of nerve fibers and permanent damage to axons and finally results in profound brain tissue loss and atrophy [7].

Many MS patients demonstrate increased susceptibility to cardiovascular diseases and impaired function of the BBB; such vascular damage not only indicates a pathology of the CNS, but also raises critical questions about the role of the BBB [8,9]. Such disruption allows inflammatory factors and immune cells to penetrate protected areas, such as the CNS, leading to a persistent state of inflammation, characterized by microglia activation and lymphocyte infiltration, thus contributing to tissue damage [10].

Moreover, neuroinflammation, marked by the accumulation and activation of immune cells within the CNS, serves as both response to and a driver of neurological damage; it plays a crucial role in the development of demyelinated plaques, whose presence is a distinctive feature of MS. Such a persistent inflammatory state poses a challenge to the clinician for distinguishing the protective responses from those that perpetuate disease progression [11].

Adding to this complexity is the role of oxidative stress, characterized by an imbalance between the generation of reactive oxygen species (ROS) and the capacity to neutralize them. In MS, oxidative stress is not merely a byproduct of neuroinflammation but a significant contributor to neuronal and axonal damage, which exacerbates the disease process [12].

Understanding the interplay between vascular damage, neuroinflammation, and oxidative stress is critical for comprehending the pathogenesis of neurodegenerative diseases. This triad of pathological processes not only coexist, but also actively contribute to the progression of existing disorders by reinforcing each other (Figure 1). To provide multifaceted therapeutic approaches for ameliorating disease progression and improving clinical outcomes, it is crucial to first understand the molecular basis of the key etiological components of the disease.

In neurological and psychiatric conditions, rehabilitation is typically focused on learning lost skills and becoming as independent as possible. Recently, many novel strategies in neurorehabilitation have been introduced, one of them being whole-body cryotherapy (WBCT), which is used in multiple sclerosis. WBCT and other cooling therapies are promising methods that can improve function and quality of life [13]. Although the neurobiological basis of WBCT in MS is not fully understood, it has been proposed that the procedure may decrease oxidative stress by enhancing antioxidative enzyme activity or partially inhibiting the generation of reactive oxygen species (ROS) [14]. Many studies have shown that exposure of the whole body to low temperatures can change the level of selected enzymes and hormones in bodily fluids.

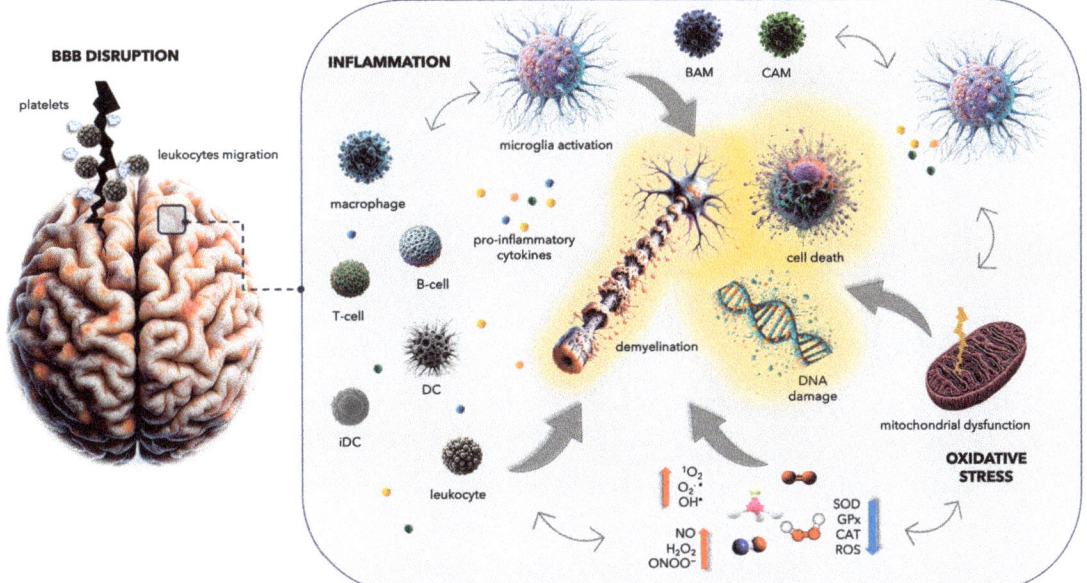

Figure 1. Multiple sclerosis (MS) manifests as inflammatory demyelination and neuronal death within the central nervous system (CNS), closely linked to blood vessel damage and heightened the permeability of the blood–brain barrier (BBB) [2]. The interaction between platelets and leukocytes entails an augmented production of pro-inflammatory cytokines and the recruitment of immune cells, including macrophages, dendritic cells (DCs), T cells, B cells, and immature monocyte-derived DCs (iDCs), traversing the disrupted BBB and initiating an inflammatory cascade. This process results in the persistent activation of microglia, collaborating with barrier-associated macrophages (BAMs) and CNS-associated macrophages (CAMs), and oxidative stress, thereby contributing to neuroinflammation and disease progression. Mitochondrial dysfunction, driven by increased reactive oxygen species (ROS), further amplifies neuronal damage [10–12]. Figure—own elaboration using elements generated by DALL·E 3, OpenAI.

Generally, evidence suggests that WBCT increases blood serum levels of adrenaline, noradrenaline, adrenocorticotropic hormone, cortisol, and testosterone and decreases certain parameters of inflammatory reactions [15]. However, no studies have yet assessed the effect of WBCT on molecular and morphological indices in patients with MS.

2. Methods

A search for peer-reviewed articles was conducted across multiple databases, including PubMed, Sage Journals, and SCOPUS, to compile relevant literature for this review. Additionally, Google Scholar was utilized to identify open-access articles. Data from authoritative sources such as clinicaltrials.gov were also incorporated into the analysis. The review encompasses 117 literature sources, comprising 64 original research studies (including case reports, clinical trials, and cohort studies) and 53 reviews (encompassing systemic reviews, literature reviews, and meta-analyses). The timeframe for the included publications ranges from 1994 to 2023, with a predominant concentration between 2019 and 2023. Identified relevant reviews underwent manual screening to ensure comprehensive coverage of pertinent references. Search terms utilized in this study encompassed a spectrum of topics relevant to multiple sclerosis, including neurodegeneration, neuroinflammation, vascular impairment, oxidative stress, and whole-body cryotherapy. Variations of these terms were employed to maximize the scope of search results. Boolean operators "AND" and "OR" were strategically applied after compiling all keywords, synonyms, and phrases to refine the search strategy and enhance result relevancy.

3. Complications in Multiple Sclerosis: From Blood–Brain Barrier Disruption to Increased Cardiovascular Disease Risk

Although MS is classified as an inflammatory demyelinating disorder of the CNS, it is intimately associated with vascular impairment, and with heightened permeability of the BBB [16]. Research has confirmed a higher susceptibility to cardiovascular diseases, notably ischemic stroke, myocardial infarction, and deep vein thrombosis, among patients with MS. Ischemic events are particularly closely linked to an intensified coagulation cascade and abnormal pro-thrombotic activity among platelets [17–24]. A population-based cohort study involving 17,418 Danish MS patients found that the disease itself to be a long-term risk factor for venous thromboembolism [25], while another analysis of 9881 MS patients found that they are over 30% more likely to die due to cardiovascular events than the general population [21]. A post-mortem analysis of 6000 Danish MS patients showed that the most common cause of death was not the disease itself, but cardiovascular diseases [24]. It has also been noted that the duration of the disease is one of the main risk factors for deep vein thrombosis [22].

A cohort study of 13,963 Danish MS patients found that the highest risk of stroke is within the first year after diagnosis and that it was most common among MS patients up to 56 years of age [22]; however, it is important to note that relapses occurring in the RRMS are often misdiagnosed as a stroke. Indeed, the opposite trend was observed in a Swedish cohort of 8281 MS patients which confirmed a positive correlation between age and risk of stroke [24]. In the later stages of the disease, the patient is typically not as fit, and a more sedentary lifestyle can elevate the risk of stroke [26]. Furthermore, stroke is strongly linked with deep venous thrombosis, the incidence of which increases by 40% in the late stage of MS [27]. Therapies for MS might also heighten the susceptibility to thromboembolic events, while disease-modifying therapies (DMTs) with anti-inflammatory properties could potentially mitigate cardiovascular risk factors [28].

It is, however, possible to reduce disease activity, influence the intensity of relapses, and treat concomitant clinical symptoms. Nevertheless, despite our more detailed knowledge about the pathomechanism of MS, the condition is characterized by a multitude of symptoms, and the possibilities for pharmacological treatment are unfortunately limited. Therefore, the key roles in treatment are played by physical activity and physiotherapy.

The increased risk of stroke, myocardial infarction, heart failure, and deep vein thrombosis observed in MS patients may all result from certain pathological mechanisms that are also implicated in cardiovascular diseases, such as oxidative stress, inflammation, and thrombotic factors (Figure 2) [29].

Pathological overactivation of blood platelets and thrombotic lesion formation within the wall of the coronary artery are widely recognized as major contributors to heart attack. Patients with acute myocardial infarction are characterized by elevated blood platelet activation and increased aggregation potential within the coronary circulation. Thrombotic occlusion of coronary vessels due to the formation of cellular aggregates can reduce or completely block blood flow [30]. Similarly, ischemic stroke can also result from the occlusion of cerebral blood vessels [31]. As the clotting cascade intensifies, excessive thrombin generation occurs; this enzyme converts soluble fibrinogen into insoluble fibrin, thus forming the clot responsible for venous thrombosis [32]. Thrombin serves as both the principal coagulation factor of the blood clotting cascade and the most potent agonist of blood platelets, thereby contributing to pro-thrombotic platelet activity [33]. However, in addition to thrombin, a number of endogenous physiological agonists are known to also activate blood platelets, with various consequences, including adhesion to the vessel wall, secretion of biologically active compounds accumulated in their numerous granules, and the generation of pro-thrombotic and pro-inflammatory microparticles. They can also increase receptor expression, which ultimately triggers the formation of platelet aggregates.

The excessive activation of blood platelets is well known to play an important role in the pathophysiology of MS [34,35]. MS patients exhibit enhanced surface receptor activity and expression on blood platelets, as well as a heightened response to platelet agonists, such as adenosine diphosphate (ADP). They are also characterized by elevated mRNA expression of the *P2RY12* gene, in both blood platelets and megakaryocytes (platelets' precursor cells), along with a higher density of P2Y12, a crucial ADP receptor, on the platelet surface. Platelets and megakaryocytes derived from patients with MS also demonstrate higher levels of fibrinogen and exhibit changes in the composition and genetic sequences of fibrinogen chains [36,37].

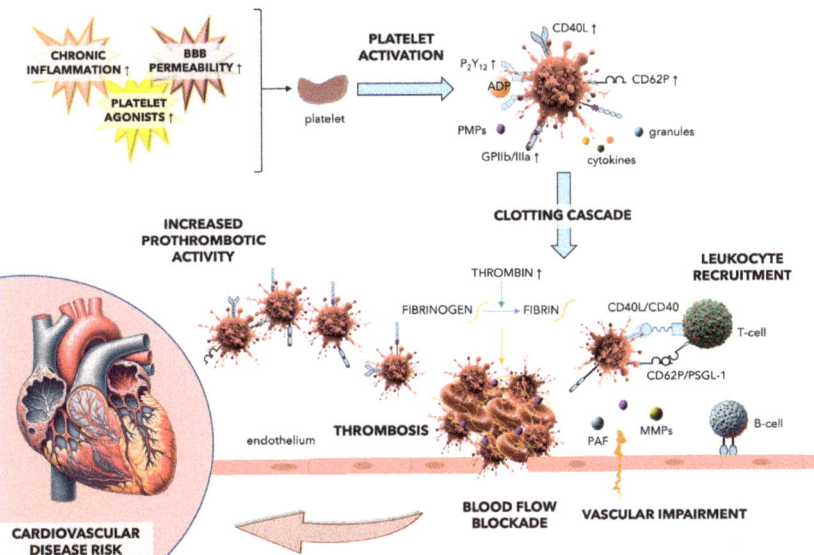

Figure 2. Multiple sclerosis (MS) pathophysiology includes chronic inflammation, blood–brain barrier (BBB) disruption, and the increased response to platelet agonists, leading to enhanced platelet activation and a predisposition towards pro-thrombotic phenotype and elevating the risk of cardiovascular disease [29]. In MS, platelets show increased expression of surface receptors, including P2RY12, CD40L, CD62P, and GPIIb/IIIa, which are essential for their activation. Once activated, platelets release molecules that trigger both pro-inflammatory and pro-thrombotic responses. The interaction between platelets, leukocytes, and endothelial cells, particularly through the CD40/CD40L and CD62P/P-selectin glycoprotein ligand (PSGL-1) pathways, exacerbates vascular impairment and activates the clotting cascade. The CD40/CD40L pathway, significant in autoimmune pathologies, enhances leukocyte adhesion and infiltration, leading to increased recruitment of immune cells to vascular injury sites [30–33]. Furthermore, the interaction between platelets and leukocytes intensifies vascular permeability involving platelet-derived microparticles (PMPs), platelet-activating factor (PAF), and matrix metalloproteinases (MMPs), disrupting endothelial junctions and promoting inflammation [30–33]. Figure—own elaboration using elements generated by DALL·E 3, OpenAI.

The inflammatory response causes plasma fibrinogen levels to rise two- to threefold [38]. Fibrinogen can modulate the inflammatory response by activating leukocytes and synthesizing pro-inflammatory mediators [39]; it can also activate glial cells, resulting in BBB dysfunction in MS patients [40]. However, Ptaszek et al. [41] report no increase in fibrinogen levels in women with MS, although a significant increase was noted in healthy women after a series of 20 WBCT sessions.

Activated blood platelets play a pivotal role in the coagulation cascade by serving as primary contributors to cellular hemostasis. Additionally, they have also been implicated in the development of neuroinflammatory processes associated with MS. The activated coagulation cascade stimulates blood platelets, which in turn amplify coagulation [42]. Therefore, the thrombin cascade also plays a significant role in the inflammatory response in MS. Studies profiling the proteome specific to the cerebrospinal fluid (CSF) found that the coagulation cascade also plays a pivotal role in MS patients with an increased burden of cortical lesions [43]. Later studies found blood platelets to be ensnared in chronic active demyelinating MS lesions, thus confirming their participation in the pathogenesis of MS through involvement in the inflammatory reaction [44]. Most importantly, a decrease in the number of platelets together with blockage of the main surface receptor GPIIb/IIIa, determining pro-thrombotic activity, inhibited the inflammation process and markedly improved symptoms in experimental autoimmune encephalomyelitis (EAE) [45].

The inflammatory response is acknowledged to play a crucial role in neuronal disorders like MS. In MS in particular, chronic inflammation and heightened pro-oxidative activity are known to be primary factors inducing excessive blood platelet activation. Blood platelets interact with immune cells to exacerbate inflammation via various inflammatory and immune pathways.

Overactivated blood platelets have a strong influence on the inflammatory response, and this is directly correlated with their increased adhesiveness to altered endothelial cells or proteins within the subendothelial layer of blood vessel walls. Moreover, stimulation increases the ability of platelets to activate both leukocytes and dendritic cells and their tendency to form aggregates with leukocytes [46,47]. It is important to note that the platelets, immune cells, and endothelial cells are all activated by reciprocal cellular interactions taking place between them. This activation has serious implications for maintaining the integrity of the blood vessel wall and contributes to the escalation of the local inflammatory response.

The interaction between blood platelets and leukocytes generates platelet-activating factor (PAF), which increases BBB permeability by interrupting endothelial junctions [48–50]. Similarly, the formation of cellular aggregates increases the production of matrix metalloproteinases (MMPs) by leukocytes, which are generally recognized as significant participants in BBB disruption [51]. MMPs are also produced by overactivated blood platelets; these share platelet-derived microparticles (PMPs), which act as a reservoir of a range of biologically active proteins [52].

Another important determinant in autoimmune disease is the CD40/CD40L platelet–leukocyte inflammatory signaling pathway. Increased levels of sCD40L, the soluble form of CD40L, a membrane glycoprotein of the TNF family, have been found in serum and CSF from MS patients [53]. Cellular interactions mediate the adhesion of circulating leukocytes to the endothelium, facilitating their recruitment and initiating their diapedesis and infiltration into the inflamed vessel. This process enables the selective recruitment of leukocytes to inflamed areas of vascular wall injury.

One of the earliest phases of the creation of new demyelination lesions is endothelial monolayer dysfunction. Briefly, a pro-inflammatory and pro-thrombotic phenotype of the endothelium increases blood platelet activation and the adhesion and subsequent migration of immune cells to the subendothelial space, resulting in vasomotor alterations [54,55]. Assuming the hypothesis that the interplay between blood platelets, leukocytes, and endothelial cells contributes to the breakdown of the BBB, this may be the pivotal initial step in certain neurological inflammatory diseases, such as MS; this process leads to the infiltration of lymphocytes and subsequent formation of inflammatory lesions in the brain [56]. The autoimmune reaction initiates a significant influx of inflammatory cells and provokes pro-inflammatory activation of microglia cells. This cascade leads to the disruption of the myelin sheath, resulting in the formation of demyelinating lesions and subsequent axonal/neuronal degeneration.

A fundamental role in the initiation and propagation of demyelinating plaque formation is believed to be played by T lymphocytes. Autoreactive T cells infiltrate the CNS and subsequently release pro-inflammatory cytokines. These cytokines activate macrophages, triggering inflammation in the white matter and the subsequent destruction of myelin [42].

In peripheral blood, under physiological conditions, the ratio of T to B cells is 9:1; however, the size of the B-cell population increases during the progression of autoimmune disease [57]. Blood platelets primarily enhance T-cell adhesion to endothelial cells, thus contributing to the formation of lymphocyte–platelet conjugates, disrupting BBB permeability. Studies indicate that T cells exhibit greater adhesive properties compared to B cells. This may suggest that T lymphocytes are most prevalent in the areas with developing inflammation; however, the B cell population represents almost 40% of all lymphocytes infiltrating the CNS structures [58,59]. The intricate relationship between MS and cardiovascular events sets the stage for a deeper exploration of neuroinflammation as a fundamental factor in MS progression.

4. Inflammatory Mechanisms in Multiple Sclerosis: Insights into Microglial Activation and CNS Immune Responses

One of the primary pathological characteristics of MS is an inflammatory process marked by the accumulation of immune cells within the CNS. In general, MS patients experience both acute and chronic inflammation, and these inflammatory processes have a crucial impact on the clinical manifestations of the disease. The acute inflammation associated with relapses leads to sudden neurological symptoms, such as muscle weakness, sensory disturbances, and visual impairments. These symptoms typically resolve partially or fully between relapses, reflecting the temporary nature of the inflammation. In contrast, the chronic inflammation observed in progressive MS contributes to a gradual decline in neurological function, leading to increasing disability over time. The accumulated damage to myelin and axons impairs the transmission of nerve impulses, gradually diminishing the ability of the brain to control muscles, senses, and cognitive processes. The chronic stage of MS is characterized by the accumulation of microglia, specialized CNS immune cells, which remain activated and contribute to the ongoing degeneration of white and grey matter of the brain [60].

One significant aspect of MS pathology is the disruption of the BBB, which allows immune cells, primarily T and B lymphocytes, to infiltrate into the brain. This leads to the development of active demyelinated plaques, the hallmark of MS, visible on magnetic resonance imaging (MRI), characterized by damaged myelin, inflammation, edema, and destruction of axons and nerve fibers [61].

Microglia play an essential role in maintaining homeostasis within the CNS. Under physiological conditions, microglia exhibit multiple, modulating functions in the brain, scavenging cellular debris, clearing apoptotic neurons, and promoting synapse formation. However, in response to injury, infection, or autoimmune processes, microglia generate an innate immune response and activate inflammatory mediators, exacerbating neuroinflammation and contributing to neurodegeneration (Figure 3) [62].

The inflammatory state in MS is characterized by both the pro-inflammatory and anti-inflammatory actions of monocyte-derived macrophages and microglia. Microglia are the innate immune cells native to the CNS, while monocyte-derived macrophages originate from peripheral blood monocytes and migrate into the CNS during inflammatory processes. Microglia can contribute to synaptic loss and cognitive decline by disrupting the homeostatic maintenance of neuronal synaptic plasticity [63]. Activated microglia and monocyte-derived macrophages intensify neuroinflammation by generating various pro-inflammatory cytokines, including tumor necrosis factor (TNF)-α and interleukins (IL)-1β and IL-6. These cytokines can also promote the differentiation of T cells into T helper (Th)17, further exacerbating the inflammatory response, and leading to neuronal damage and synaptic loss [64]. Nevertheless, the cells also play a vital role in tissue repair and recovery, clearing away debris and dead cells, and promoting oligodendrocyte differentiation and remyelination, which are essential for restoring myelin sheaths and restoring neural function [65,66]. Anti-inflammatory microglia express transforming growth factor (TGF)-β and cytokines such as IL-4 and IL-10, which can decrease the inflammatory response and promote tissue repair. The equilibrium between these two activations is crucial for preserving brain homeostasis [67].

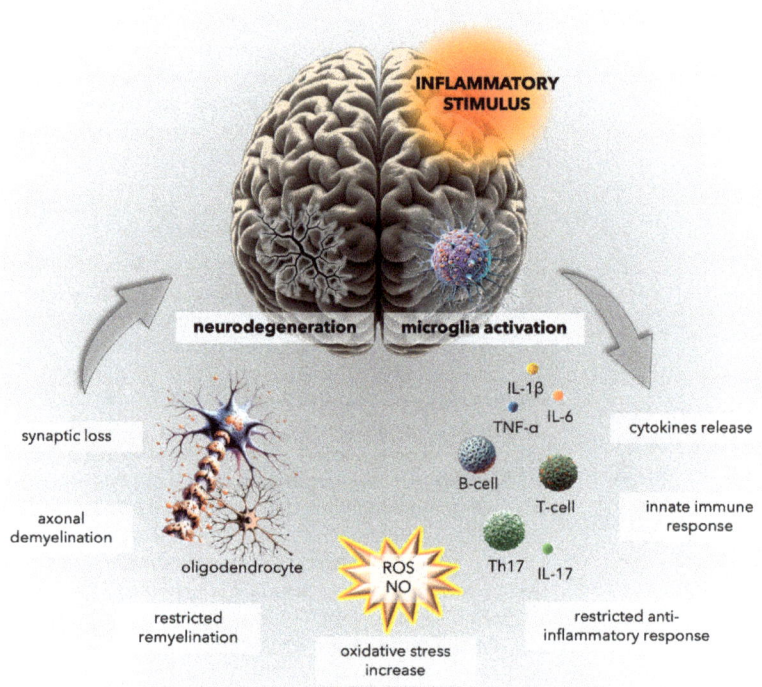

Figure 3. The balance between pro-inflammatory and anti-inflammatory activity of microglia is crucial for maintaining a balance between myelin loss and oligodendrocyte differentiation and remyelination. However, in the chronic stage of multiple sclerosis (MS), microglia accumulate and remain activated, contributing to white and grey matter degeneration [62]. The pro-inflammatory phenotype of microglia promotes the innate immune response, differentiation of T cells into T helper (Th)17 cells, generation of pro-inflammatory cytokines (e.g., tumor necrosis factor (TNF)-α, interleukin (IL)-1β, IL-6, IL-17), and reactive oxygen species (ROS) and nitric oxide (NO), all leading to synaptic loss and neurodegeneration [63–67]. Figure—own elaboration using elements generated by DALL·E 3, OpenAI.

In addition to microglia, barrier-associated macrophages (BAMs) and CNS dendritic cells (DCs) play critical roles in CNS immunity. Their ability to rapidly sense damage signals and modulate the immune response makes them crucial for maintaining CNS homeostasis and orchestrating the delicate balance between neuroinflammation and repair. During autoimmune-mediated neuroinflammation, the BBB becomes compromised, allowing immune cells from the peripheral circulation, including DCs, to enter the CNS [68]. BAMs interact with the BBB and monitor the constant molecular exchange between the bloodstream and the CNS; these are located in the non-parenchymal regions of the CNS, primarily in the meninges, choroid, and perivascular spaces, which all act as critical entry points for immune cells into the CNS [69,70]. BAMs actively participate in the neuroimmune response and communicate with astrocytes, the star-shaped glial cells that support neurons and contribute to maintaining the integrity of the BBB [71,72].

Early studies have shown that immature monocyte-derived DCs (iDCs) are more efficient at traversing the inflamed BBB than mature DCs. This is likely due to their ability to adhere more effectively to activated endothelial cells. Moreover, the adhesion between iDCs and BBB endothelial cells is mediated by adhesion molecules, including vascular (V)CAM-1, platelet endothelial (PE)CAM-1, intercellular adhesion molecule (ICAM)-1, and ICAM-2. While iDCs are more effective in passing the BBB, mature DCs are more selective in their crossing. Studies have shown that mature DCs are only affected by ICAM-1 [73]. This suggests that mature DCs require more specific signals to cross the BBB, perhaps indicating that they are only recruited in a severe state of CNS damage. CD18 and the DC-specific intracellular adhesion molecule-3-grabbing non-integrin (SIGN), expressed on both immature and mature DCs, also contribute to this process [74].

E- and P-selectins are adhesion molecules that play a crucial role in leukocyte recruitment during inflammation. However, it has been found that despite their elevated expression at the BBB during neuroinflammation, E- and P-selectins are not necessary for leukocyte recruitment across the BBB or the development of EAE [73,74]. Even so, it remains unclear whether selectins are essential for DC recruitment across the BBB, with current evidence being contradictory [75,76].

MS presents a multifaceted challenge for clinicians. It requires a comprehensive approach, balancing the need to prevent relapses, slow disease progression, effectively manage acute relapses and symptoms, and minimize the adverse effects of medications to manage the various aspects of the disease. Understanding the role of inflammation in MS has paved the way for the development of effective therapeutic strategies aimed at alleviating neuroinflammation, promoting tissue regeneration, and preventing neurodegeneration. Modern MS treatments aim to suppress the immune response and reduce the frequency and severity of relapses, slowing the progression of the disease and improving overall outcomes for patients.

The inflammation associated with MS may stimulate the respiratory burst system in activated microglia, raising ROS levels and thus increasing oxidative stress. ROS have been implicated as mediators of demyelination and axonal damage. It is assumed that the resulting free-radical-mediated tissue destruction may be prevented by antioxidants, which may also inhibit some of the early pro-inflammatory events and the trafficking of cells into the CNS [77]. It is hence recommended to support the mechanisms that can limit the severity of oxidative stress when treating diseases such as MS. One common approach is WBCT, which has been found to be very well tolerated by patients. A study of WBCT of MS patients by Bryczkowska et al. [78] found key antioxidant enzymes to act as reducing factors that neutralize the oxidative compounds before they can cause any damage to various biomolecules [79].

5. Oxidative Stress in Multiple Sclerosis: Unraveling the Complex Interplay

Persistent neuroinflammatory processes not only inflict direct damage to myelin sheaths and axonal structures but also create a milieu conducive to another critical aspect of MS pathology: oxidative stress. This alteration shifts the balance between the production of ROS and the effectiveness of endogenous antioxidant defense systems, thereby promoting neuronal damage and contributing to the progression of MS. Understanding the interaction between inflammation and oxidative damage is crucial for elucidating the pathophysiological underpinnings of MS.

5.1. General Facts about Oxidative Damage in MS

Oxidative stress is a key aspect of the pathophysiology of MS, resulting from a lack of balance between the production of ROS and the activation of antioxidant protection mechanisms, which is primarily influenced by the aberrant levels of the free radical scavenging enzymes [80]. Within the CNS, persistent inflammation and disrupted redox equilibrium impair brain plasticity, resulting in gradual demyelination and impaired neuronal signaling. These factors constitute the primary driver of psycho-motor disability. Oxidative stress is known to be associated with increased damage to myelin and axons in MS, and therefore, it almost certainly contributes to the observed clinical symptoms [81]. Furthermore, excess ROS production might trigger increased T-cell activation through an arachidonic acid cascade or inflict harm upon the BBB or myelin sheath, either directly or indirectly.

Despite the presence of natural antioxidant mechanisms, CNS cells, especially neurons and oligodendrocytes, are not entirely shielded against excessive ROS production. Indeed, the brain consumes 20% more oxygen than other organs, rendering it particularly susceptible to oxidative stress. Furthermore, brain cells are rich in polyunsaturated fatty acids with lower regenerative capacity [82], which additionally makes them more susceptible to oxidative damage.

Overproduction of highly reactive free radicals, including nitric oxide (NO), peroxynitrite (ONOO−), singlet oxygen (O_2), superoxide anion ($O_2\bullet-$), hydrogen peroxide (H_2O_2), and hydroxyl radicals (OH•) [83], can lead to harmful protein oxidation, lipid peroxidation, nucleic acid damage, antioxidant enzyme inhibition, and programmed cell death pathway activation [84]. NO is a reactive nitrogen species (RNS) consisting of a free radical possessing an unpaired electron; it is a key regulator of blood flow and synaptic transmission [85]. Serum NO level is significantly higher in RRMS patients during relapse ($p < 0.0001$) [86]. The rapid reaction between NO and $O_2\bullet-$ produces short-lived RNS, particularly highly reactive ONOO−, which may prompt oxidative/nitrative alterations in a diverse range of biomolecules [87]. Excessive NO production by immune cells induces hypoxia, hindering electron transport in the mitochondrial respiratory chain. This incomplete oxygen reduction triggers substantial ROS synthesis, altering mitochondrial structure and function and ultimately increasing oxidative stress [88]. Siotto et al. indicate elevated oxidative stress in RRMS patients with low levels of disability [89]. Moreover, clinical investigations have revealed increased oxidative stress in the bloodstream of patients with MS, characterized by dysregulated superoxide dismutase (SOD) [90] and glutathione (GSH) activity [91].

5.2. Mitochondrial Dysfunction in MS

Numerous human studies have provided compelling evidence indicative of mitochondrial dysfunction in patients with MS [92–94]. In mammalian cells, mitochondria represent a substantial source of ROS, and any impairment in the functionality of the respiratory chain could influence cell survival [95]. Persistent neuroinflammatory stimuli in MS disrupt neuroaxonal homeostasis, resulting in heightened oxidative stress marked by increased levels of ROS and mitochondrial damage. Such disruption increases excitotoxicity and disrupts the balance in neurotrophic factors needed to maintain neurons and oligodendrocytes [96]. The resultant impairment compromises mitochondrial functionality, exacerbating ROS generation and thus diminishing energy production efficiency. In this state, the cell is incapable of providing the necessary energy levels within demyelinated axons. As reduced ATP production reaches a critical point, ionic homeostasis becomes increasingly imbalanced, triggering the activation of apoptosis mechanisms [97,98].

Although ROS can damage mitochondria by altering their protein and lipid content, their predominant impact is observed on mitochondrial DNA, where they inactivate promoters and suppress mitochondrial gene expression. It is assumed that increased generation of ROS in mitochondria, encompassing species with prolonged half-life, such as H_2O_2 or lipid hydroperoxide, particularly may precipitate mitochondrial dysfunction, disrupting biological processes and contributing to various metabolic diseases [99].

Furthermore, previous studies suggest a reduction in peroxisome proliferator-activated receptor-gamma coactivator (PGC)-1α levels, a transcriptional factor crucial for regulating mitochondrial function; this decline is notably evident in the pyramidal neurons in SPMS and PPMS. This reduction in PGC-1α was correlated with the diminished expression of key components in mitochondrial machinery, such as oxidative phosphorylation (OXPHOS) subunits and antioxidants. These findings were confirmed with a functional model employing neuronal cells, which demonstrated a correlation between these alterations and increased ROS production [100].

Moreover, an independent study found that elevated ROS levels adversely impact the binding capacity of nuclear factor erythroid 2-related factor (NRF)-2, a transcription factor governing electron transport chain (ETC) proteins in SPMS patients, even within seemingly normal regions of the gray matter cortex [101]. In progressive MS patients (including 14 SPMS and 5 PPMS patients), heightened ROS production in the CNS was linked to an increase in the number of mitochondria in axons and astrocytes. Higher levels of ROS have been correlated with the translation of mitochondrial proteins in both active and inactive MS lesions; this is evidenced by heightened expression of proteins originating from the mitochondrial ETC complex IV and elevated levels of the mitochondrial stress marker mtHSP70 compared to controls [100].

A study comparing 10 post-mortem brains from individuals with MS (including 9 with SPMS and 1 with PPMS) revealed distinct alterations in the MS cortex in comparison to the control group. Notable differences in both nuclear DNA and mitochondrial (mt)DNA transcripts were observed between the groups. Furthermore, functional analysis conducted on identical samples revealed diminished activity in complexes I and III from neurons localized in the motor cortex of patients with MS; this was accompanied by a decline in GABAergic synaptic elements [102]. A separate study involving 13 SPMS patients identified significant mtDNA deletions in neurons, with some of these mutations being specific to the subunits of complex IV [103].

5.3. Genetic Factors Potentially Responsible for Oxidative Stress in MS

There has been a growing interest in the genetic predisposition to generating free radicals and the occurrence of MS. Evidence suggests that genetic factors, including single-nucleotide polymorphisms (SNPs) in genes encoding enzymes involved in oxidative stress pathways, play a pivotal role in determining treatment outcomes for MS.

The *NOX3* gene, located on chromosome 6q25.1, is responsible for synthesizing NADPH oxidase 3 (NOX3), an enzyme primarily found in the plasma membrane of the lung and cerebral cortex. NOX3 facilitates the generation of $O_2\bullet-$ through a single-electron reduction of O_2, with NADPH serving as the electron donor [104]. NOX3-generated ROS are particularly common in oligodendrocyte precursor cells, where they influence their differentiation and sensitivity to oxidative stress. It has been proposed that NOX3 generation stimulates oligodendrocyte maturation in MS patients [105]. Carlström et al. [86] report a significant association between the G allele of the rs6919626 (G > A,T) polymorphism in the *NOX3* gene and a decrease in ROS production by monocytes following ex vivo stimulation ($p = 0.057$) in a study of 564 RRMS patients in Sweden. This allele was also linked to a diminished response to dimethyl fumarate [106].

The *GSTP1* gene, located on chromosome 11 in the q13.2 region, is responsible for encoding the glutathione S-transferase P protein, an antioxidative enzyme that facilitates the merging of endogenous GSH. This enzyme is implicated in the modulation of MS progression, as disease advancement appears correlated with oxidative stress resulting from inflammation [107]. One extensively investigated polymorphism associated with varied responses to natalizumab is rs1695 (A > G, Ile105Val) [108]. A study on the rs1695 polymorphism found an improvement in disability among RRMS patients harboring the A allele ($\chi^2 = 0.031$; df = 1; $p = 0.861$) [108].

The *NQO1* gene, located on chromosome 16 in region q22.1, is responsible for producing an antioxidative enzyme known as NAD(P)H quinone oxidoreductase (NOQO1). Its function is to catalyze the double-electron reduction of quinones, thereby impeding their involvement in the redox cycle and ROS production [109]. One study found the rs1800566 polymorphism (C > T, Pro187Ser) to correlate with the reaction to natalizumab in RRMS patients; the identified association was particularly noticeable in MS patients possessing the C allele ($\chi^2 = 3.320$; df = 1; $p = 0.068$) [108].

WBCT offers promise for treating various disorders. WBCT is currently being used to relieve symptoms in diseases affecting the musculoskeletal system and the nervous system, such as MS. The application of low-temperature stimuli to the entire body is known to influence the autonomic, endocrine, circulatory, neuromuscular, and immunological systems [110]. Indeed, Capodaglio et al. [111] report that WBCT is an effective anti-inflammatory and antioxidant treatment that minimizes secondary tissue damage by reducing the production of pro-inflammatory and oxidative substances.

Attempts should be made to rehabilitate patients with MS throughout the course of the disease, not only during hospitalization. Such rehabilitation should be multidisciplinary and address both motor function and mental status. The rehabilitation protocol itself should be individualized and include physical rehabilitation intended to reduce spasticity and improve balance and posture [112]. Many studies underline the need for continued research into the effectiveness of different physiotherapeutic methods and types of therapies; however, current studies indicate that an effective approach is based on a combination of pharmacological treatment and physiotherapy.

It is known that ROS play an important role in demyelination [41], and hence, oxidative stress is believed to be one of the key factors involved in the pathogenesis of MS. Indeed, patients with MS show tend to present higher oxidative stress indices, as well as greater DNA failure [113]. Studies indicate that a course of at least 10 WBCT sessions can improve antioxidant potential: although MS patients usually demonstrate higher oxidative stress than healthy subjects, this value decreases after WBCT. While further research is clearly needed, WBCT appears to be an effective method of improving the antioxidant capacity of the body [114].

6. Whole-Body Cryotherapy (WBCT): Antioxidant Effects and Clinical Implications

The treatment approaches for MS include pharmacological interventions and various methods of physical medicine and rehabilitation. The latest research highlights the importance of exercise as a key therapy that can improve the functional status of MS patients. However, about 60–80% of MS patients are heat-sensitive, and exposure to a warm environment could potentially result in a transient exacerbation of symptoms. Therefore, WBCT and cooling therapies are very promising methods that can reduce fatigue and improve functional status and quality of life [13].

Recent clinical investigations indicate that WBCT has an antioxidant effect in MS patients resulting in improvements in plasma total antioxidative status, SOD, and uric acid levels [41,115]. However, there is a need to conduct more extensive clinical trials involving larger cohorts of participants and with consistent protocols. In Poland, WBCT is widely applied; according to National Health Fund data, 14,239 of the total 641,737 covered cryochamber therapy services were performed each year with MS patients during 2010–2019, representing about 2.3–2.5% of the total.

The molecular mechanisms responsible for the effectiveness of cryotherapy in minimizing oxidative damage remain unclear. Nevertheless, some studies have indicated that the induction of hypothermia may play a role in partially inhibiting ROS generation [14].

It has been proposed that long-term WBCT decreases oxidative stress by enhancing antioxidative enzyme activity. Repeated exposure to acute cold temperatures over several months may induce adaptive mechanisms, potentially contributing to body hardening. This adaptation to cold stimuli is believed to enhance protection against oxidative stress [116].

Siems et al. [117] discovered that regular winter swimming or intense endurance exercise increased enzymatic protection, suggesting activation of the antioxidant defense. Our studies showed that MS patients treated with three cycles of 10 exposures in a cryogenic chamber increased total antioxidant status (TAS) (an indicator of redox status) in plasma and improved disease symptoms. Moreover, SOD and CAT activities were further enhanced during WBCT sessions using melatonin supplementation (10 mg daily), without affecting TAS levels. The combined approach showed promise, emphasizing the need for further research on the antioxidative mechanisms of WBCT in MS treatment [96].

7. Conclusions

Our analysis confirms that the progression of MS is characterized by a critical convergence of vascular impairment, neuroinflammation, and oxidative stress, which form an intricate interplay. It is important to consider that MS manifests not as a singularly defined neurological disorder but rather as a spectrum of intertwined pathological processes.

A pivotal factor in the pathophysiology of MS is vascular impairment, particularly the disruption of the BBB. This disruption facilitates the infiltration of autoreactive immune cells in the CNS, thereby setting the stage for sustained neuroinflammation. The resulting inflammatory milieu, characterized by activated microglia and infiltrating lymphocytes, contributes to the demyelination and degeneration of the axons that are pathological features of MS. The pro-inflammatory factors released in this environment further perpetuate BBB permeability, creating a vicious cycle of inflammation and vascular compromise.

A critical role is also played by oxidative stress, which serves as both a consequence and a driver of neuroinflammation and vascular damage. Excessive production of ROS in this milieu causes direct damage to cellular elements, including DNA, proteins, and lipids. This oxidative damage not only exacerbates demyelination but also impairs remyelination processes, crucial for CNS repair. Mitochondrial dysfunction, particularly in neuronal cells, underscores the significance of oxidative injury in MS. The complex interrelation between oxidative stress and inflammatory and vascular pathology represents a multifaced aspect of MS pathogenesis.

This understanding calls for a holistic approach to the management and treatment of the disease, where therapeutic strategies should be multi-targeted and personalized, addressing the specific needs and pathophysiological profiles of individual patients. Incorporating modalities such as WBCT, which involves the application of extremely cold temperatures to affected areas, can aid in reducing inflammation and promoting vascular health. Additionally, WBCT can complement rehabilitative efforts for individuals recovering from a stroke, helping to improve motor function and overall well-being. Thus, the integration of WBCT into holistic therapies and rehabilitation programs for MS patients can offer promising avenues for comprehensive care and management of the condition.

Author Contributions: Conceptualization, A.D., E.D.M. and J.S.; writing—original draft preparation, A.D., E.D.M., M.S. and J.S.; writing—review and editing, A.D., E.D.M., K.M. and J.S.; figures, K.M. All authors have read and agreed to the published version of the manuscript.

Funding: This research received no external funding.

Institutional Review Board Statement: Not applicable.

Informed Consent Statement: Not applicable.

Data Availability Statement: No new data were created or analyzed in this study. Data sharing is not applicable to this article.

Acknowledgments: The figures within this manuscript were generated in part with DALL·E 3, an AI system that can create realistic images and art from a description in natural language, developed by OpenAI (Chat GTP 4.0). Upon generating particular elements by DALL·E 3, the author designed and made the final figures and takes responsibility for this publication.

Conflicts of Interest: The authors declare no conflicts of interest.

References

1. Ng, P.; Murray, S.; Hayes, S.M. Clinical decision-making in multiple sclerosis: Challenges reported internationally with emerging treatment complexity. *Mult. Scler. Relat. Disord.* **2015**, *4*, 320–328. [CrossRef] [PubMed]
2. Filippi, M.; Bar-Or, A.; Piehl, F.; Preziosa, P.; Solari, A.; Vukusic, S.; Rocca, M.A. Multiple sclerosis. *Nat. Rev. Dis. Primers* **2018**, *4*, 43. [CrossRef] [PubMed]
3. Ziemssen, T.; Kern, R.; Thomas, K. Multiple sclerosis: Clinical profiling and data collection as prerequisite for personalized medicine approach. *BMC Neurol.* **2016**, *16*, 124. [CrossRef] [PubMed]

4. Lublin, F.D.; Reingold, S.C. Defining the clinical course of multiple sclerosis: Results of an international survey. National Multiple Sclerosis Society (USA) Advisory Committee on Clinical Trials of New Agents in Multiple Sclerosis. *Neurology* **1996**, *46*, 907–911. [CrossRef] [PubMed]
5. Lassmann, H. Multiple Sclerosis Pathology. *Cold Spring Harb. Perspect. Med.* **2018**, *8*, a028936. [CrossRef] [PubMed]
6. Ontaneda, D.; Fox, R.J. Progressive multiple sclerosis. *Curr. Opin. Neurol.* **2015**, *28*, 237–243. [CrossRef] [PubMed]
7. Kutzelnigg, A.; Lassmann, H. Pathology of multiple sclerosis and related inflammatory demyelinating diseases. *Handb. Clin. Neurol.* **2014**, *122*, 15–58. [CrossRef] [PubMed]
8. Palladino, R.; Marrie, R.A.; Majeed, A.; Chataway, J. Evaluating the Risk of Macrovascular Events and Mortality among People with Multiple Sclerosis in England. *JAMA Neurol.* **2020**, *77*, 820–828. [CrossRef] [PubMed]
9. Cashion, J.M.; Young, K.M.; Sutherland, B.A. How does neurovascular unit dysfunction contribute to multiple sclerosis? *Neurobiol. Dis.* **2023**, *178*, 106028. [CrossRef]
10. Papiri, G.; D'Andreamatteo, G.; Cacchiò, G.; Alia, S.; Silvestrini, M.; Paci, C.; Luzzi, S.; Vignini, A. Multiple Sclerosis: Inflammatory and Neuroglial Aspects. *Curr. Issues Mol. Biol.* **2023**, *45*, 94. [CrossRef]
11. Zhang, W.; Xiao, D.; Mao, Q.; Xia, H. Role of neuroinflammation in neurodegeneration development. *Signal Transduct. Target. Ther.* **2023**, *8*, 267. [CrossRef] [PubMed]
12. Pegoretti, V.; Swanson, K.A.; Bethea, J.R.; Probert, L.; Eisel, U.L.M.; Fischer, R. Inflammation and Oxidative Stress in Multiple Sclerosis: Consequences for Therapy Development. *Oxidative Med. Cell. Longev.* **2020**, *2020*, 7191080. [CrossRef] [PubMed]
13. Miller, E.; Kostka, J.; Włodarczyk, T.; Dugué, B. Whole-body cryostimulation (cryotherapy) provides benefits for fatigue and functional status in multiple sclerosis patients. A case–control study. *Acta Neurol. Scand.* **2016**, *134*, 420–426. [CrossRef] [PubMed]
14. Alva, N.; Palomeque, J.; Carbonell, T. Oxidative stress and antioxidant activity in hypothermia and rewarming: Can RONS modulate the beneficial effects of therapeutic hypothermia? *Oxid. Med. Cell Longev.* **2013**, *2013*, 957054. [CrossRef] [PubMed]
15. Banfi, G.; Melegati, G.; Barassi, A.; Dogliotti, G.; Melzi d'Eril, G.; Dugué, B.; Corsi, M.M. Effects of whole-body cryotherapy on serum mediators of inflammation and serum muscle enzymes in athletes. *J. Therm. Biol.* **2009**, *34*, 55–59. [CrossRef]
16. Schreiner, T.G.; Romanescu, C.; Popescu, B.O. The Blood-Brain Barrier-A Key Player in Multiple Sclerosis Disease Mechanisms. *Biomolecules* **2022**, *12*, 538. [CrossRef] [PubMed]
17. Jain, S. Role of interleukin-17 signaling pathway in the interaction between multiple sclerosis and acute myocardial infarction. *Mult. Scler. Relat. Disord.* **2022**, *58*, 103515. [CrossRef] [PubMed]
18. Yang, F.; Hu, T.; He, K.; Ying, J.; Cui, H. Multiple Sclerosis and the Risk of Cardiovascular Diseases: A Mendelian Randomization Study. *Front. Immunol.* **2022**, *13*, 861885. [CrossRef] [PubMed]
19. Ghoshouni, H.; Shafaei, B.; Farzan, M.; Hashemi, S.M.; Afshari-Safavi, A.; Ghaffary, E.M.; Mohammadzamani, M.; Shaygannejad, V.; Shamloo, A.S.; Mirmosayyeb, O. Multiple sclerosis and the incidence of venous thromboembolism: A systematic review and meta-analysis. *J. Thromb. Thrombolysis* **2023**, *56*, 463–473. [CrossRef]
20. Setyawan, J.; Mu, F.; Yarur, A.; Zichlin, M.L.; Yang, H.; Fernan, C.; Billmyer, E.; Downes, N.; Azimi, N.; Strand, V. Risk of Thromboembolic Events and Associated Risk Factors, Including Treatments, in Patients with Immune-mediated Diseases. *Clin. Ther.* **2021**, *43*, 1392–1407.e1391. [CrossRef]
21. Brønnum-Hansen, H.; Koch-Henriksen, N.; Stenager, E. Trends in survival and cause of death in Danish patients with multiple sclerosis. *Brain* **2004**, *127*, 844–850. [CrossRef] [PubMed]
22. Christiansen, C.F.; Christensen, S.; Farkas, D.K.; Miret, M.; Sørensen, H.T.; Pedersen, L. Risk of arterial cardiovascular diseases in patients with multiple sclerosis: A population-based cohort study. *Neuroepidemiology* **2010**, *35*, 267–274. [CrossRef] [PubMed]
23. Christensen, S.; Farkas, D.K.; Pedersen, L.; Miret, M.; Christiansen, C.F.; Sorensen, H.T. Multiple sclerosis and risk of venous thromboembolism: A population-based cohort study. *Neuroepidemiology* **2012**, *38*, 76–83. [CrossRef] [PubMed]
24. Jadidi, E.; Mohammadi, M.; Moradi, T. High risk of cardiovascular diseases after diagnosis of multiple sclerosis. *Mult. Scler.* **2013**, *19*, 1336–1340. [CrossRef] [PubMed]
25. Koch-Henriksen, N.; Brønnum-Hansen, H.; Stenager, E. Underlying cause of death in Danish patients with multiple sclerosis: Results from the Danish Multiple Sclerosis Registry. *J. Neurol. Neurosurg. Psychiatry* **1998**, *65*, 56–59. [CrossRef]
26. Wang, Z.; Jin, X.; Liu, Y.; Wang, C.; Li, J.; Tian, L.; Teng, W. Sedentary behavior and the risk of stroke: A systematic review and dose-response meta-analysis. *Nutr. Metab. Cardiovasc. Dis.* **2022**, *32*, 2705–2713. [CrossRef] [PubMed]
27. Arpaia, G.; Bavera, P.M.; Caputo, D.; Mendozzi, L.; Cavarretta, R.; Agus, G.B.; Milani, M.; Ippolito, E.; Cimminiello, C. Risk of deep venous thrombosis (DVT) in bedridden or wheelchair-bound multiple sclerosis patients: A prospective study. *Thromb. Res.* **2010**, *125*, 315–317. [CrossRef]
28. Sternberg, Z.; Leung, C.; Sternberg, D.; Li, F.; Karmon, Y.; Chadha, K.; Levy, E. The prevalence of the classical and non-classical cardiovascular risk factors in multiple sclerosis patients. *CNS Neurol. Disord. Drug Targets* **2013**, *12*, 104–111. [CrossRef]
29. Saluk-Bijak, J.; Dziedzic, A.; Bijak, M. Pro-Thrombotic Activity of Blood Platelets in Multiple Sclerosis. *Cells* **2019**, *8*, 110. [CrossRef]
30. Stojkovic, S.; Wadowski, P.P.; Haider, P.; Weikert, C.; Pultar, J.; Lee, S.; Eichelberger, B.; Hengstenberg, C.; Wojta, J.; Panzer, S.; et al. Circulating MicroRNAs and Monocyte-Platelet Aggregate Formation in Acute Coronary Syndrome. *Thromb. Haemost.* **2021**, *121*, 913–922. [CrossRef]
31. Bacigaluppi, M.; Semerano, A.; Gullotta, G.S.; Strambo, D. Insights from thrombi retrieved in stroke due to large vessel occlusion. *J. Cereb. Blood Flow. Metab.* **2019**, *39*, 1433–1451. [CrossRef] [PubMed]

32. Hulshof, A.M.; Hemker, H.C.; Spronk, H.M.H.; Henskens, Y.M.C.; Ten Cate, H. Thrombin-Fibrin(ogen) Interactions, Host Defense and Risk of Thrombosis. *Int. J. Mol. Sci.* **2021**, *22*, 2590. [CrossRef] [PubMed]
33. Muravlev, I.A.; Dobrovolsky, A.B.; Antonova, O.A.; Khaspekova, S.G.; Alieva, A.K.; Pevzner, D.V.; Mazurov, A.V. Effects of Antiplatelet Drugs on Platelet-Dependent Coagulation Reactions. *Biomolecules* **2023**, *13*, 1124. [CrossRef] [PubMed]
34. Orian, J.M.; D'Souza, C.S.; Kocovski, P.; Krippner, G.; Hale, M.W.; Wang, X.; Peter, K. Platelets in Multiple Sclerosis: Early and Central Mediators of Inflammation and Neurodegeneration and Attractive Targets for Molecular Imaging and Site-Directed Therapy. *Front. Immunol.* **2021**, *12*, 620963. [CrossRef] [PubMed]
35. Dziedzic, A.; Morel, A.; Miller, E.; Bijak, M.; Sliwinski, T.; Synowiec, E.; Ceremuga, M.; Saluk-Bijak, J. Oxidative Damage of Blood Platelets Correlates with the Degree of Psychophysical Disability in Secondary Progressive Multiple Sclerosis. *Oxidative Med. Cell. Longev.* **2020**, *2020*, 2868014. [CrossRef] [PubMed]
36. Bijak, M.; Olejnik, A.; Rokita, B.; Morel, A.; Dziedzic, A.; Miller, E.; Saluk-Bijak, J. Increased level of fibrinogen chains in the proteome of blood platelets in secondary progressive multiple sclerosis patients. *J. Cell Mol. Med.* **2019**, *23*, 3476–3482. [CrossRef] [PubMed]
37. Dziedzic, A.; Miller, E.; Saluk-Bijak, J.; Niwald, M.; Bijak, M. The Molecular Aspects of Disturbed Platelet Activation through ADP/P2Y(12) Pathway in Multiple Sclerosis. *Int. J. Mol. Sci.* **2021**, *22*, 6572. [CrossRef]
38. Sen, U.; Tyagi, N.; Patibandla, P.K.; Dean, W.L.; Tyagi, S.C.; Roberts, A.M.; Lominadze, D. Fibrinogen-induced endothelin-1 production from endothelial cells. *Am. J. Physiol. Cell Physiol.* **2009**, *296*, C840–C847. [CrossRef] [PubMed]
39. Jennewein, C.; Tran, N.; Paulus, P.; Ellinghaus, P.; Eble, J.A.; Zacharowski, K. Novel aspects of fibrin(ogen) fragments during inflammation. *Mol. Med.* **2011**, *17*, 568–573. [CrossRef]
40. Davalos, D.; Kyu Ryu, J.; Merlini, M.; Baeten, K.M.; Le Moan, N.; Petersen, M.A.; Deerinck, T.J.; Smirnoff, D.S.; Bedard, C.; Hakozaki, H.; et al. Fibrinogen-induced perivascular microglial clustering is required for the development of axonal damage in neuroinflammation. *Nat. Commun.* **2012**, *3*, 1227. [CrossRef]
41. Ptaszek, B.; Teległów, A.; Adamiak, J.; Głodzik, J.; Podsiadło, S.; Mucha, D.; Marchewka, J.; Halski, T. Effect of Whole-Body Cryotherapy on Morphological, Rheological and Biochemical Indices of Blood in People with Multiple Sclerosis. *J. Clin. Med.* **2021**, *10*, 2833. [CrossRef] [PubMed]
42. Rawish, E.; Nording, H.; Münte, T.; Langer, H.F. Platelets as Mediators of Neuroinflammation and Thrombosis. *Front. Immunol.* **2020**, *11*, 2560. [CrossRef] [PubMed]
43. Magliozzi, R.; Hametner, S.; Facchiano, F.; Marastoni, D.; Rossi, S.; Castellaro, M.; Poli, A.; Lattanzi, F.; Visconti, A.; Nicholas, R.; et al. Iron homeostasis, complement, and coagulation cascade as CSF signature of cortical lesions in early multiple sclerosis. *Ann. Clin. Transl. Neurol.* **2019**, *6*, 2150–2163. [CrossRef] [PubMed]
44. Langer, H.F.; Chavakis, T. Platelets and neurovascular inflammation. *Thromb. Haemost.* **2013**, *110*, 888–893. [CrossRef] [PubMed]
45. Langer, H.F.; Choi, E.Y.; Zhou, H.; Schleicher, R.; Chung, K.J.; Tang, Z.; Göbel, K.; Bdeir, K.; Chatzigeorgiou, A.; Wong, C.; et al. Platelets contribute to the pathogenesis of experimental autoimmune encephalomyelitis. *Circ. Res.* **2012**, *110*, 1202–1210. [CrossRef] [PubMed]
46. Morel, A.; Bijak, M.; Miller, E.; Rywaniak, J.; Miller, S.; Saluk, J. Relationship between the Increased Haemostatic Properties of Blood Platelets and Oxidative Stress Level in Multiple Sclerosis Patients with the Secondary Progressive Stage. *Oxidative Med. Cell. Longev.* **2015**, *2015*, 240918. [CrossRef] [PubMed]
47. Cognasse, F.; Duchez, A.C.; Audoux, E.; Ebermeyer, T.; Arthaud, C.A.; Prier, A.; Eyraud, M.A.; Mismetti, P.; Garraud, O.; Bertoletti, L.; et al. Platelets as Key Factors in Inflammation: Focus on CD40L/CD40. *Front. Immunol.* **2022**, *13*, 825892. [CrossRef]
48. Dehghani, T.; Panitch, A. Endothelial cells, neutrophils and platelets: Getting to the bottom of an inflammatory triangle. *Open Biol.* **2020**, *10*, 200161. [CrossRef] [PubMed]
49. Midgley, A.; Barakat, D.; Braitch, M.; Nichols, C.; Nebozhyn, M.; Edwards, L.J.; Fox, S.C.; Gran, B.; Robins, R.A.; Showe, L.C.; et al. PAF-R on activated T cells: Role in the IL-23/Th17 pathway and relevance to multiple sclerosis. *Immunobiology* **2021**, *226*, 152023. [CrossRef]
50. Marchio, P.; Guerra-Ojeda, S.; Vila, J.M.; Aldasoro, M.; Victor, V.M.; Mauricio, M.D. Targeting Early Atherosclerosis: A Focus on Oxidative Stress and Inflammation. *Oxid. Med. Cell Longev.* **2019**, *2019*, 8563845. [CrossRef]
51. Gresele, P.; Falcinelli, E.; Momi, S.; Petito, E.; Sebastiano, M. Platelets and Matrix Metalloproteinases: A Bidirectional Interaction with Multiple Pathophysiologic Implications. *Hamostaseologie* **2021**, *41*, 136–145. [CrossRef] [PubMed]
52. Kassassir, H.; Papiewska-Pająk, I.; Kryczka, J.; Boncela, J.; Kowalska, M.A. Platelet-derived microparticles stimulate the invasiveness of colorectal cancer cells via the p38MAPK-MMP-2/MMP-9 axis. *Cell Commun. Signal* **2023**, *21*, 51. [CrossRef]
53. Masuda, H.; Mori, M.; Uchida, T.; Uzawa, A.; Ohtani, R.; Kuwabara, S. Soluble CD40 ligand contributes to blood-brain barrier breakdown and central nervous system inflammation in multiple sclerosis and neuromyelitis optica spectrum disorder. *J. Neuroimmunol.* **2017**, *305*, 102–107. [CrossRef]
54. Marcos-Ramiro, B.; Oliva Nacarino, P.; Serrano-Pertierra, E.; Blanco-Gelaz, M.A.; Weksler, B.B.; Romero, I.A.; Couraud, P.O.; Tuñón, A.; López-Larrea, C.; Millán, J.; et al. Microparticles in multiple sclerosis and clinically isolated syndrome: Effect on endothelial barrier function. *BMC Neurosci.* **2014**, *15*, 110. [CrossRef] [PubMed]
55. Beckman, J.D.; DaSilva, A.; Aronovich, E.; Nguyen, A.; Nguyen, J.; Hargis, G.; Reynolds, D.; Vercellotti, G.M.; Betts, B.; Wood, D.K. JAK-STAT inhibition reduces endothelial prothrombotic activation and leukocyte-endothelial proadhesive interactions. *J. Thromb. Haemost.* **2023**, *21*, 1366–1380. [CrossRef]

56. Balasa, R.; Barcutean, L.; Mosora, O.; Manu, D. Reviewing the Significance of Blood-Brain Barrier Disruption in Multiple Sclerosis Pathology and Treatment. *Int. J. Mol. Sci.* **2021**, *22*, 8370. [CrossRef]
57. Engelhardt, B.; Ransohoff, R.M. The ins and outs of T-lymphocyte trafficking to the CNS: Anatomical sites and molecular mechanisms. *Trends Immunol.* **2005**, *26*, 485–495. [CrossRef] [PubMed]
58. Wimmer, I.; Tietz, S.; Nishihara, H.; Deutsch, U.; Sallusto, F.; Gosselet, F.; Lyck, R.; Muller, W.A.; Lassmann, H.; Engelhardt, B. PECAM-1 Stabilizes Blood-Brain Barrier Integrity and Favors Paracellular T-Cell Diapedesis Across the Blood-Brain Barrier during Neuroinflammation. *Front. Immunol.* **2019**, *10*, 711. [CrossRef] [PubMed]
59. Kuznik, B.I.; Vitkovsky, Y.A.; Gvozdeva, O.V.; Solpov, A.V.; Magen, E. Lymphocyte-platelet crosstalk in Graves' disease. *Am. J. Med. Sci.* **2014**, *347*, 206–210. [CrossRef]
60. Dong, Y.; Yong, V.W. When encephalitogenic T cells collaborate with microglia in multiple sclerosis. *Nat. Rev. Neurol.* **2019**, *15*, 704–717. [CrossRef]
61. Lassmann, H. Pathogenic Mechanisms Associated with Different Clinical Courses of Multiple Sclerosis. *Front. Immunol.* **2018**, *9*, 3116. [CrossRef] [PubMed]
62. Borst, K.; Dumas, A.A.; Prinz, M. Microglia: Immune and non-immune functions. *Immunity* **2021**, *54*, 2194–2208. [CrossRef] [PubMed]
63. Salter, M.W.; Stevens, B. Microglia emerge as central players in brain disease. *Nat. Med.* **2017**, *23*, 1018–1027. [CrossRef] [PubMed]
64. Vogel, D.Y.; Vereyken, E.J.; Glim, J.E.; Heijnen, P.D.; Moeton, M.; van der Valk, P.; Amor, S.; Teunissen, C.E.; van Horssen, J.; Dijkstra, C.D. Macrophages in inflammatory multiple sclerosis lesions have an intermediate activation status. *J. Neuroinflammation* **2013**, *10*, 35. [CrossRef] [PubMed]
65. Trapp, B.D.; Peterson, J.; Ransohoff, R.M.; Rudick, R.; Mörk, S.; Bö, L. Axonal transection in the lesions of multiple sclerosis. *N. Engl. J. Med.* **1998**, *338*, 278–285. [CrossRef]
66. Sosa, R.A.; Murphey, C.; Ji, N.; Cardona, A.E.; Forsthuber, T.G. The kinetics of myelin antigen uptake by myeloid cells in the central nervous system during experimental autoimmune encephalomyelitis. *J. Immunol.* **2013**, *191*, 5848–5857. [CrossRef] [PubMed]
67. Smith, A.M.; Park, T.I.; Aalderink, M.; Oldfield, R.L.; Bergin, P.S.; Mee, E.W.; Faull, R.L.M.; Dragunow, M. Distinct characteristics of microglia from neurogenic and non-neurogenic regions of the human brain in patients with Mesial Temporal Lobe Epilepsy. *Front. Cell Neurosci.* **2022**, *16*, 1047928. [CrossRef] [PubMed]
68. Arjmandi, A.; Liu, K.; Dorovini-Zis, K. Dendritic cell adhesion to cerebral endothelium: Role of endothelial cell adhesion molecules and their ligands. *J. Neuropathol. Exp. Neurol.* **2009**, *68*, 300–313. [CrossRef] [PubMed]
69. Mrdjen, D.; Pavlovic, A.; Hartmann, F.J.; Schreiner, B.; Utz, S.G.; Leung, B.P.; Lelios, I.; Heppner, F.L.; Kipnis, J.; Merkler, D.; et al. High-Dimensional Single-Cell Mapping of Central Nervous System Immune Cells Reveals Distinct Myeloid Subsets in Health, Aging, and Disease. *Immunity* **2018**, *48*, 380–395.e386. [CrossRef]
70. Goldmann, T.; Wieghofer, P.; Jordão, M.J.; Prutek, F.; Hagemeyer, N.; Frenzel, K.; Amann, L.; Staszewski, O.; Kierdorf, K.; Krueger, M.; et al. Origin, fate and dynamics of macrophages at central nervous system interfaces. *Nat. Immunol.* **2016**, *17*, 797–805. [CrossRef]
71. Utz, S.G.; See, P.; Mildenberger, W.; Thion, M.S.; Silvin, A.; Lutz, M.; Ingelfinger, F.; Rayan, N.A.; Lelios, I.; Buttgereit, A.; et al. Early Fate Defines Microglia and Non-Parenchymal Brain Macrophage Development. *Cell* **2020**, *181*, 557–573.e518. [CrossRef] [PubMed]
72. Dermitzakis, I.; Theotokis, P.; Evangelidis, P.; Delilampou, E.; Evangelidis, N.; Chatzisavvidou, A.; Avramidou, E.; Manthou, M.E. CNS Border-Associated Macrophages: Ontogeny and Potential Implication in Disease. *Curr. Issues Mol. Biol.* **2023**, *45*, 272. [CrossRef] [PubMed]
73. Sathiyanadan, K.; Coisne, C.; Enzmann, G.; Deutsch, U.; Engelhardt, B. PSGL-1 and E/P-selectins are essential for T-cell rolling in inflamed CNS microvessels but dispensable for initiation of EAE. *Eur. J. Immunol.* **2014**, *44*, 2287–2294. [CrossRef] [PubMed]
74. Döring, A.; Wild, M.; Vestweber, D.; Deutsch, U.; Engelhardt, B. E- and P-Selectin Are Not Required for the Development of Experimental Autoimmune Encephalomyelitis in C57BL/6 and SJL Mice. *J. Immunol.* **2007**, *179*, 8470. [CrossRef]
75. Kerfoot, S.M.; Kubes, P. Overlapping roles of P-selectin and alpha 4 integrin to recruit leukocytes to the central nervous system in experimental autoimmune encephalomyelitis. *J. Immunol.* **2002**, *169*, 1000–1006. [CrossRef] [PubMed]
76. Wang, J.; Yang, B.; Weng, Q.; He, Q. Targeting Microglia and Macrophages: A Potential Treatment Strategy for Multiple Sclerosis. *Front. Pharmacol.* **2019**, *10*, 286. [CrossRef] [PubMed]
77. Gilgun-Sherki, Y.; Melamed, E.; Offen, D. The role of oxidative stress in the pathogenesis of multiple sclerosis: The need for effective antioxidant therapy. *J. Neurol.* **2004**, *251*, 261–268. [CrossRef] [PubMed]
78. Bryczkowska, I.; Radecka, A.; Knyszyńska, A.; Łuczak, J.; Lubkowska, A. Effect of whole body cryotherapy treatments on antioxidant enzyme activity and biochemical parameters in patients with multiple sclerosis. *Fam. Med. Prim. Care Rev.* **2018**, *20*, 214–217. [CrossRef]
79. Dugué, B.; Smolander, J.; Westerlund, T.; Oksa, J.; Nieminen, R.; Moilanen, E.; Mikkelsson, M. Acute and long-term effects of winter swimming and whole-body cryotherapy on plasma antioxidative capacity in healthy women. *Scand. J. Clin. Lab. Invest.* **2005**, *65*, 395–402. [CrossRef]
80. Pizzino, G.; Irrera, N.; Cucinotta, M.; Pallio, G.; Mannino, F.; Arcoraci, V.; Squadrito, F.; Altavilla, D.; Bitto, A. Oxidative Stress: Harms and Benefits for Human Health. *Oxid. Med. Cell Longev.* **2017**, *2017*, 8416763. [CrossRef]

81. Correale, J.; Marrodan, M.; Ysrraelit, M.C. Mechanisms of Neurodegeneration and Axonal Dysfunction in Progressive Multiple Sclerosis. *Biomedicines* **2019**, *7*, 14. [CrossRef] [PubMed]
82. Jové, M.; Mota-Martorell, N.; Obis, È.; Sol, J.; Martín-Garí, M.; Ferrer, I.; Portero-Otín, M.; Pamplona, R. Lipid Adaptations against Oxidative Challenge in the Healthy Adult Human Brain. *Antioxidants* **2023**, *12*, 177. [CrossRef] [PubMed]
83. Collin, F. Chemical Basis of Reactive Oxygen Species Reactivity and Involvement in Neurodegenerative Diseases. *Int. J. Mol. Sci.* **2019**, *20*, 2407. [CrossRef] [PubMed]
84. Tobore, T.O. Oxidative/Nitroxidative Stress and Multiple Sclerosis. *J. Mol. Neurosci.* **2021**, *71*, 506–514. [CrossRef] [PubMed]
85. Beckhauser, T.F.; Francis-Oliveira, J.; De Pasquale, R. Reactive Oxygen Species: Physiological and Physiopathological Effects on Synaptic Plasticity. *J. Exp. Neurosci.* **2016**, *10*, 23–48. [CrossRef] [PubMed]
86. Abdel Naseer, M.; Rabah, A.M.; Rashed, L.A.; Hassan, A.; Fouad, A.M. Glutamate and Nitric Oxide as biomarkers for disease activity in patients with multiple sclerosis. *Mult. Scler. Relat. Disord.* **2020**, *38*, 101873. [CrossRef]
87. Di Meo, S.; Reed, T.T.; Venditti, P.; Victor, V.M. Role of ROS and RNS Sources in Physiological and Pathological Conditions. *Oxid. Med. Cell Longev.* **2016**, *2016*, 1245049. [CrossRef]
88. D'Aiuto, N.; Hochmann, J.; Millán, M.; Di Paolo, A.; Bologna-Molina, R.; Sotelo Silveira, J.; Arocena, M. Hypoxia, acidification and oxidative stress in cells cultured at large distances from an oxygen source. *Sci. Rep.* **2022**, *12*, 21699. [CrossRef] [PubMed]
89. Siotto, M.; Filippi, M.M.; Simonelli, I.; Landi, D.; Ghazaryan, A.; Vollaro, S.; Ventriglia, M.; Pasqualetti, P.; Rongioletti, M.C.A.; Squitti, R.; et al. Oxidative Stress Related to Iron Metabolism in Relapsing Remitting Multiple Sclerosis Patients with Low Disability. *Front. Neurosci.* **2019**, *13*, 86. [CrossRef]
90. Tasset, I.; Agüera, E.; Sánchez-López, F.; Feijóo, M.; Giraldo, A.; Cruz, A.; Luna, F.; Túnez, I. Peripheral oxidative stress in relapsing-remitting multiple sclerosis. *Clin. Biochem.* **2012**, *45*, 440–444. [CrossRef]
91. Gironi, M.; Borgiani, B.; Mariani, E.; Cursano, C.; Mendozzi, L.; Cavarretta, R.; Saresella, M.; Clerici, M.; Comi, G.; Rovaris, M.; et al. Oxidative Stress Is Differentially Present in Multiple Sclerosis Courses, Early Evident, and Unrelated to Treatment. *J. Immunol. Res.* **2014**, *2014*, 961863. [CrossRef] [PubMed]
92. Leurs, C.E.; Podlesniy, P.; Trullas, R.; Balk, L.; Steenwijk, M.D.; Malekzadeh, A.; Piehl, F.; Uitdehaag, B.M.; Killestein, J.; van Horssen, J.; et al. Cerebrospinal fluid mtDNA concentration is elevated in multiple sclerosis disease and responds to treatment. *Mult. Scler.* **2018**, *24*, 472–480. [CrossRef]
93. Nakajima, H.; Amano, W.; Kubo, T.; Fukuhara, A.; Ihara, H.; Azuma, Y.-T.; Tajima, H.; Inui, T.; Sawa, A.; Takeuchi, T. Glyceraldehyde-3-phosphate dehydrogenase aggregate formation participates in oxidative stress-induced cell death. *J. Biol. Chem.* **2009**, *284*, 34331–34341. [CrossRef]
94. Sadeghian, M.; Mastrolia, V.; Rezaei Haddad, A.; Mosley, A.; Mullali, G.; Schiza, D.; Sajic, M.; Hargreaves, I.; Heales, S.; Duchen, M.R.; et al. Mitochondrial dysfunction is an important cause of neurological deficits in an inflammatory model of multiple sclerosis. *Sci. Rep.* **2016**, *6*, 33249. [CrossRef] [PubMed]
95. Clemente-Suárez, V.J.; Redondo-Flórez, L.; Beltrán-Velasco, A.I.; Ramos-Campo, D.J.; Belinchón-deMiguel, P.; Martinez-Guardado, I.; Dalamitros, A.A.; Yáñez-Sepúlveda, R.; Martín-Rodríguez, A.; Tornero-Aguilera, J.F. Mitochondria and Brain Disease: A Comprehensive Review of Pathological Mechanisms and Therapeutic Opportunities. *Biomedicines* **2023**, *11*, 2488. [CrossRef]
96. Barcelos, I.P.d.; Troxell, R.M.; Graves, J.S. Mitochondrial Dysfunction and Multiple Sclerosis. *Biology* **2019**, *8*, 37. [CrossRef]
97. Zorov, D.B.; Juhaszova, M.; Sollott, S.J. Mitochondrial reactive oxygen species (ROS) and ROS-induced ROS release. *Physiol. Rev.* **2014**, *94*, 909–950. [CrossRef] [PubMed]
98. Zorova, L.D.; Popkov, V.A.; Plotnikov, E.Y.; Silachev, D.N.; Pevzner, I.B.; Jankauskas, S.S.; Babenko, V.A.; Zorov, S.D.; Balakireva, A.V.; Juhaszova, M.; et al. Mitochondrial membrane potential. *Anal. Biochem.* **2018**, *552*, 50–59. [CrossRef]
99. Giorgi, C.; Marchi, S.; Simoes, I.C.M.; Ren, Z.; Morciano, G.; Perrone, M.; Patalas-Krawczyk, P.; Borchard, S.; Jędrak, P.; Pierzynowska, K.; et al. Mitochondria and Reactive Oxygen Species in Aging and Age-Related Diseases. *Int. Rev. Cell Mol. Biol.* **2018**, *340*, 209–344. [CrossRef]
100. Witte, M.E.; Bø, L.; Rodenburg, R.J.; Belien, J.A.; Musters, R.; Hazes, T.; Wintjes, L.T.; Smeitink, J.A.; Geurts, J.J.; De Vries, H.E.; et al. Enhanced number and activity of mitochondria in multiple sclerosis lesions. *J. Pathol.* **2009**, *219*, 193–204. [CrossRef]
101. Pandit, A.; Vadnal, J.; Houston, S.; Freeman, E.; McDonough, J. Impaired regulation of electron transport chain subunit genes by nuclear respiratory factor 2 in multiple sclerosis. *J. Neurol. Sci.* **2009**, *279*, 14–20. [CrossRef]
102. Dutta, R.; McDonough, J.; Yin, X.; Peterson, J.; Chang, A.; Torres, T.; Gudz, T.; Macklin, W.B.; Lewis, D.A.; Fox, R.J.; et al. Mitochondrial dysfunction as a cause of axonal degeneration in multiple sclerosis patients. *Ann. Neurol.* **2006**, *59*, 478–489. [CrossRef]
103. Campbell, G.R.; Ziabreva, I.; Reeve, A.K.; Krishnan, K.J.; Reynolds, R.; Howell, O.; Lassmann, H.; Turnbull, D.M.; Mahad, D.J. Mitochondrial DNA deletions and neurodegeneration in multiple sclerosis. *Ann. Neurol.* **2011**, *69*, 481–492. [CrossRef]
104. Vermot, A.; Petit-Härtlein, I.; Smith, S.M.E.; Fieschi, F. NADPH Oxidases (NOX): An Overview from Discovery, Molecular Mechanisms to Physiology and Pathology. *Antioxidants* **2021**, *10*, 890. [CrossRef]
105. Accetta, R.; Damiano, S.; Morano, A.; Mondola, P.; Paternò, R.; Avvedimento, E.V.; Santillo, M. Reactive Oxygen Species Derived from NOX3 and NOX5 Drive Differentiation of Human Oligodendrocytes. *Front. Cell Neurosci.* **2016**, *10*, 146. [CrossRef] [PubMed]
106. Carlström, K.E.; Ewing, E.; Granqvist, M.; Gyllenberg, A.; Aeinehband, S.; Enoksson, S.L.; Checa, A.; Badam, T.V.S.; Huang, J.; Gomez-Cabrero, D.; et al. Therapeutic efficacy of dimethyl fumarate in relapsing-remitting multiple sclerosis associates with ROS pathway in monocytes. *Nat. Commun.* **2019**, *10*, 3081. [CrossRef]

107. Singhal, S.S.; Singh, S.P.; Singhal, P.; Horne, D.; Singhal, J.; Awasthi, S. Antioxidant role of glutathione S-transferases: 4-Hydroxynonenal, a key molecule in stress-mediated signaling. *Toxicol. Appl. Pharmacol.* **2015**, *289*, 361–370. [CrossRef] [PubMed]
108. Alexoudi, A.; Zachaki, S.; Stavropoulou, C.; Gavrili, S.; Spiliopoulou, C.; Papadodima, S.; Karageorgiou, C.E.; Sambani, C. Possible Implication of GSTP1 and NQO1 Polymorphisms on Natalizumab Response in Multiple Sclerosis. *Ann. Clin. Lab. Sci.* **2016**, *46*, 586–591. [PubMed]
109. Pey, A.L.; Megarity, C.F.; Timson, D.J. NAD(P)H quinone oxidoreductase (NQO1): An enzyme which needs just enough mobility, in just the right places. *Biosci. Rep.* **2019**, *39*, BSR20180459. [CrossRef] [PubMed]
110. Louis, J.; Theurot, D.; Filliard, J.R.; Volondat, M.; Dugué, B.; Dupuy, O. The use of whole-body cryotherapy: Time- and dose-response investigation on circulating blood catecholamines and heart rate variability. *Eur. J. Appl. Physiol.* **2020**, *120*, 1733–1743. [CrossRef]
111. Capodaglio, P.; Cremascoli, R.; Piterà, P.; Fontana, J.M. Whole-Body Cryostimulation: A Rehabilitation Booster. *J. Rehabil. Med. Clin. Commun.* **2022**, *5*, 2810. [CrossRef] [PubMed]
112. Ghaidar, D.; Sippel, A.; Riemann-Lorenz, K.; Kofahl, C.; Morrison, R.; Kleiter, I.; Schmidt, S.; Dettmers, C.; Schulz, H.; Heesen, C. Experiences of persons with multiple sclerosis with rehabilitation—A qualitative interview study. *BMC Health Serv. Res.* **2022**, *22*, 770. [CrossRef] [PubMed]
113. Lu, F.; Selak, M.; O'Connor, J.; Croul, S.; Lorenzana, C.; Butunoi, C.; Kalman, B. Oxidative damage to mitochondrial DNA and activity of mitochondrial enzymes in chronic active lesions of multiple sclerosis. *J. Neurol. Sci.* **2000**, *177*, 95–103. [CrossRef] [PubMed]
114. Miller, E.; Mrowicka, M.; Malinowska, K.; Mrowicki, J.; Saluk-Juszczak, J.; Kędziora, J. Effects of whole-body cryotherapy on a total antioxidative status and activities of antioxidative enzymes in blood of depressive multiple sclerosis patients. *World J. Biol. Psychiatry* **2011**, *12*, 223–227. [CrossRef]
115. Lubkowska, A.; Radecka, A.; Knyszyńska, A.; Łuczak, J. Effect of whole-body cryotherapy treatments on the functional state of patients with MS (multiple sclerosis) in a Timed 25-Foot Walk Test and Hand Grip Strength Test. *Pomeranian J. Life Sci.* **2019**, *65*, 46–49. [CrossRef]
116. Siqueira, A.F.; Vieira, A.; Ramos, G.V.; Marqueti, R.C.; Salvini, T.F.; Puntel, G.O.; Durigan, J.L.Q. Multiple cryotherapy applications attenuate oxidative stress following skeletal muscle injury. *Redox Rep.* **2017**, *22*, 323–329. [CrossRef]
117. Siems, W.G.; van Kuijk, F.J.; Maass, R.; Brenke, R. Uric acid and glutathione levels during short-term whole body cold exposure. *Free Radic. Biol. Med.* **1994**, *16*, 299–305. [CrossRef]

Disclaimer/Publisher's Note: The statements, opinions and data contained in all publications are solely those of the individual author(s) and contributor(s) and not of MDPI and/or the editor(s). MDPI and/or the editor(s) disclaim responsibility for any injury to people or property resulting from any ideas, methods, instructions or products referred to in the content.

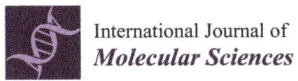

Article

The Relevance of Reperfusion Stroke Therapy for miR-9-3p and miR-9-5p Expression in Acute Stroke—A Preliminary Study

Daria Gendosz de Carrillo [1,2,*], Olga Kocikowska [1,3], Małgorzata Rak [1], Aleksandra Krzan [4,5], Sebastian Student [3,6], Halina Jędrzejowska-Szypułka [1], Katarzyna Pawletko [1,7] and Anetta Lasek-Bal [4,5]

1. Department of Physiology, Faculty of Medicine, Medical University of Silesia in Katowice, 40-752 Katowice, Poland; olga.kocikowska@sum.edu.pl (O.K.); hszypulka@sum.edu.pl (H.J.-S.); kpawletko@sum.edu.pl (K.P.)
2. Department of Histology and Cell Pathology, Faculty of Medical Sciences in Zabrze, Medical University of Silesia in Katowice, 40-752 Katowice, Poland
3. Department of Engineering and Systems Biology, Faculty of Automatic Control, Electronics and Computer Science, Silesian University of Technology, 44-100 Gliwice, Poland; sebastian.student@polsl.pl
4. Department of Neurology, School of Health Sciences, Medical University of Silesia in Katowice, 40-752 Katowice, Poland; aleksandra.krzan@sum.edu.pl (A.K.); alasek@gcm.pl (A.L.-B.)
5. Department of Neurology, Upper-Silesian Medical Center of the Silesian Medical University, 40-752 Katowice, Poland
6. Biotechnology Centre, Silesian University of Technology, 44-100 Gliwice, Poland
7. Department for Experimental Medicine, Medical University of Silesia in Katowice, 40-752 Katowice, Poland
* Correspondence: dgendosz@sum.edu.pl

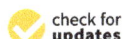

Citation: Gendosz de Carrillo, D.; Kocikowska, O.; Rak, M.; Krzan, A.; Student, S.; Jędrzejowska-Szypułka, H.; Pawletko, K.; Lasek-Bal, A. The Relevance of Reperfusion Stroke Therapy for miR-9-3p and miR-9-5p Expression in Acute Stroke—A Preliminary Study. Int. J. Mol. Sci. 2024, 25, 2766. https://doi.org/10.3390/ijms25052766

Academic Editor: Aurel Popa-Wagner

Received: 23 January 2024
Revised: 21 February 2024
Accepted: 22 February 2024
Published: 27 February 2024

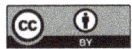

Copyright: © 2024 by the authors. Licensee MDPI, Basel, Switzerland. This article is an open access article distributed under the terms and conditions of the Creative Commons Attribution (CC BY) license (https://creativecommons.org/licenses/by/4.0/).

Abstract: Reperfusion stroke therapy is a modern treatment that involves thrombolysis and the mechanical removal of thrombus from the extracranial and/or cerebral arteries, thereby increasing penumbra reperfusion. After reperfusion therapy, 46% of patients are able to live independently 3 months after stroke onset. MicroRNAs (miRNAs) are essential regulators in the development of cerebral ischemia/reperfusion injury and the efficacy of the applied treatment. The first aim of this study was to examine the change in serum miRNA levels via next-generation sequencing (NGS) 10 days after the onset of acute stroke and reperfusion treatment. Next, the predictive values of the bioinformatics analysis of miRNA gene targets for the assessment of brain ischemic response to reperfusion treatment were explored. Human serum samples were collected from patients on days 1 and 10 after stroke onset and reperfusion treatment. The samples were subjected to NGS and then validated using qRT-PCR. Differentially expressed miRNAs (DEmiRNAs) were used for enrichment analysis. Hsa-miR-9-3p and hsa-miR-9-5p expression were downregulated on day 10 compared to reperfusion treatment on day 1 after stroke. The functional analysis of miRNA target genes revealed a strong association between the identified miRNA and stroke-related biological processes related to neuroregeneration signaling pathways. Hsa-miR-9-3p and hsa-miR-9-5p are potential candidates for the further exploration of reperfusion treatment efficacy in stroke patients.

Keywords: stroke; reperfusion treatment; miRNA; NGS; hsa-miR-9-3p; hsa-miR-9-5p; enrichment analysis; GO; KEGG

1. Introduction

Stroke is one of the leading causes of death and long-term disabilities in adults worldwide. The Global Burden of Diseases report states that the number of strokes increased worldwide between 1990 and 2019, particularly in the population of patients under the age of 65 [1]. The modern reperfusion treatment (RT) of ischemic stroke allows for lysis and/or the removal of thrombus from the closed lumen of the carotid or cerebral arteries via intravenous thrombolysis with the *IV* RT-plasminogen activator (rt-PA), and/or mechanical thrombectomy (MT). These methods increase the likelihood of penumbra reperfusion, which occurs in the ischemic region around the heart of the brain infarct. RT (i.e., IV rt-PA and MT) aims to preserve as many hypoxic cells as possible in this zone, including neuronal, endothelial, and glial cells.

In 2015, a randomized trial confirmed the efficacy and safety of MT in patients with stroke. Notably, 3 months after performing MT in the acute phase of stroke, 46% of patients were living independently, compared to 26.5% in the conservative treatment group from the trial [2]. Recent studies and meta-analyses have highlighted MT as an important treatment modality for stroke due to its potential to increase the length of the therapeutic window [3,4]. Now, physicians perform MT up to 24 h after stroke onset, according to the patient's clinical and radiological profile, improving their chances of clinical success.

Based on the results of the meta-analysis, the use of MT in stroke patients results in the recanalization of more than 80% of the arteries that underwent the intervention and a return to full patient independence in approximately 45% of patients within 3 months after stroke. However, this means that a significant post-stroke neurological deficit remains in half of the patients, including some of those who have favorable angiographic results after MT. This reveals that a significant proportion of patients have futile recanalization (as their angiogram showed recanalization). There are likely many factors that influence the clinical outcome of thrombectomy. The unfavorable prognostic parameters identified in the subpopulation of endovascularly treated stroke patients include the following: older age, diabetes mellitus, severe neurological deficit on the first day of stroke, and a low ASPECTS scale score [5–8]. Regardless, up to 9% of patients reocclude within 48 h after complete recanalization. Identifying parameters that reduce the clinical benefit of MT can improve therapeutic strategies and ultimately better guide stroke reperfusion treatment. The search for the optimal qualifying tools for stroke treatment has been ongoing for years. Using patients' miRNA profiles when selecting them for MT might help neurologists reduce the risk of failure and improve the clinical effects of MT.

In the age of emerging personalized medicine, biochemical and molecular biomarkers are being investigated to improve prognostic value with respect to the course of stroke and post-stroke disability. Therefore, many studies are focused on discovering miRNAs for use as potential biomarkers for stroke diagnosis and prognosis. Most of them involve the extraction of differentially expressed miRNAs (DEmiRNAs) from large-scale expression profiles, such as next-generation sequencing (NGS) data. The discovery of DEmiRNAs allows miRNAs with significant changes in expression levels, which have the potential to become biomarkers, and those with insignificant changes to be distinguished. Therefore, by examining the patient's miRNA profile in the first hours and days after ischemic stroke, one could predict which processes (i.e., neuroprotection or neurodegeneration) will predominate in that patient [9–13]. Understanding specific molecular processes associated with restoring blood flow in hypoxic areas and the mechanisms underlying reperfusion injury could help predict clinical deficits in patients who have suffered an ischemic stroke.

The presented study is the first to report on changes in miRNA expression in the acute phase of stroke in patients who have undergone endovascular treatment. The clinical status of patients can change over several hours and days after the onset of a stroke. Therefore, we analyzed how reperfusion treatment affects the miRNA profile 10 days after stroke onset. Next, we used the results of the statistical NGS data to search for target genes of DEmiRNAs, which we validated using qRT-PCR. Then, we performed a functional analysis of the target genes to find out which metabolic pathways they are involved in. To identify and understand the biological role of miRNAs, we analyzed how reperfusion-induced changes in the miRNA expression profile might affect estimated targets (ETs) and how these changes might relate to ischemic stroke treatment.

2. Results

2.1. Study Design

We analyzed circulating miRNA in serum samples from stroke patients on days 1 and 10 after stroke onset to find differentially regulated miRNAs and perform the enrichment analysis of significant miRNA gene targets. Figure 1 presents the study design. Table 1 summarizes the detailed clinical characteristics of the patients included in the NGS study, and Table 2 summarizes the detailed clinical characteristics of the patients included in the RT-qPCR validation study.

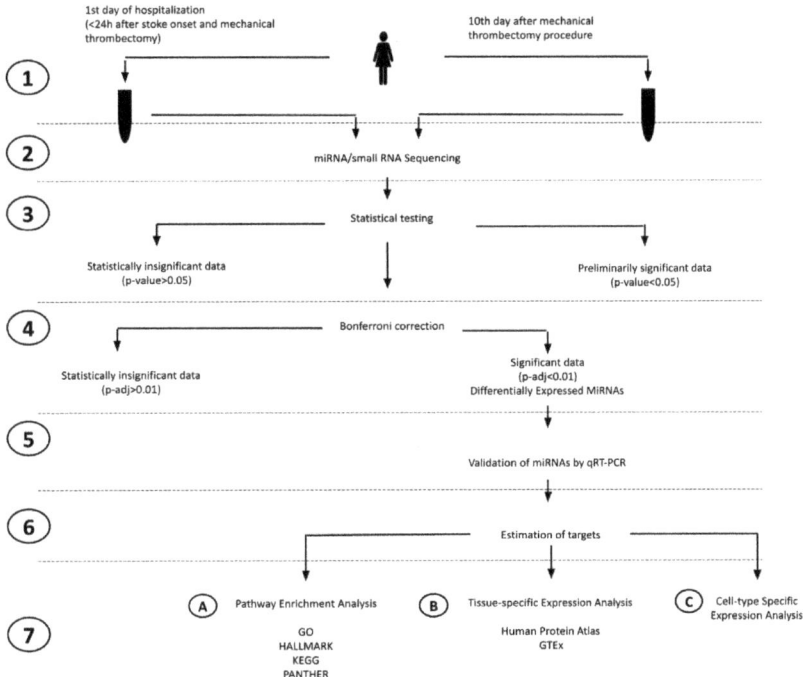

Figure 1. Study overview flowchart. The flowchart illustrates the key steps of our study as follows: (1) blood collection and serum separation, (2) miRNA/small RNA sequencing, (3) statistical testing (Exact Test), (4) Bonferroni correction, (5) miRNAs using qRT-PCR on a larger patient group and the statistical testing of qRT-PCR data, (6) estimation of gene targets based on MSigDB, (7A) GSEA (gene set enrichment analysis), (7B) TSEA (Tissue-Specific Expression Analysis), and (7C) CSEA (cell-type-specific expression analysis).

Table 1. Characteristics of the patients included in the NGS study.

Parameter	Patients, n = 5
Age, mean., med. [ref.]	66.6, 64 [50–82]
Occluded artery	
MCA right	3 (60%)
ICA left	2 (40%)
rtPA	4 (80%)
OCSP_TACI	5 (100%)
TOAST_A	3 (60%)
TOAST_C	2 (40%)
MT	
Stent retriever	4 (80%)
Aspiration	1 (20%)
Stroke onset–groin puncture, mean [ref.] min.	270 [210–360]
TICI	
1	0

Table 1. *Cont.*

Parameter	Patients, n = 5
1a	0
2b	2 (40%)
3	3 (60%)
AF	2 (40%)
AH	5 (100%)
DM	2 (40%)
CAD	2 (40%)
PAD	1 (20%)
LD	1 (20%)
RBC_1	$4.32 \times 10^6/\mu L$ [4.00–5.00]
WBC_1	$10.72 \times 10^3/\mu L$ [4.00–10.00]
Lymphocyte_1	$1.89 \times 10^3/\mu L$ [1.00–4.50]
Neutrophile_1	$8.39 \times 10^3/\mu L$ [2.00–6.14]
Basophile_1	$0.03 \times 10^3/\mu L$ [0.00–0.10]
Eosinophile_1	$0.08 \times 10^3/\mu L$ [0.05–0.50]
PLT_1	$197 \times 10^3/\mu L$ [135–350]
HCT_1	35.88% [36.00–47.00]
Hb_1	12.24 g/dL [12.00–16.00]
Creatinine	0.57 mg/dL [0.51–0.95]
eGFR	89 mL/min/1.73 m^2 [>60]
CRP	13.0 mg/l [<5.0]
RBC_10	$4.20 \times 10^6/\mu L$ [4.00–5.00]
WBC_10	$8.83 \times 10^6/\mu L$ [4.00–10.00]
PLT_10	$320 \times 10^3/\mu L$ [135–350]
HCT_10	36.20% [36.00–47.00]
Hb_10	12.35 g/dL [12.00–16.00]
Smoking	1 (20%)
NIHSS_1 med. [ref.]	13 [5–19]
NIHSS_2	13 [6–18]
NIHSS_10	8 [0–16]
mRS_dis	3 [0–4]
mRS_3m	3 [0–5]
Parameter	**Patients, n = 5**
Age, mean., med. [ref.]	66.6, 64 [50–82]
Occluded artery	
MCA right	3 (60%)
ICA left	2 (40%)
rtPA	4 (80%)
OCSP_TACI	5 (100%)
TOAST_A	3 (60%)
TOAST_C	2 (40%)
MT	
Stent retriever	4 (80%)
Aspiration	1 (20%)
Stroke onset–groin puncture, mean [ref.] min.	270 [210–360]

Table 1. Cont.

Parameter	Patients, n = 5
TICI	
1	0
1a	0
2b	2 (40%)
3	3 (60%)
AF	2 (40%)
AH	5 (100%)
DM	2 (40%)
CAD	2 (40%)
PAD	1 (20%)
LD	1 (20%)
RBC_1	$4.32 \times 10^6/\mu L$ [4.00–5.00]
WBC_1	$10.72 \times 10^3/\mu L$ [4.00–10.00]
Lymphocyte_1	$1.89 \times 10^3/\mu L$ [1.00–4.50]
Neutrophile_1	$8.39 \times 10^3/\mu L$ [2.00–6.14]
Basophile_1	$0.03 \times 10^3/\mu L$ [0.00–0.10]
Eosinophile_1	$0.08 \times 10^3/\mu L$ [0.05–0.50]
PLT_1	$197 \times 10^3/\mu L$ [135–350]
HCT_1	35.88% [36.00–47.00]
Hb_1	12.24 g/dL [12.00–16.00]
Creatinine	0.57 mg/dL [0.51–0.95]
eGFR	89 mL/min/1.73 m^2 [>60]
CRP	13.0 mg/l [<5.0]
RBC_10	$4.20 \times 10^6/\mu L$ [4.00–5.00]
WBC_10	$8.83 \times 10^6/\mu L$ [4.00–10.00]
PLT_10	$320 \times 10^3/\mu L$ [135–350]
HCT_10	36.20% [36.00–47.00]
Hb_10	12.35 g/dL [12.00–16.00]
Smoking	1 (20%)
NIHSS_1 med. [ref.]	13 [5–19]
NIHSS_2	13 [6–18]
NIHSS_10	8 [0–16]
mRS_dis	3 [0–4]
mRS_3m	3 [0–5]

ICA—internal carotid artery, MCA—middle cerebral artery, rtPA—recombinant tissue plasminogen activator, OCSP—Oxfordshire Community Stroke Project, TACI—total anterior cerebral artery, TOAST—trial of ORG 10172 in acute stroke treatment, TOAST_A—atherosclerosis, TOAST_C—cor, MT—mechanical thrombectomy, AF—atrial fibrillation, AH—arterial hypertension, DM—diabetes mellitus, CAD—coronary artery disease, PAD—peripheral artery disease, LD—lipid disorders, RBC_1—red blood cells on the 1st day, RBC_10—red blood cells on the 10th day, WBC_1—white blood cells on the 1st day, WBC_10—white blood cells on the 10th day, PLT_1—platelets on the 1st day, PLT_10—platelets on the 10th day, HCT_1—hematocrit on the 1st day, HCT_10—hematocrit on the 10th day, Hb_1—hemoglobin on the 1st day, Hb_10—hemoglobin on the 10th day, eGFR_1—estimated glomerular filtration rate on the 1st day, eGFR_10—estimated glomerular filtration rate on the 10th day, CRP_1—C-reactive protein on the 1st day, CRP_10—C-reactive protein on the 10th day, NIHSS—National Institutes of Health Stroke Scale, NIHSS_1—NIHSS on the 1st day, NIHSS_2—NIHSS on the 2nd day, NIHSS_10—NIHSS on the 10th day, mRS—modified Rankin Scale, mRS_dis—mRS at discharge, and mRS_3m—mRS on the 90th day. For laboratory tests, values in the square [ ] brackets indicate reference values for the presented parameter. In other cases, the square [ ] brackets enclose the lowest and highest value for a given parameter assessed in patients included in the study.

Table 2. Characteristics of the patients included in the RT-qPCR study.

Parameter	Patients, n = 38
Age, mean., med. [ref.]	66.6, 64 [50–82]
Occluded artery	
MCA right	7 (18.42%)
MCA left	20 (52.63%)
ICA left	4 (10.53%)
PCA left	1 (2.63%)
VA right	1 (2.63%)
No occlusion	5 (13.16%)
rtPA	28 (73.7%)
OCSP_TACI	12 (31.58%)
OCSP_PACI	21 (55.26%)
OCSP_LACI	3 (7.89%)
OCSP_POCI	2 (5.26%)
TOAST_A	14 (36.84%)
TOAST_C	11 (28.95%)
TOAST_S	11 (28.95%)
TOAST_U	2 (5.26%)
MT	
Stent retriever	18 (47.37%)
Aspiration	8 (21.05%)
Stroke onset–groin puncture, mean [ref.] min.	282 [145–360]
TICI	
0	2 (5.26%)
2C	1 (2.63%)
3	23 (60.53%)
AF	16 (42.11%)
AH	36 (94.74%)
DM	16 (42.11%)
CAD	17 (44.74%)
PAD	14 (36.84%)
LD	23 (60.52%)
RBC_1	$4{,}03 \times 10^6/\mu L$ [4.00–5.00]
WBC_1	$8{,}44 \times 10^3/\mu L$ [4.00–10.00]
Lymphocyte_1	$1.36 \times 10^3/\mu L$ [1.00–4.50]
Neutrophile_1	$6.09 \times 10^3/\mu L$ [2.00–6.14]
Basophile_1	$0.03 \times 10^3/\mu L$ [0.00–0.10]
Eosinophile_1	$0.04 \times 10^3/\mu L$ [0.05–0.50]
PLT_1	$201 \times 10^3/\mu L$ [135–350]
HCT_1	36.95% [36.00–47.00]
Hb_1	12.9 g/dL [12.00–16.00]
creatinine	0.87 mg/dL [0.51–0.95]

Table 2. Cont.

Parameter	Patients, n = 38
eGFR	83 mL/min/1.73 m2 [>60]
CRP	9.4 mg/L [<5.0]
RBC_10	$4.06 \times 10^6/\mu L$ [4.00–5.00]
WBC_10	$7.8 \times 10^6/\mu L$ [4.00–10.00]
PLT_10	$228 \times 10^3/\mu L$ [135–350]
HCT_10	36.75% [36.00–47.00]
Hb_10	12.6 g/dL [12.00–16.00]
Smoking	12 (31.59%)
Statins	15 (39.5%)
ASA	9 (23.7%)
DAPT	3 (7.9%)
VKA	5 (13.16%)
NIHSS_1 med. [ref.]	12 [1–28]
NIHSS_2	4.5 [0–28]
NIHSS_10	2 [0–24]
mRS_dis	2 [0–6]
mRS_3m	2 [0–6]

ICA—internal carotid artery, MCA—middle cerebral artery, PCA—posterior cerebral artery, rtPA—recombinant tissue plasminogen activator, OCSP—Oxfordshire Community Stroke Project, TACI—total anterior cerebral artery, PACI—partial anterior cerebral artery, LACI—lacunar infarct, POCI—posterior circulation infarct, TOAST—trial of ORG 10172 in acute stroke treatment, TOAST_A—atherosclerosis, TOAST_C—cardioembolism, TOAST_S—small vessel occlusion, TOAST_U—unknow/others origin of stroke, MT—mechanical thrombectomy, AF—atrial fibrillation, AH—arterial hypertension, DM—diabetes mellitus, CAD—coronary artery disease, PAD—peripheral artery disease, LD—lipid disorders, RBC_1—red blood cells on the 1st day, RBC_10—red blood cells on the 10th day, WBC_1—white blood cells on the 1st day, WBC_10—white blood cells on the 10th day, PLT_1—platelets on the 1st day, PLT_10—platelets on the 10th day, HCT_1—hematocrit on the 1st day, HCT_10—hematocrit on the 10th day, Hb_1—hemoglobin on the 1st day, Hb_10—hemoglobin on the 10th day, eGFR_1—estimated glomerular filtration rate on the 1st day, eGFR_10—estimated glomerular filtration rate on the 10th day, CRP_1—C-reactive protein on the 1st day, CRP_10—C-reactive protein on the 10th day, Statins prior to stroke event (atorvastatin or rosuvastatin), ASA—aspirin, DAPT dual antiplatelet therapy (clopidogrel and aspirin), VKA—warfrin, NIHSS—National Institutes of Health Stroke Scale, NIHSS_1—NIHSS on the 1st day, NIHSS_2—NIHSS on the 2nd day, NIHSS_10—NIHSS on the 10th day, mRS—modified Rankin Scale, mRS_dis—mRS at discharge, and mRS_3m—mRS on the 90th day. For laboratory tests, values in the square [ ] brackets indicate reference values for the presented parameter. In other cases, the square [ ] brackets enclose the lowest and highest value for a given parameter assessed in patients included in the study.

2.2. NGS miRNA Discovery

We used NGS analysis to find DEmiRNAs in the serum of stroke patients between day 10 after the reperfusion procedure and day 1 after stroke onset. Because of the small sample set mentioned above and the variations that might be due to individual differences, we assumed errors in categories I and II (the occurrence of false positives and false negatives). Therefore, we applied a larger confidence range to avoid potentially removing significant preliminary data. We found 30 preliminary significant miRNAs ($p < 0.05$) in a dataset of 2632 miRNAs. In total, 18 miRNAs had an upregulated expression, and 12 had a downregulated expression (Figure 2). After correction for multiple tests (Bonferroni correction, p-adjusted < 0.05) 3 significant and downregulated miRNAs emerged from 30 preliminary significant miRNA: hsa-miR-9-3p ($p = 1.78 \times 10^{-7}$), hsa-miR-9-5p ($p = 5.54 \times 10^{-9}$), and hsa-miR-129-5p ($p = 7.37 \times 10^{-5}$). These miRNAs were used in further target prediction and enrichment analysis (Figure 3).

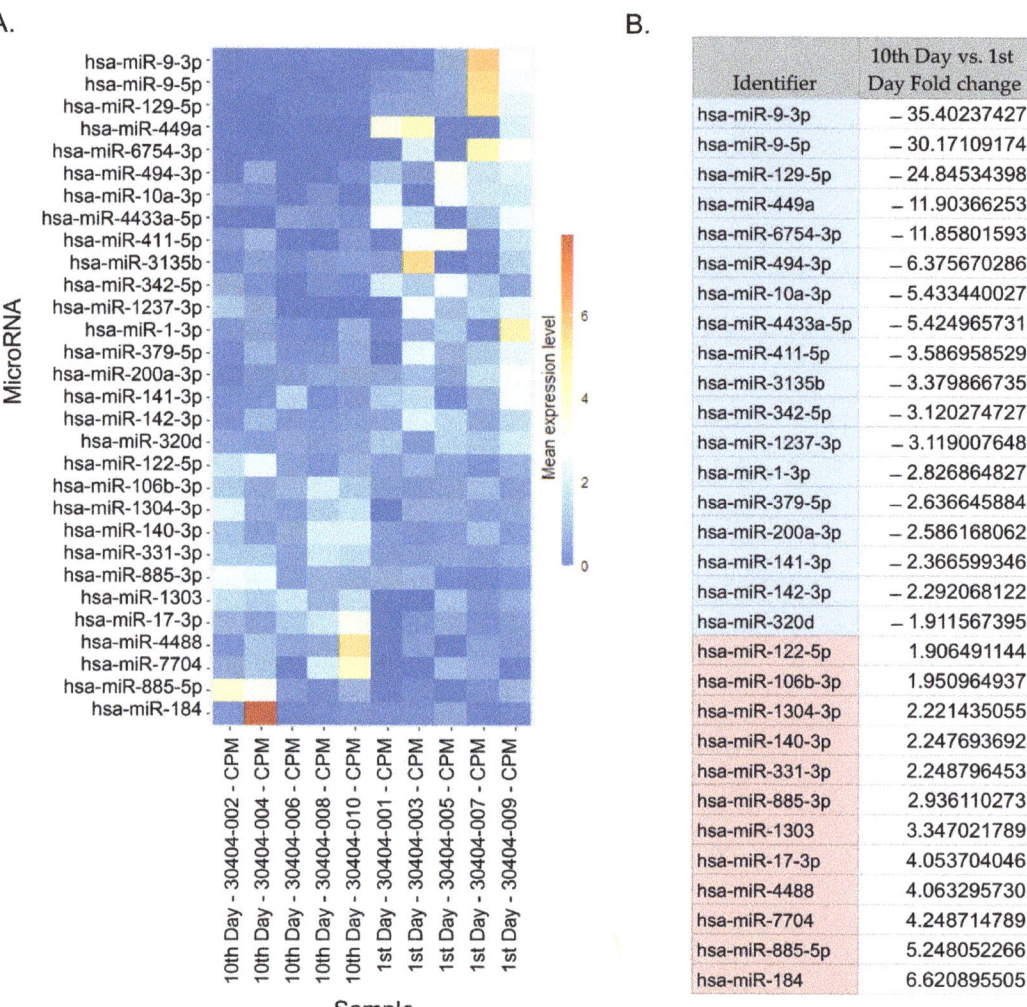

Figure 2. DEmiRNAs. (**A**) A heatmap depicting preliminary significant miRNAs based on a normalized expression. The heatmap shows the fold change in miRNA expression from the lowest to highest for samples between day 10 after reperfusion and day 1 after stroke onset. The sample description indicates the time of sample collection (i.e., an odd number indicates the sample was collected on day 1 post-stroke, and an even-numbered sample was collected on day 10). (**B**) A table listing the preliminary significant miRNAs and their fold change values. The top three scores in the table are the following DEmiRNAs: hsa-miR-9-3p, hsa-miR-9-5p, and hsa-miR-129-5p.

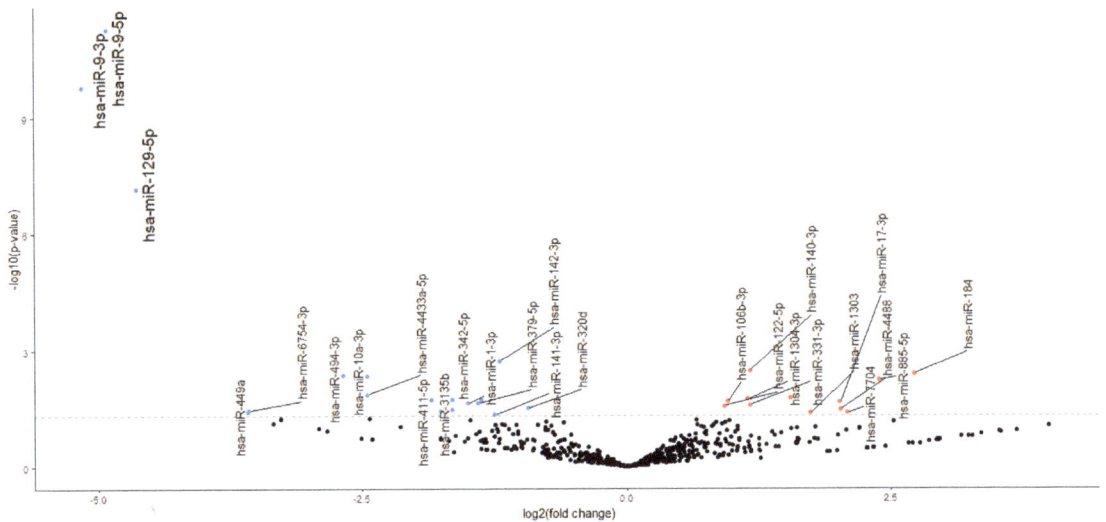

Figure 3. Volcano plot. Expression changes in preliminary significant miRNAs are presented in the volcano plot. Red dots indicate increased expression (12 preliminary significant miRNAs), and blue dots indicate decreased expression (18 preliminary significant miRNAs). Larger font indicates the following 3 significant DEmiRNAs: hsa-miR-9-5p, hsa-miR-3-5p, and hsa-miR-129-5p.

2.3. DE-miRNAs Validation

We performed the validation of the following three significantly downregulated DEmiRNAs from NGS statistical analysis: miR-9-3p, miR-9-5p, and miR-129-5p (Figure 4). The levels of miR-9-3p and miR-9-5p significantly decreased between day 10 and day 1 after stroke. However, the miR-129-5p level did not reach statistical significance.

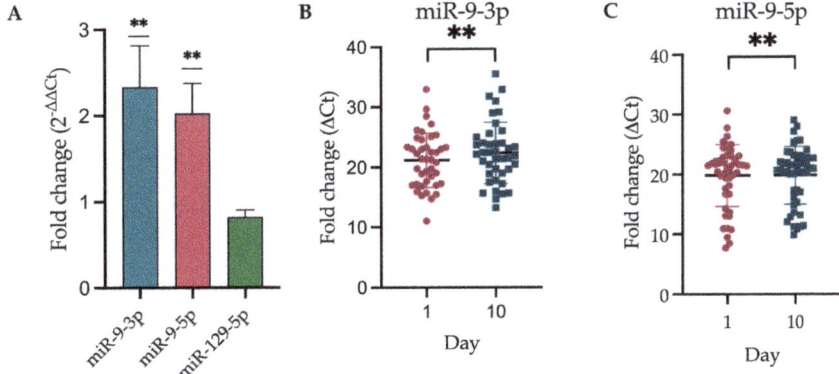

Figure 4. Expression level of DEmiRNAs according to Livak's method. (**A**) Histogram representing the fold change, $2^{-\Delta\Delta Ct}$, for validated miRNAs. (**B,C**) Dot plots representing individual values for miR-9-3p and miR-9-5p, the level of which was significantly different between day 10 (turquoise dots) and day 1 (magenta dots) (normalized against UniSp6). $\Delta Ct = Ct$ (target miRNA) $- Ct$ (control miRNA); ** p-value < 0.01 (one sample t-test, $\mu = 1$), miR-9-3p p-value = 0.0087 and miR-9-5p p-value = 0.0046.

The results of the Spearman correlation are presented in Figure 5. We did not find any significant correlation between the level of miR-9-3p ($r = -0.13$) or miR-9-5p ($r = -0.15$)

on day 10 after stroke occurrence and the patient's functional status on day 90 following a stroke as per the mRS scale [14].

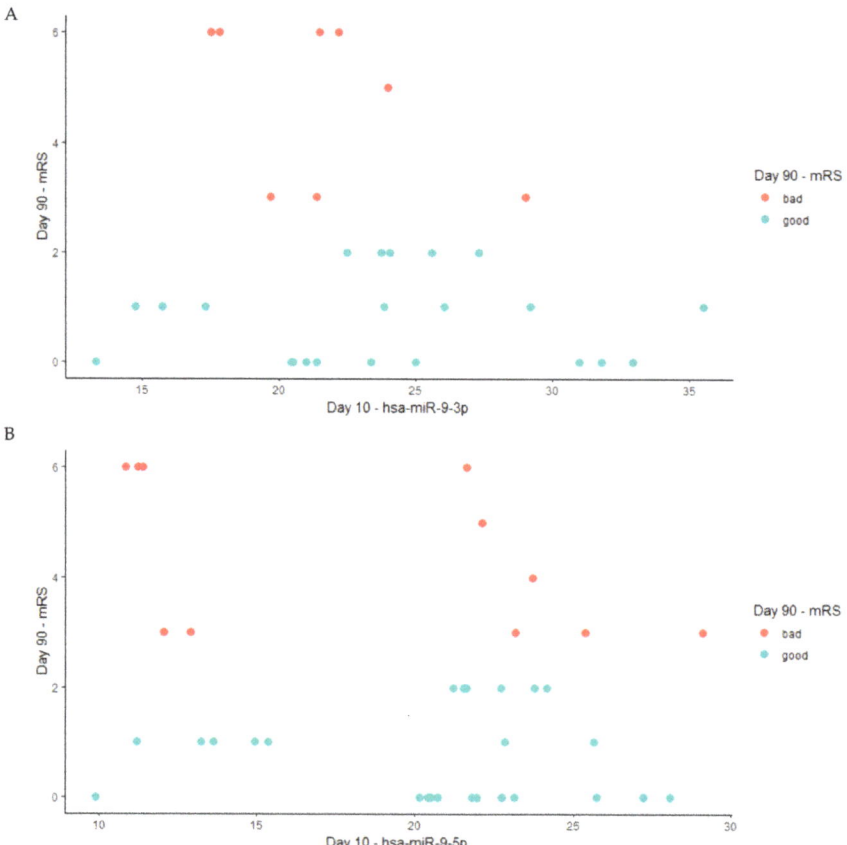

Figure 5. The Spearman correlation between the levels of miRNA on the 10th day after a stroke and the patient's functional outcome on day 90, where red dots present data for patients with bad functional outcomes based on the mRS (3–6) and blue dots present data for patients with good functional outcomes based on mRS (0–2). (**A**) hsa-miRNA-9-3p (Spearman, r = −0.13); (**B**) hsa-miR-9-5p (Spearman, r = −0.15).

2.4. miRNA Target Prediction for DEmiRNAs

Based on the target prediction analysis in the MSigDB database, we distinguished 1117 gene targets affected by DEmiRNAs [15]. Then, we restricted the number of targets to those shared between DEmiRNAs (Figure 6). For hsa-miR-9-5p and hsa-miR-9-3p, we found the following 32 common targets: ACOT7, ATP11A, C21orf91, CAPZA1, CCSER2, CPEB3, DCBLD2, DCUN1D4, DR1, ENPEP, FAM126B, FAM91A1, FOXG1, HIC2, HIPK3, ICMT, ID4, IGF2BP3, KITLG, MAP3K1, MFSD14A, MICAL2, ONECUT1, ONECUT2, POU2F1, POU3F2, PRTG, REST, SMARCE1, TGFBR2, ZBTB41, ZDHHC21. The hsa-miR-129-5p and hsa-miR-9-3p shared the following 22 common targets: ACSL4, AUTS2, BICD2, HAPLN1, HIPK2, IFT80, IGF1, MINAR1, NEXMIF, NRXN1, PIK3R1, SCAI, SESTD1, SOX4, STIM2, TENT4B, VASH2, WNK3, YIPF5, ZFHX3, ZNF281, ZNF704. Hsa-miR-129-5p and hsa-miR-9-5p shared 23 common targets: AMMECR1, ARID1B, CHMP2B, CLOCK, DSE, FRYL, GALNT1, HIPK1, LMNA, NFIC, PAK3, PDE12, PGRMC2, POU2F2, PSD3, PWWP3B, RBMS3, SBNO1, TENM1, UBASH3B, UNC80, VGLL4, ZBTB20). Hsa-miR-9-3p, hsa-miR-9-5p, and hsa-miR-129-5p shared the following four common targets: CREB5, OTUD7B, PCDH7, and PHIP. For further DEmiRNA gene target analysis, we chose four common targets, CREB5, OTUD7B, PCDH7, and PHIP, because gene co-targeting analyses show that miRNAs synergistically regulate cohorts of genes that participate in similar processes [15,16].

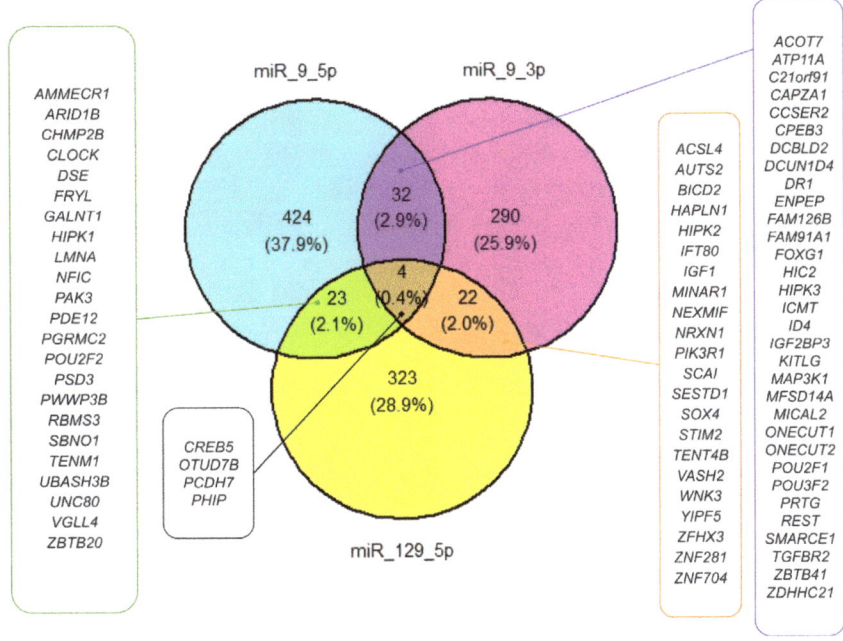

Figure 6. DEmiRNA ETs. The Venn diagram presents the ETs selected for DEmiRNAs. Targets shared by miR-9-5p and miR-129-5p, miR-9-3p and miR-129-5p, and miR-9-3p and miR-9-5p are shown in green-, orange-, and purple-framed boxes, respectively. Targets shared by miR-9-3p, miR-9-5p, and miR-129-5p are presented in a black-framed box.

Given the large absolute values of DEmiRNA fold changes and their impact on previously mentioned targets, we used all targets in the enrichment analysis.

2.5. Pathway Enrichment for DEmiRNAs' Targets Based on GO, HALLMARK, KEGG, and PANTHER Databases

Analysis using the GO database showed that the ETs and DEmiRNAs were enriched in biological processes (BP), including cellular component (CC) morphogenesis, cell morphogenesis, neuron development, neuron differentiation, the generation of neurons, cellular responses to endogenous stimulus, and neurogenesis pathways (Figure 7A). Enrichment results identified up to 180 genes affected in these signaling pathways due to the DEmiRNAs. For CCs, the ETs were enriched in the transcription regulator complex, the perinuclear region of cytoplasm, and cell body pathways with up to 130 genes affected by DEmiRNAs (Figure 7B). We observed the effect of DEmiRNAs on their targets in the synaptic membrane, the neuronal cell body, the axon, and the post-synapse cellular compartment.

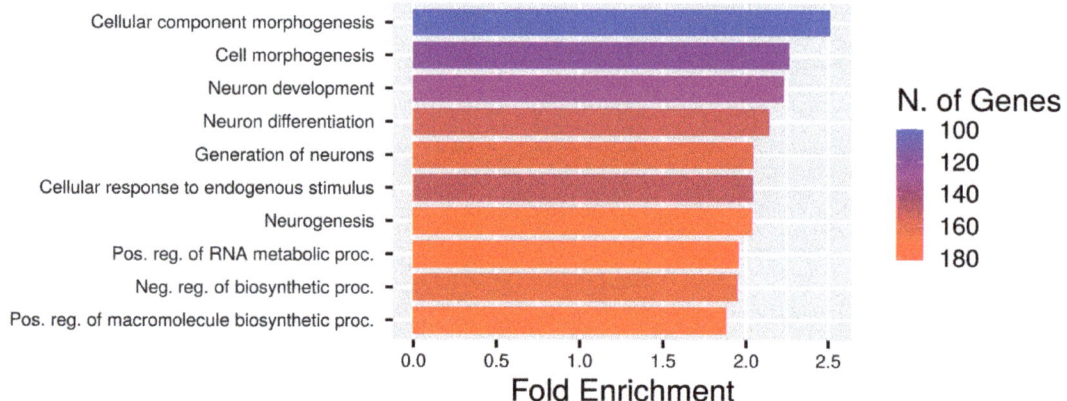
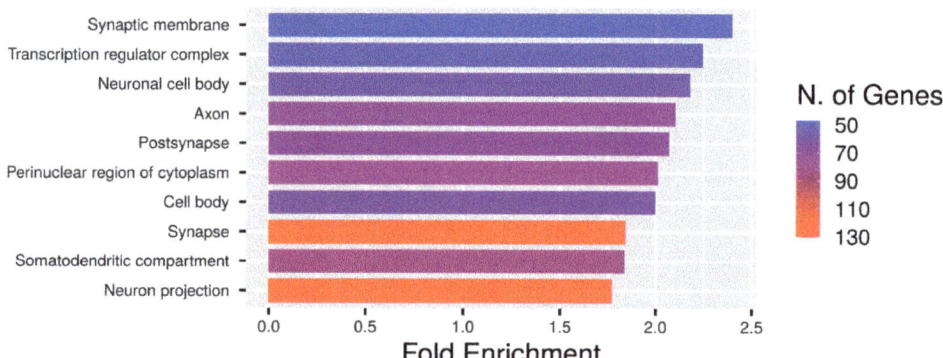

Figure 7. GO, BP, and CC analyses. (**A**) GO enrichment analysis of target genes regulated by significant DEmiRNAs. The diagram presents the top 10 target gene terms in BP pathways. (**B**) GO enrichment analysis of target genes regulated by significant miRNAs. The diagram presents the top 10 target gene terms in CC signaling pathways [16].

Pathway enrichment analysis using the HALLMARK database showed that ETs primarily augmented in HALLMARK were the apical surface, protein secretion, UV response DN (down-regulated genes), apical junction, PI3K AKT MTOR signaling, hypoxia, and mitotic spindle pathways. DEmiRNAs' targets were present within KRAS signaling up (genes up-regulated by KRAS activation), IL2 STAT5 signaling, and the myogenesis pathways (Figure 8A).

Pathway enrichment analyses using the KEGG database showed that ETs were expressed in the longevity-regulating pathway, dilated cardiomyopathy, miRNAs in cancer, cellular senescence, and signaling pathways regulating the pluripotency of stem cells (Figure 8B).

Pathway enrichment analysis using the PANTHER database showed DEmiRNA targets involved in axon guidance mediated by netrin, the p38 MAPK pathway, Ras pathway, p53 pathway, PDGF signaling pathway, endothelin signaling pathway, integrin signaling pathway, TGF-beta signaling pathway, and angiogenesis pathway (Figure 8C).

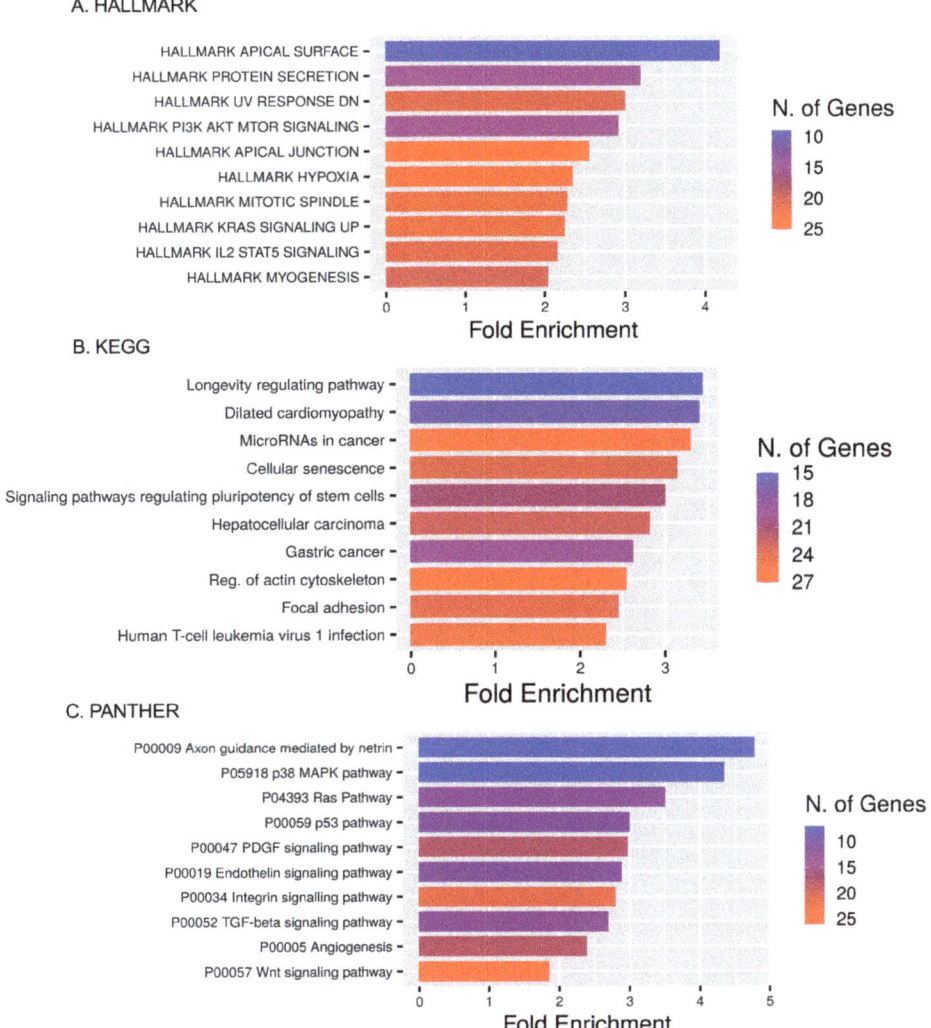

Figure 8. HALLMARK, KEGG, and PANTHER analyses. (**A**) The top 10 target gene terms in BP pathways for the HALLMARK enrichment analysis of target genes regulated by DEmiRNAs. (**B**) The top 10 target gene terms in CC pathways for the KEGG enrichment analysis of target genes regulated by significant miRNAs. (**C**) The top 10 target gene terms for the PANTHER enrichment analysis of target genes regulated by significant miRNAs.

2.6. Tissue-Specific Expression Analysis (TSEA) and Cell-Type-Specific Expression Analysis (CSEA)

TSEA for DEmiRNA targets based on the Human Protein Atlas for pooled targets of miR-9-3p, miR-9-5p, and miR-129-5p (Figure 9A) demonstrated a fold change value greater than one in the gallbladder, placenta, cerebral cortex, prostate, adrenal gland, heart muscle, cervix, uterine and adipose tissue, which referred to weak enrichment. However, the Benjamin–Hochberg correction only demonstrated significant enrichment in the cerebral cortex. Although some fold changes for individual DEmiRNA TSEAs are greater than one, the Benjamini–Hochberg correction showed no significance.

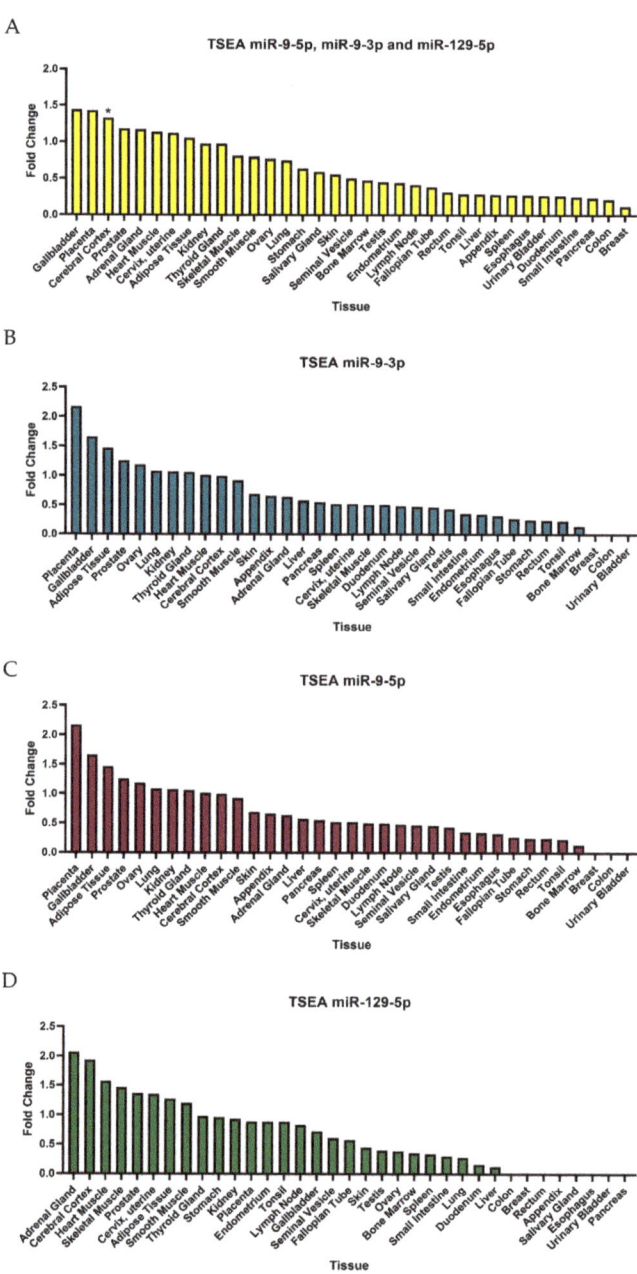

Figure 9. TSEA based on Human Protein Atlas. (**A**) Tissue-specific expression for all three DEmiRNAs. (**B**) TSEA for miR-9-3p. (**C**) TSEA for miR-9-5p. (**D**) TSEA for miR-129-5p. * The data show significance (p-value < 0.05) for summed targets of DEmiRNAs for the cerebral cortex; however, no data showed the significance of TSEA for separate targets of miRNAs.

The TSEA for targets of DEmiRNAs based on RNA-Seq data from GTEx (Figure 10A) showed significant enrichment in the nerve, muscle, blood vessels, and adipose tissues. The *p*-value suggested a strong association in nerve, muscle, and blood vessel tissues.

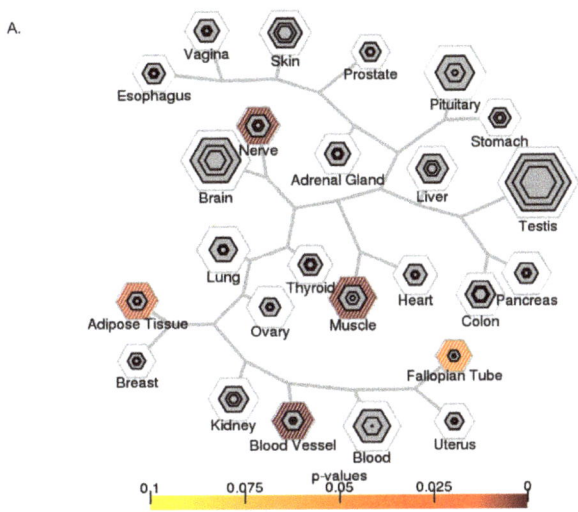

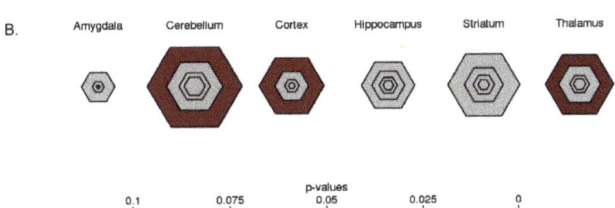

Figure 10. Specific expression analysis. (**A**) TSEA based on GTEx (http://genetics.wustl.edu/jdlab/tsea/#, accessed on 6 June 2023). Significant enrichment in nerve, muscle, blood vessels, and adipose tissues. (**B**) CSEA based on data from the Brainspan collection (http://genetics.wustl.edu/jdlab/csea-tool-2/, accessed on 6 June 2023). Significant enrichment in the cerebellum, cortex, and thalamus.

CSEA for human brain cells and DEmiRNA targets (Figure 10B) showed significant enrichment in the cerebellum, cortex, and thalamus. Enrichment for CSEA was qualified as significant based on the *p*-value.

3. Discussion

MT is a recently developed treatment and has been used as a very efficient therapy for large vessel occlusion stroke. Currently, RT-PA is the main method of treating cerebral infarction. However, due to the short time window (4.5 h), its application is restricted to only a limited number of patients receiving thrombolytic therapy. Endovascular treatment (i.e., MT) increases the recanalization rate of occluded large vessels and prolongs the time window for stroke intervention (up to 24 h) compared to rt-PA. The biological mechanism behind its effectiveness has not yet been fully explored. Various miRNAs have been shown to be elevated or decreased in a stroke. These studies have been mostly advantageous for the prognosis or diagnosis of strokes, but none of them focused on miRNA relevance in stroke therapy effectiveness, its role in patient enrollment to a certain type of endovascular recanalization treatment, or the patient's recovery rate. More comprehensive studies investigating the miRNA profile are needed to evaluate the effects of reperfusion treatment.

The research project presented here aimed to show whether the reperfusion therapy affected miRNA between the beginning and the end of the acute post-stroke phase, and we believe our preliminary results help to fill a significant knowledge gap. MiRNAs are a representative class of non-coding RNA molecules that mediate neurological alterations before, during, and after an ischemic stroke. Several miRNAs have been proposed as potential biomarkers for ischemic stroke to support the process of stroke risk assessment and the early detection of the disease [17,18]. However, we know very little about the impact of therapy on the miRNA profile and recovery prognosis. In this paper, we integrated preliminary miRNA NGS data from stroke patients after reperfusion treatment with detailed bioinformatics analyses. We identified 30 DEmiRNAs ($p < 0.05$), but after Bonferroni correction, we narrowed down the potential DEmiRNAs to the following 3: miR-9-3p, miR-9-5p, and miR-129-5p. The qRT-PCR validation confirmed the significant downregulation of identified miR-9-3p and miR-9-5p but did not obtain statistical significance for miR-129-5p. Human studies on serum from stroke patients [19], serum exosomes [20], or cerebral spinal fluid (CSF) [21] found elevated levels of miR-9-5p in acute ischemic stroke patients compared to those in healthy individuals. Wang et al. found a pronounced correlation between miR-9-5p upregulation and poor outcomes in patients after stroke. Increased miR-9 has been identified as a potential biomarker for diabetes complicated with stroke [22]. CSF shows elevated levels of miR-9-3p and miR-9-5p after subarachnoid hemorrhage, and these miRNAs are associated with a poor neurological outcome of delayed cerebral ischemia [23]. The analysis of serum from patients after traumatic brain injury (TBI) [24] revealed increased levels of miR-9-3p after TBI compared to the controls. Bioinformatic analysis revealed that miR-9-3p was significantly enriched in the brain compared to other tissues in patients with TBI [24]. In another study, elevated serum levels of exosomal miR-9 were positively correlated with the stroke severity scale and infarct volume [20]. Beske et al. showed that increased plasma levels of miR-9-3p were associated with unfavorable neurological outcomes following out-of-hospital cardiac arrest, and they reported peak levels of miR-9-3p 48 h after cardiac arrest [25]. The temporal analysis of altered miRNA in human stroke showed that miR-129-5p was upregulated and unique to the post-stroke recovery period [26]. We believe that the downregulated expression of miR-9 family members via reperfusion treatment confirms that miR-9-3p and miR-9-5p may have a functional value. Based on the functional analysis we performed here, we suggest that reperfusion treatment itself by reducing the levels of miR-9-3p and miR-9-5p affects the dependent metabolic pathways engaged in neuroprotection and, therefore, may influence the neuroprotective mechanisms in stroke patients.

Target prediction analysis revealed that DEmiRNAs regulate the following four common genes: *CREB5*, *OTUD7B*, *PCDH7*, and *PHIP*. *CREB5* is a cyclic AMP (cAMP)-responsive element binding protein (CREB) that belongs to the family of leucine zipper transcription factors. *CREB5* is specific for brain tissue (white matter) and is expressed in many regions of the brain, such as the thalamus, basal ganglia, hypothalamus, or medulla oblongata. Additionally, *CREB5* is found in various neuronal cells but mainly in oligodendrocytes. In the nervous system, growth factors (e.g., NGF, BDNF), hypoxia, oxidative, or glutamate stressors trigger the robust phosphorylation of CREB and CRE-mediated genes in neurons, which regulate a wide range of processes, including the proliferation, growth, and survival of neuronal precursors, and the synaptic connectivity of developing neurons [27,28]. The list of CREB target genes includes genes that control neurotransmission, cell morphology, signal transduction, transcription, and metabolism. Brain damage in stroke eliminates the somatosensory body map in the brain, and recovery from stroke involves the reorganization of the surviving cortical areas in adjacent motor and ectopic somatosensory regions [29–31]. Treadmill exercise improved short-term memory via the ERK-Akt-CREB-BDNF signaling pathway and resulted in the inhibition of apoptosis in the hippocampus of ischemia-affected gerbils [32]. CREB takes part in learning and memory consolidation through its involvement in adult hippocampal neurogenesis [33]. The downregulation of DEmiRNAs by reperfusion treatment may accelerate the CREB-mediated remapping mechanisms of sensorimotor functions associated with better recovery in human stroke [34]. Inflammation is another important factor in brain ischemia. Cerebral ischemic injury and the reperfusion of blood flow cause an inflammatory cascade, including oxidative stress, excitotoxicity, inflammatory cell infiltration, and the release of toxic inflammatory mediators that further contribute to neural tissue damage and cell death. CREB5 is associated with the immune system, where it plays various roles. CREB primarily promotes anti-inflammatory immune responses through the inhibition of NF-κB functions, induction of IL-10, and generation of Tregs. However, depending on the context, these responses can have a protective or pathogenic effect on the tissue [35]. We found that CREB5 is enriched in neutrophils, but its detailed function in these cells is still unknown. Though another member of the CREB family, CREB1 is responsible for neutrophil activation and pro-inflammatory cytokine production [36]. Neutrophils play a significant role in post-stroke pathology, where they promote blood–brain barrier disruption, cerebral edema, cellular injury, and neurological impairment. Anti-neutrophil therapy targets neutrophil activation, recruitment, and adhesion, as well as the release of proteases, ROS, and cytokines. However, early human studies face challenges, suggesting that the selective targeting of neutrophils may be required [37,38]. Several properties of neutrophils are protective, and thus, their antimicrobial, anti-inflammatory, and neuroprotective functions may be important to preserve tissue remodeling and repair during nerve cell recovery [39] in patients with stroke [40].

The next DEmiRNA target we discovered was the OUT domain-containing 7B (*OTUD7B*), called Cezanne, as a multifunctional deubiquitylate [41]. OTUD7B plays a diverse role in cancer and vascular diseases. Similarly, OTUD7B controls many important signaling pathways, including the inhibition of the NF-KB-mediated inflammatory response and restraining pro-inflammatory transcription in response to TNF receptor (TNFR) signaling [42,43]. In cardiovascular research, Cezanne has been implicated in scar formation, cell survival, the regulation of hypoxia, arterial remodeling, and neovascularization [44]. In the penumbra region, many neurons undergo reversible degeneration because of the supply of collateral circulation. This process provides the possibility to rescue the neurons and neurovascular unit via reperfusion treatment. The immediate restoration of local blood flow promotes the formation of new blood vessels in the ischemic region, which is not only necessary to rescue degenerated neurons but also provides a good microenvironment for neural stem cell survival, proliferation, and remodeling for functional repair. However, not much is known about the role of Cezanne in cerebral ischemic injury. Recently, Cheng et al. investigated the role of Cezanne-SIRT6-DNA DSB signaling pathways in I/R-induced ischemic brain injury in rats. The inhibition of Cezanne increased SIRT6 levels and conferred neuroprotection after cerebral ischemia injury in rats and in cultured neurons after OGD insult [45]. However, clinical research data showed that the prognosis of patients with a high density of new capillaries in the brain region affected by cerebral ischemia injury is significantly better than that of patients with a low density of new capillaries [46].

In the penumbra region, many neurons undergo reversible degeneration because of the supply of collateral circulation. This process provides the possibility to rescue the neurons and neurovascular unit by reperfusion treatment. The immediate restoration of local blood flow promotes the formation of new blood vessels in the ischemic region, which is not only necessary to rescue degenerated neurons but also provides a good microenvironment for neural stem cell survival, proliferation, and remodeling for functional repair. The prognosis of patients with a high density of new capillaries in the brain region affected by cerebral ischemia injury is significantly better than that of patients with a low density of new capillaries [46].

Another DEmiRNA target was *PCDH7*, which belongs to the non-clustered protocadherin PCDHδ1 subfamily and is termed brain–heart (BH)-protocadherin due to its predominant expression in the brain and heart [47]. In the brain, PCDH7 is produced in neurons and astrocytes [48], where it modulates axon/dendrite morphology. At the molecular level, PCDH7 is present in the excitatory synaptic cleft [49–53]. Although most studies on PCDH7 have focused on its role in cancer [50], some studies in recent years have linked PCDH7 to central nervous system disorders [53]. MeCP2 binds to the promoter region of *PCDH7* and downregulates its mRNA level, suggesting that the dysregulation of these molecules may be related to the neuronal and synaptic dysfunction observed in the brains of patients with Rett syndrome [54]. Genome-wide association studies have linked *PCDH7* to epilepsy, shorter sleep [55], and antipsychotic treatment responses in schizophrenic patients [56]. In hypertensive African Americans who suffer from a higher stroke burden due to hypertension, *PCDH7* is a plausible genetic determinant for stroke incidence [57].

The last target of DEmiRNA identified in this study was the *PHIP* gene, which encodes the pleckstrin homology domain interacting protein, which is involved in multiple biological processes, including cancer pathogenesis [58–60], cell cycle control [61] and metabolism [62]. Studies on *PHIP*-mutant mice [63] and mouse embryonic stem cells demonstrated that PHIP is dispensable for neurogenesis but is essential for postnatal growth and survival. However, *PHIP*'s chromatin binding is disrupted in neurodevelopmental disorders [64]. Loss-of-function mutations in the *PHIP* gene are associated with the neurodevelopmental disorder Chung–Jansen syndrome [65], which includes dysmorphic features, cognitive dysfunction, aberrant behavior, childhood-onset obesity, and severe childhood obesity related to the inhibition of pro-opiomelanocortin (POMC) expression: a neuropeptide that suppresses appetite [62].

Further tissue (TSEA) and cell (CSEA) enrichment analyses demonstrated that DEM targets are specific to brain cells in the cerebellum, cortex, and thalamus. The GO analysis of BPs and CCs revealed that targets were involved in neurogenesis (e.g., the generation of neurons) and neuronal differentiation (e.g., CC morphogenesis and neuron development). Analyses performed using the HALLMARK and PANTHER databases are consistent with stroke pathology. HALLMARK showed significant enrichment for DEmiRNAs in several pathways, including hypoxia [66], inflammation [67] (HALLMARK: Interleukin 2 STAT 5 signaling), the blood–brain barrier [68] (HALLMARK: apical surface, apical junction), cell growth and metabolism [69] (HALLMARK: PI3K AKT mTOR signaling), and cell proliferation [70] (HALLMARK: Mitotic spindle). PANTHER scores overlapped some of the above-mentioned metabolic pathways discovered in the GO and HALLMARK databases (e.g., axon guidance mediated by netrin). Several enrichment scores were similar for the PANTHER, GO, and HALLMARK databases, including the p38 MAPK pathway [71], RAS pathway [72], p53 pathway [73], PDGF signaling pathway [74], endothelin signaling pathway [75], integrin signaling pathway [76], TGF-beta signaling pathway, and angiogenesis [77].

KEGG enrichment analyses for DE genes revealed significant metabolic pathways related to longevity-regulating signaling pathways, which encompass genes regulating autophagy, mitochondrial activity, or oxidative stress and may trigger cellular senescence pathways, leading to irreversible cellular arrest. Conversely, DE genes retain the potential for self-renewal and differentiation by activating pathways that regulate stem cell pluripotency, focal adhesion, and the actin cytoskeleton in the nervous system. The prevailing conclusion is that stroke is a polygenic condition. Reperfusion treatment affected the miRNA profile of stroke patients and elicited the expression of targets commonly associated with dilated cardiomyopathy, cancer (hepatocellular carcinoma and gastric cancer), and human T-cell leukemia virus 1. These diseases are risk factors for stroke and indicators of poor post-stroke outcomes. Cardiomyopathy, associated with the macro- and microstructural remodeling of the heart cavities, affects systemic hemodynamic factors and could be the source of systemic embolism. Neoplasm disease is associated with a pro-thrombotic state and is one of the leading causes of embolic stroke. The association between brain ischemia and cancer is multifactorial and bidirectional. Furthermore, the mechanism of brain ischemia in cancer patients may be polyetiological. Tumors can release circulating microparticles into the bloodstream and increase the concentration of procoagulant factors, including factor X. Tumors can release mucins that activate platelets and endothelial cells through the binding of P- and L-selectin [78]. Cancers stimulate neutrophils to release de-condensed chromatin, forming neutrophil extracellular traps (NETs), which promote inflammation and thrombosis [79]. In particular, brain tumors can overexpress podoplanin, which is a transmembrane sialoglycoprotein and a potent activator of platelet aggregation [80].

Limitations

Our study has a few limitations. First, the limited number of patients (total n = 43) and the small group size of the validated group (n = 38) could be responsible for the non-significant outcome for miR-129-5p or lack of correlation between the levels of miRNAs on day 10 and the patient's functional outcome on day 90 in the mRS scale. The individual variations in patients, like the patient's medication dosage, economic situation, rehabilitation, and the patient's mental condition between day 10 and day 90 may significantly affect the functional outcome evaluation on day 90. As a result, it may mask the biological effect of tested miRNA on the patient's functional outcome in the presented preliminary study. Therefore, further studies should be performed on a bigger cohort of patients, together with subgrouping patients according to their TICI (thrombolysis in cerebral infraction) scores. Second, the target estimation research was based on the recently published data package but did not include the most recent studies. The estimated targets for miRNA 9-3p and miR9-5p were enriched by the analysis of the OMIC databases and need further in situ revalidation. Therefore, further investigations are needed to demonstrate the importance of reperfusion treatment for molecular processes in ischemic cerebral tissue.

4. Materials and Methods

This study included patients hospitalized in the Upper Silesian Medical Center of the Silesian Medical University in Katowice between 2020 and 2022 due to stroke. The patients suffered from an ischemic stroke due to large vessel occlusion and were treated with reperfusion treatment within six hours of ischemic stroke onset.

4.1. Study Population

During the study period, 443 stroke patients were treated with reperfusion therapy (MT and/or RT-PA) at our Comprehensive Stroke Center. Among these patients, we selected a group of 63 individuals. Based on the inclusion criteria, we initially included 31 patients in the study and finally qualified 5 patients for the NGS study (Table 1). Later, we qualified an additional 38 patients for the RT-qPCR study (Table 2).

Inclusion criteria are as follows: (1) 50–85 years of age, (2) patient's first ever symptomatic ischemic stroke diagnosed according to the WHO definition and head CT and/or MRI result, (3) informed consent to participate in the study (with limitations in verbalizing their consent, a written declaration was provided by two people: a family representative and/or staff member uninvolved in the study's course), (4) a pre-stroke status of 0–2 mRankin, (5) no history of intracranial hemorrhage and no other severe and/or disabling neurological disorders, and (6) the onset of symptoms up to 24 h prior to study enrollment. Exclusion criteria are as follows: (1) hemorrhagic transformation of stroke lesion, (2) pregnancy, (3) alcohol abuse/chronic use of a psychostimulant, (4) chronic infection/active neoplastic disease, (5) brain tumor, (6) history of a transient ischemic attack (TIA) or stroke, (7) renal/hepatic failure, or (8) surgery in the last three months. Table 1 summarizes the characteristics of the patients included in the study.

4.2. Sampling of Serum

Blood samples (5 mL) were collected twice from each patient by venipuncture into serum separator tubes (BD) on days 1 and 10 after the stroke's onset. After incubation at room temperature for 30–45 min to allow clotting, the samples were then centrifuged at $1940 \times g$ for 10 min at room temperature. The supernatant was collected and pipetted into aliquots (500 µL). The samples were stored at $-80\ °C$ until further NGS and qRT-PCR analyses.

4.3. Library Preparation and Sequencing of miRNA/Small RNA-Seq from Serum

The Exiqon Genomics Services performed RNA extraction from the serum and small RNA sequencing (Hilden, Germany; $n = 5$). For 5 patients, 2 samples of 500 µL serum aliquot tubes (10 in total) were shipped to the Qiagen center (Hilden, Germany). The qPCR assay evaluated the quality of the tested samples. First, the expression levels of the samples were tested to see if the miRNA expressions were within the expected range for the miRNA content (hsa-miR-103a-3p, hsa-miR-191-5p, hsa-miR-451a, hsa-miR-23a-3p, and hsa-miR-30c-5p miRNAs are expressed in biofluids such as serum and plasma). The samples were then screened for the inhibition of enzymatic reactions (spike in control UniSp6) and potential hemolysis (miR23a-miR451a) [81]. The expression levels of the samples were within the expected range of miRNA content, and no inhibition or hemolysis was observed. The preparation of the small RNA library was then performed using the QIASeq miRNA library kit, including unique molecular identifiers (UMIs) for Illumina NGS systems (performed at the Qiagen center, Hilden, Germany). The single-end sequencing of 75 bp reads (50 bp in target and 25 bp for UMIs) was performed at a depth of 20 M, with one sample/lane in the Illumina Next-Seq 550.

4.4. Quantification of miRNAs and Differential Expression Analysis of miRNA

The raw fastq files acquired from small RNA-Seq were first manually inspected with FastQC (v. 0.11.3) to check the overall quality of the sequencing data. The fastq files were then uploaded to the Qiagen Geneglobe data analysis center (DAC), which is the web platform to analyze data from Qiagen's QIASeq NGS library kits (https://geneglobe.qiagen.com/in/analyze/ (accessed on 15 September 2019). The primary quantification of read counts in the DAC was performed through the following three steps: (i) trimming the 3′-adapter and low-quality bases using cutadapt, (ii) identifying the insert sequences and UMIs (reads with <16 bp insert sequences or <10 bp UMI sequences were discarded), and (iii) aligning the processed reads to the human reference genome GRCh38 with a sequential alignment strategy using bowtie (with a perfect match to miRBase mature, miRBase hairpin, non-coding RNA, mRNA, and other RNAs, and ultimately a second mapping to miRBase mature, where up to 2 mismatches were tolerated). The annotation of miRNAs was performed with miRBase (v. 21). After primary quantification, we performed a differential expression analysis for miRNAs with DESeq2 (v. 1.22.2) in the R environment (v. 3.5.3). Data were visualized with R (v. 3.5.3). The mean expression levels were used for subsequent analysis. Preliminary statistical analysis was performed using the 'Exact Test' for two group comparisons [82]. Group 1 comprised samples acquired from patients on their 1st day (<24 h) after stroke, and group 2's samples were from the same patients on the 10th day after reperfusion treatment. Sample description denoted the time of sample collection. An odd number signified that the sample was collected on day 1 after the stroke, and even-numbered samples were collected on day 10. We selected preliminarily significant miRNAs based on the 'Exact Test' ($p < 0.05$) and excluded the miRNAs that did not present a change in the mean expression level (the fold change for miRNAs was equal to 0) from further analysis. We conducted additional statistical tests on the remaining data with the Bonferroni test (p-adjusted < 0.01). Further analysis was performed on miRNAs that met the criteria of the Bonferroni correction (DEmiRNAs).

4.5. DE-miRNAs Validaton

Total miRNA was extracted from serum plasma samples of 38 stroke patients treated with reperfusion treatment using the GeneMATRIX Universal RNA/miRNA Purification Kit (E3599; EURx) according to the product's instructions. The synthesis of cDNA was performed using the miRCURY LNA RT Kit (339340; Qiagen) with a total reaction volume of 10 µL, including 0.5 µL of UniSp6 and 10 ng/µL of miRNA. The expression level of DE-miRNAs was detected using RT PCR Mix SYBR (2008; A&A Biotechnology, Gdańsk, Poland), with cDNA as a template and the miRCURY LNA miRNA PCR assay. The mix reaction contained 6 µL of cDNA, 7 µL of SYBR Green, 1 µL of the primer (Table 3), and

1 µL of ddH$_2$O. A 2-step cycling qPCR protocol (95 °C for 2 min followed by 60 cycles at 95 °C for 10 s and 56 °C for 60 s) was conducted using the CFX Opus 96 Real-Time PCR System (Bio-Rad, Hercules, CA, USA). The relative expression of each miRNA was normalized to UniSP6 by a relative quantitative method. The miRNA primer sequence is presented in Table 3.

Table 3. miR-9-3p, miR-9-5p, miR-129-5p primer sequences.

miRNA	Sequence
miR-9-3p	5′AUAAAGCUAGAUAACCGAAAGU
miR-9-5p	5′UCUUUGGUUAUCUAGCUGUAUGA
miR-129-5p	5′CUUUUUGCGGUCUGGGCUUGC

miRNA levels were measured relative to UniSp6 levels, which served as an internal control. Relative miRNA levels were calculated using the comparative Ct method and expressed using the Livak method as fold changes relative to control samples [83]. Next, we used one sample t-test (µ = 1) to assess the statistical significance of $2^{-\Delta\Delta Ct}$ values. Differences at $p < 0.05$ were considered to be statistically significant.

Additionally, we performed the Spearman correlation between the level of miR-9-3p or miR-9-5p and the functional status on day 90 following stroke as per the modified Rankin Scale (mRS) [14].

4.6. Target Estimation Based on NGS Analysis and Enrichment Analysis

Based on the DEmiRNAs, we performed the target estimation [84]. First, we created a list of DEmiRNA targets using the molecular signatures database (MsigDB, category = "C3", subcategory = "MIR: MIRDB") (v. 7.5.1) [85,86]. To assess the number of individual and shared targets for DEmiRNAs, a Venn diagram was constructed [87].

Assuming that the DEmiRNA targets were significant, we performed an enrichment analysis (ShinyGO 0.80) for which we used HALLMARK [82,88], Gene Ontology (GO) [89,90], the Protein Analysis Through Evolutionary Relationships (PANTHER) classification system [88,89], and the Kyoto Encyclopedia of Genes and Genomes (KEGG) [91,92] databases. The p-value for the enrichment analysis was calculated by comparing the observed frequency of an annotation term with the frequency expected by chance [93]. The cut-off for significant pathways affected by targets of DEmiRNAs was set at $p < 0.05$ [82,88]. In the following evaluation, a fold change greater than or equal to 2 was assumed to be significant, according to Fold-Change-Specific Enrichment Analysis (FSEA) [94].

4.7. Tissue-Specific Expression Analysis (TSEA) and Cell-Type-Specific Expression Analysis (CSEA)

In addition to enrichment through the HALLMARK, KEGG, PANTHER, and GO databases, we performed the tissue-specific analysis of DEmiRNAs targets based on the Human Protein Atlas and Genotype-Tissue Expression (GTEx) projects. First, we used RNA-seq data from the Human Protein Atlas project for tissue enrichment [95]. Second, we used GTEx to perform tissue-specific expression analysis (TSEA), where the list of targets affected by DEmiRNAs [96,97] was checked for overlapping transcripts enriched in a particular tissue using Fisher's Exact Test with a Benjamini–Hochberg correction.

To find cell populations likely to be affected by altered DEmiRNA levels in the adult human brain, we performed cell-type-specific expression analysis (CSEA). In this analysis, we used data from the Brainspan collection to indicate transcripts enriched in specific regions of the human brain [98].

The interpretation of TSEA and CSEA plots is given as follows (): the dendrogram skeleton depicts an approximation of the hierarchical clustering of tissues based on gene expression. The size of the outer hexagon is proportional to the number of transcripts enriched in a particular tissue at the least stringent threshold of pSI < 0.05. The size of the concentric hexagons is proportional to the number of transcripts enriched in a particular tissue at the more stringent threshold (0.001, 0.001, 0.0001 from the outermost to the innermost). A heatmap color scheme is added at the appropriate hexagon to depict the significance of Fisher's Exact Test. Note that any significance in the outermost hexagon is hashed to reflect that the transcript lists are less specific at this threshold [99].

5. Conclusions

We discovered a significant decrease in hsa-miR-9-3p and hsa-miR-9-5p expression during the acute phase of stroke in patients treated with reperfusion treatment. Bioinformatic analysis showed that the negative regulation of hsa-miR-9-3p and hsa-miR-9-5p can promote neuroregeneration in treated stroke patients. Thus, we believe our data advances knowledge on the biological mechanism behind the efficacy of reperfusion treatment and points to the miRNA involved in reperfusion treatment efficacy as well as their target genes *CREB5*, *OTUD7B*, *PCDH7*, and *PHIP*, and proteins encoded by these target genes in the neuroprotective role of reperfusion treatment in stroke treatment. Our findings respond to the urgent need to further investigate the significance of miRNA in the development of a treatment strategy for acute stroke intervention.

Author Contributions: D.G.d.C., H.J.-S. and A.L.-B. conceived the study. D.G.d.C., O.K. and M.R. wrote the manuscript. A.K. collected samples. D.G.d.C. and O.K. collected data. O.K. and S.S. analyzed data. M.R. validated data. D.G.d.C., O.K., A.K. and H.J.-S. interpreted data. K.P., H.J.-S. and A.L.-B. reviewed the manuscript. All authors have read and agreed to the published version of the manuscript.

Funding: The Medical University of Silesia grants PCN-1-196/N/9/Z and PCN-1-204/N/2/0 and the Silesian University of Technology grant 02/040/BKM23/1044 supported this work.

Institutional Review Board Statement: We conducted this study in accordance with the Declaration of Helsinki and this study was approved by the Ethics Committee of the Medical University of Silesia on 04.02.2020 (No PCN/0022/KB1/14/20).

Informed Consent Statement: Informed consent was obtained from every subject involved in this study.

Data Availability Statement: Data is contained within the article.

Conflicts of Interest: The authors declare no conflicts of interest.

References

1. Murray, C.J.L.; Afshin, A.; Alam, T.; Ashbaugh, C.; Barthelemy, C.; Biehl, M.; Brauer, M.; Compton, K.; Cromwell, E.; Dandona, L.; et al. Global Burden of 369 Diseases and Injuries in 204 Countries and Territories, 1990–2019: A Systematic Analysis for the Global Burden of Disease Study 2019. *Lancet* **2020**, *396*, 1204–1222. [CrossRef]
2. Goyal, M.; Menon, B.K.; van Zwam, W.H.; Dippel, D.W.J.; Mitchell, P.J.; Demchuk, A.M.; Dávalos, A.; Majoie, C.B.L.M.; van der Lugt, A.; de Miquel, M.A.; et al. Endovascular Thrombectomy after Large-Vessel Ischaemic Stroke: A Meta-Analysis of Individual Patient Data from Five Randomised Trials. *Lancet* **2016**, *387*, 1723–1731. [CrossRef]
3. Albers, G.W.; Marks, M.P.; Kemp, S.; Christensen, S.; Tsai, J.P.; Ortega-Gutierrez, S.; McTaggart, R.A.; Torbey, M.T.; Kim-Tenser, M.; Leslie-Mazwi, T.; et al. Thrombectomy for Stroke at 6 to 16 Hours with Selection by Perfusion Imaging. *N. Engl. J. Med.* **2018**, *378*, 708–718. [CrossRef] [PubMed]
4. Jovin, T.G.; Saver, J.L.; Ribo, M.; Pereira, V.; Furlan, A.; Bonafe, A.; Baxter, B.; Gupta, R.; Lopes, D.; Jansen, O.; et al. Diffusion-Weighted Imaging or Computerized Tomography Perfusion Assessment with Clinical Mismatch in the Triage of Wake up and Late Presenting Strokes Undergoing Neurointervention with Trevo (DAWN) Trial Methods. *Int. J. Stroke* **2017**, *12*, 641–652. [CrossRef] [PubMed]
5. Kim, J.T.; Liebeskind, D.S.; Jahan, R.; Menon, B.K.; Goyal, M.; Nogueira, R.G.; Pereira, V.M.; Gralla, J.; Saver, J.L. Impact of Hyperglycemia According to the Collateral Status on Outcomes in Mechanical Thrombectomy. *Stroke* **2018**, *49*, 2706–2714. [CrossRef] [PubMed]
6. Goyal, N.; Tsivgoulis, G.; Pandhi, A.; Dillard, K.; Katsanos, A.H.; Magoufis, G.; Chang, J.J.; Zand, R.; Hoit, D.; Safouris, A.; et al. Admission Hyperglycemia and Outcomes in Large Vessel Occlusion Strokes Treated with Mechanical Thrombectomy. *J. Neurointerv. Surg.* **2018**, *10*, 112–117. [CrossRef]
7. Broocks, G.; Kemmling, A.; Aberle, J.; Kniep, H.; Bechstein, M.; Flottmann, F.; Leischner, H.; Faizy, T.D.; Nawabi, J.; Schön, G.; et al. Elevated Blood Glucose Is Associated with Aggravated Brain Edema in Acute Stroke. *J. Neurol.* **2020**, *267*, 440–448. [CrossRef]

8. Zhang, Y.H.; Shi, M.C.; Wang, Z.X.; Li, C.; Sun, M.Y.; Zhou, J.; Zhang, W.B.; Huo, L.W.; Wang, S.C. Factors Associated with Poor Outcomes in Patients Undergoing Endovascular Therapy for Acute Ischemic Stroke Due to Large-Vessel Occlusion in Acute Anterior Circulation: A Retrospective Study. *World Neurosurg.* **2021**, *149*, e128–e134. [CrossRef]
9. Vemuganti, R. All's Well That Transcribes Well: Non-Coding RNAs and Post-Stroke Brain Damage. *Neurochem. Int.* **2013**, *63*, 438–449. [CrossRef]
10. Long, G.; Wang, F.; Li, H.; Yin, Z.; Sandip, C.; Lou, Y.; Wang, Y.; Chen, C.; Wang, D.W. Circulating MiR-30a, MiR-126 and Let-7b as Biomarker for Ischemic Stroke in Humans. *BMC Neurol.* **2013**, *13*, 178. [CrossRef]
11. Shah, J.S.; Soon, P.S.; Marsh, D.J. Comparison of Methodologies to Detect Low Levels of Hemolysis in Serum for Accurate Assessment of Serum MicroRNAs. *PLoS ONE* **2016**, *11*, e0153200. [CrossRef]
12. Robinson, M.D.; Smyth, G.K. Moderated Statistical Tests for Assessing Differences in Tag Abundance. *Bioinformatics* **2007**, *23*, 2881–2887. [CrossRef]
13. Motameny, S.; Wolters, S.; Nürnberg, P.; Schumacher, B. Next Generation Sequencing of MiRNAs—Strategies, Resources and Methods. *Genes* **2010**, *1*, 70–84. [CrossRef]
14. Weisscher, N.; Vermeulen, M.; Roos, Y.B.; de Haan, R.J. What Should Be Defined as Good Outcome in Stroke Trials; a Modified Rankin Score of 0–1 or 0–2? *J. Neurol.* **2008**, *255*, 867–874. [CrossRef]
15. Bejleri, J.; Jirström, E.; Donovan, P.; Williams, D.J.; Pfeiffer, S. Diagnostic and Prognostic Circulating MicroRNA in Acute Stroke: A Systematic and Bioinformatic Analysis of Current Evidence. *J. Stroke* **2021**, *23*, 162. [CrossRef] [PubMed]
16. Gennarino, V.A.; D'Angelo, G.; Dharmalingam, G.; Fernandez, S.; Russolillo, G.; Sanges, R.; Mutarelli, M.; Belcastro, V.; Ballabio, A.; Verde, P.; et al. Identification of MicroRNA-Regulated Gene Networks by Expression Analysis of Target Genes. *Genome Res.* **2012**, *22*, 1163–1172. [CrossRef]
17. Deng, Y.; Huang, P.; Zhang, F.; Chen, T. Association of MicroRNAs With Risk of Stroke: A Meta-Analysis. *Front. Neurol.* **2022**, *13*, 865265. [CrossRef]
18. Eyileten, C.; Wicik, Z.; De Rosa, S.; Mirowska-Guzel, D.; Soplinska, A.; Indolfi, C.; Jastrzebska-Kurkowska, I.; Czlonkowska, A.; Postula, M. Cells MicroRNAs as Diagnostic and Prognostic Biomarkers in Ischemic Stroke-A Comprehensive Review and Bioinformatic Analysis. *Cells* **2018**, *7*, 249. [CrossRef]
19. Wang, Q.; Wang, F.; Fu, F.; Liu, J.; Sun, W.; Chen, Y. Diagnostic and Prognostic Value of Serum MiR-9-5p and MiR-128-3p Levels in Early-Stage Acute Ischemic Stroke. *Clinics* **2021**, *76*, e2958. [CrossRef] [PubMed]
20. Ji, Q.; Ji, Y.; Peng, J.; Zhou, X.; Chen, X.; Zhao, H.; Xu, T.; Chen, L.; Xu, Y. Increased Brain-Specific MiR-9 and MiR-124 in the Serum Exosomes of Acute Ischemic Stroke Patients. *PLoS ONE* **2016**, *11*, e0163645. [CrossRef] [PubMed]
21. Sorensen, S.S.; Nygaard, A.-B.; Carlsen, A.L.; Heegaard, N.H.H.; Bak, M.; Christensen, T. Elevation of Brain-Enriched MiRNAs in Cerebrospinal Fluid of Patients with Acute Ischemic Stroke. *Biomark. Res.* **2017**, *5*, 24. [CrossRef] [PubMed]
22. Abdelaleem, O.O.; Shaker, O.G.; Mohamed, M.M.; Ahmed, T.I.; Elkhateeb, A.F.; Abdelghaffar, N.K.; Ahmed, N.A.; Khalefa, A.A.; Hemeda, N.F.; Mahmoud, R.H. Differential Expression of Serum TUG1, LINC00657, MiR-9, and MiR-106a in Diabetic Patients with and without Ischemic Stroke. *Front. Mol. Biosci.* **2022**, *8*, 1382. [CrossRef] [PubMed]
23. Bache, S.; Rasmussen, R.; Wolcott, Z.; Rossing, M.; Møgelvang, R.; Tolnai, D.; Hassager, C.; Forman, J.L.; Køber, L.; Nielsen, F.C.; et al. Elevated MiR-9 in Cerebrospinal Fluid Is Associated with Poor Functional Outcome After Subarachnoid Hemorrhage. *Transl. Stroke Res.* **2020**, *11*, 1243–1252. [CrossRef]
24. O'Connell, G.C.; Smothers, C.G.; Winkelman, C. Bioinformatic Analysis of Brain-Specific MiRNAs for Identification of Candidate Traumatic Brain Injury Blood Biomarkers. *Brain Inj.* **2020**, *34*, 965–974. [CrossRef]
25. Beske, R.P.; Bache, S.; Abild Stengaard Meyer, M.; Kjærgaard, J.; Bro-Jeppesen, J.; Obling, L.; Olsen, M.H.; Rossing, M.; Nielsen, F.C.; Møller, K.; et al. MicroRNA-9-3p: A Novel Predictor of Neurological Outcome after Cardiac Arrest. *Eur. Heart J. Acute Cardiovasc. Care* **2022**, *11*, 609–616. [CrossRef]
26. Sepramaniam, S.; Tan, J.-R.; Tan, K.-S.; DeSilva, D.; Tavintharan, S.; Woon, F.-P.; Wang, C.-W.; Yong, F.-L.; Karolina, D.-S.; Kaur, P.; et al. Circulating MicroRNAs as Biomarkers of Acute Stroke. *Int. J. Mol. Sci.* **2014**, *15*, 1418–1432. [CrossRef] [PubMed]
27. Lonze, B.E.; Ginty, D.D. Function and Regulation of CREB Family Transcription Factors in the Nervous System. *Neuron* **2002**, *35*, 605–623. [CrossRef]
28. Kitagawa, K. CREB and CAMP Response Element-Mediated Gene Expression in the Ischemic Brain. *FEBS J.* **2007**, *274*, 3210–3217. [CrossRef]
29. Harrison, T.C.; Silasi, G.; Boyd, J.D.; Murphy, T.H. Displacement of Sensory Maps and Disorganization of Motor Cortex after Targeted Stroke in Mice. *Stroke* **2013**, *44*, 2300–2306. [CrossRef]
30. Brown, C.E.; Aminoltejari, K.; Erb, H.; Winship, I.R.; Murphy, T.H. In Vivo Voltage-Sensitive Dye Imaging in Adult Mice Reveals That Somatosensory Maps Lost to Stroke Are Replaced over Weeks by New Structural and Functional Circuits with Prolonged Modes of Activation within Both the Peri-Infarct Zone and Distant Sites. *J. Neurosci.* **2009**, *29*, 1719–1734. [CrossRef]
31. Caracciolo, L.; Marosi, M.; Mazzitelli, J.; Latifi, S.; Sano, Y.; Galvan, L.; Kawaguchi, R.; Holley, S.; Levine, M.S.; Coppola, G.; et al. CREB Controls Cortical Circuit Plasticity and Functional Recovery after Stroke. *Nat. Commun.* **2018**, *9*, 2250. [CrossRef] [PubMed]
32. Lee, S.-S.; Kim, C.-J.; Shin, M.-S.; Lim, B.-V.; Lee, S.-S.; Kim, C.-J.; Shin, M.-S.; Lim, B.-V. Treadmill Exercise Ameliorates Memory Impairment through ERK-Akt-CREB-BDNF Signaling Pathway in Cerebral Ischemia Gerbils. *J. Exerc. Rehabil.* **2020**, *16*, 49–57. [CrossRef]

33. Ortega-Martínez, S. A New Perspective on the Role of the CREB Family of Transcription Factors in Memory Consolidation via Adult Hippocampal Neurogenesis. *Front. Mol. Neurosci.* **2015**, *8*, 46. [CrossRef] [PubMed]
34. Cramer, S.C. Repairing the Human Brain after Stroke: I. Mechanisms of Spontaneous Recovery. *Ann. Neurol.* **2008**, *63*, 272–287. [CrossRef] [PubMed]
35. Wen, A.Y.; Sakamoto, K.M.; Miller, L.S. The Role of the Transcription Factor CREB in Immune Function. *J. Immunol.* **2010**, *185*, 6413–6419. [CrossRef] [PubMed]
36. Ai, Z.; Udalova, I.A. Transcriptional Regulation of Neutrophil Differentiation and Function during Inflammation. *J. Leukoc. Biol.* **2020**, *107*, 419–430. [CrossRef]
37. Sherman, D.; Bes, A.; Easton, J.D.; Hacke, W.; Kaste, M.; Polmar, S.H.; Zivin, J.A.; Clark, W.; Schneider, D.; Whisnant, J.; et al. Use of Anti-ICAM-1 Therapy in Ischemic Stroke: Results of the Enlimomab Acute Stroke Trial. *Neurology* **2001**, *57*, 1428–1434. [CrossRef]
38. Krams, M.; Lees, K.R.; Hacke, W.; Grieve, A.P.; Orgogozo, J.-M.; Ford, G.A.; ASTIN Study Investigators. Acute Stroke Therapy by Inhibition of Neutrophils (ASTIN): An Adaptive Dose-Response Study of UK—279,276 in Acute Ischemic Stroke. *Stroke* **2003**, *34*, 2543–2548. [CrossRef]
39. Sakai, S.; Shichita, T. Inflammation and Neural Repair after Ischemic Brain Injury. *Neurochem. Int.* **2019**, *130*, 104316. [CrossRef]
40. Jickling, G.C.; Liu, D.; Ander, B.P.; Stamova, B.; Zhan, X.; Sharp, F.R. Targeting Neutrophils in Ischemic Stroke: Translational Insights from Experimental Studies. *J. Cereb. Blood Flow Metab.* **2015**, *35*, 888–901. [CrossRef]
41. Evans, P.C.; Smith, T.S.; Lai, M.-J.; Williams, M.G.; Burke, D.F.; Heyninck, K.; Kreike, M.M.; Beyaert, R.; Blundell, T.L.; Kilshaw, P.J. A Novel Type of Deubiquitinating Enzyme. *J. Biol. Chem.* **2003**, *278*, 23180–23186. [CrossRef] [PubMed]
42. Enesa, K.; Zakkar, M.; Chaudhury, H.; Luong, L.A.; Rawlinson, L.; Mason, J.C.; Haskard, D.O.; Dean, J.L.E.; Evans, P.C. NF-ΚB Suppression by the Deubiquitinating Enzyme Cezanne: A NOVEL NEGATIVE FEEDBACK LOOP IN PRO-INFLAMMATORY SIGNALING. *J. Biol. Chem.* **2008**, *283*, 7036–7045. [CrossRef]
43. Ji, Y.; Cao, L.; Zeng, L.; Zhang, Z.; Xiao, Q.; Guan, P.; Chen, S.; Chen, Y.; Wang, M.; Guo, D. The N-terminal Ubiquitin-associated Domain of Cezanne Is Crucial for Its Function to Suppress NF-κB Pathway. *J. Cell. Biochem.* **2018**, *119*, 1979–1991. [CrossRef] [PubMed]
44. Zhang, J.; Zha, Y.; Jiao, Y.; Li, Y.; Wang, J.; Zhang, S. OTUD7B (Cezanne) Ameliorates Fibrosis after Myocardial Infarction via FAK-ERK/P38 MAPK Signaling Pathway. *Arch. Biochem. Biophys.* **2022**, *724*, 109266. [CrossRef] [PubMed]
45. Cheng, J.; Fan, Y.-Q.; Jiang, H.-X.; Chen, S.-F.; Chen, J.; Liao, X.-Y.; Zou, Y.-Y.; Lan, H.; Cui, Y.; Chen, Z.-B.; et al. Transcranial Direct-Current Stimulation Protects against Cerebral Ischemia-Reperfusion Injury through Regulating Cezanne-Dependent Signaling. *Exp. Neurol.* **2021**, *345*, 113818. [CrossRef]
46. Sinden, J.D.; Hicks, C.; Stroemer, P.; Vishnubhatla, I.; Corteling, R. Human Neural Stem Cell Therapy for Chronic Ischemic Stroke: Charting Progress from Laboratory to Patients. *Stem Cells Dev.* **2017**, *26*, 933–947. [CrossRef]
47. Yoshida, K.; Yoshitomo-Nakagawa, K.; Seki, N.; Sasaki, M.; Sugano, S. Cloning, Expression Analysis, and Chromosomal Localization of BH-Protocadherin (PCDH7), a Novel Member of the Cadherin Superfamily. *Genomics* **1998**, *49*, 458–461. [CrossRef]
48. Zamanian, J.L.; Xu, L.; Foo, L.C.; Nouri, N.; Zhou, L.; Giffard, R.G.; Barres, B.A. Genomic Analysis of Reactive Astrogliosis. *J. Neurosci.* **2012**, *32*, 6391–6410. [CrossRef] [PubMed]
49. Hayashi, S.; Takeichi, M. Emerging Roles of Protocadherins: From Self-Avoidance to Enhancement of Motility. *J. Cell Sci.* **2015**, *128*, 1455–1464. [CrossRef] [PubMed]
50. Redies, C.; Vanhalst, K.; Roy, F. van δ-Protocadherins: Unique Structures and Functions. *Cell. Mol. Life Sci.* **2005**, *62*, 2840–2852. [CrossRef]
51. Kim, S.-Y.; Yasuda, S.; Tanaka, H.; Yamagata, K.; Kim, H. Non-Clustered Protocadherin. *Cell Adh. Migr.* **2011**, *5*, 97–105. [CrossRef]
52. Loh, K.H.; Stawski, P.S.; Draycott, A.S.; Udeshi, N.D.; Lehrman, E.K.; Wilton, D.K.; Svinkina, T.; Deerinck, T.J.; Ellisman, M.H.; Stevens, B.; et al. Proteomic Analysis of Unbounded Cellular Compartments: Synaptic Clefts. *Cell* **2016**, *166*, 1295–1307.e21. [CrossRef]
53. Wang, Y.; Kerrisk Campbell, M.; Tom, I.; Foreman, O.; Hanson, J.E.; Sheng, M. PCDH7 Interacts with GluN1 and Regulates Dendritic Spine Morphology and Synaptic Function. *Sci. Rep.* **2020**, *10*, 10951. [CrossRef]
54. Miyake, K.; Hirasawa, T.; Soutome, M.; Itoh, M.; Goto, Y.; Endoh, K.; Takahashi, K.; Kudo, S.; Nakagawa, T.; Yokoi, S.; et al. The Protocadherins, PCDHB1 and PCDH7, Are Regulated by MeCP2 in Neuronal Cells and Brain Tissues: Implication for Pathogenesis of Rett Syndrome. *BMC Neurosci.* **2011**, *12*, 81. [CrossRef] [PubMed]
55. Ollila, H.M.; Kettunen, J.; Pietiläinen, O.; Aho, V.; Silander, K.; Kronholm, E.; Perola, M.; Lahti, J.; Räikkönen, K.; Widen, E.; et al. Genome-Wide Association Study of Sleep Duration in the Finnish Population. *J. Sleep Res.* **2014**, *23*, 609–618. [CrossRef] [PubMed]
56. Yu, H.; Yan, H.; Wang, L.; Li, J.; Tan, L.; Deng, W.; Chen, Q.; Yang, G.; Zhang, F.; Lu, T.; et al. Five Novel Loci Associated with Antipsychotic Treatment Response in Patients with Schizophrenia: A Genome-Wide Association Study. *Lancet Psychiatry* **2018**, *5*, 327–338. [CrossRef] [PubMed]
57. Armstrong, N.D.; Srinivasasainagendra, V.; Patki, A.; Tanner, R.M.; Hidalgo, B.A.; Tiwari, H.K.; Limdi, N.A.; Lange, E.M.; Lange, L.A.; Arnett, D.K.; et al. Genetic Contributors of Incident Stroke in 10,700 African Americans With Hypertension: A Meta-Analysis from the Genetics of Hypertension Associated Treatments and Reasons for Geographic and Racial Differences in Stroke Studies. *Front. Genet.* **2021**, *12*, 781451. [CrossRef] [PubMed]
58. de Semir, D.; Bezrookove, V.; Nosrati, M.; Dar, A.A.; Wu, C.; Shen, J.; Rieken, C.; Venkatasubramanian, M.; Miller, J.R.; Desprez, P.-Y.; et al. PHIP as a Therapeutic Target for Driver-Negative Subtypes of Melanoma, Breast, and Lung Cancer. *Proc. Natl. Acad. Sci. USA* **2018**, *115*, E5766–E5775. [CrossRef] [PubMed]

59. Bezrookove, V.; Nosrati, M.; Miller, J.R.; De Semir, D.; Dar, A.A.; Vosoughi, E.; Vaquero, E.; Sucker, A.; Lazar, A.J.; Gershenwald, J.E.; et al. Role of Elevated PHIP Copy Number as a Prognostic and Progression Marker for Cutaneous Melanoma. *Clin. Cancer Res.* **2018**, *24*, 4119–4125. [CrossRef] [PubMed]
60. Jang, S.M.; Nathans, J.F.; Fu, H.; Redon, C.E.; Jenkins, L.M.; Thakur, B.L.; Pongor, L.S.; Baris, A.M.; Gross, J.M.; O'Neill, M.J.; et al. The RepID–CRL4 Ubiquitin Ligase Complex Regulates Metaphase to Anaphase Transition via BUB3 Degradation. *Nat. Commun.* **2020**, *11*, 24. [CrossRef]
61. Marenne, G.; Hendricks, A.E.; Perdikari, A.; Bounds, R.; Payne, F.; Keogh, J.M.; Lelliott, C.J.; Henning, E.; Pathan, S.; Ashford, S.; et al. Exome Sequencing Identifies Genes and Gene Sets Contributing to Severe Childhood Obesity, Linking PHIP Variants to Repressed POMC Transcription. *Cell Metab.* **2020**, *31*, 1107–1119.e12. [CrossRef]
62. Li, S.; Francisco, A.B.; Han, C.; Pattabiraman, S.; Foote, M.R.; Giesy, S.L.; Wang, C.; Schimenti, J.C.; Boisclair, Y.R.; Long, Q. The Full-Length Isoform of the Mouse Pleckstrin Homology Domain-Interacting Protein (PHIP) Is Required for Postnatal Growth. *FEBS Lett.* **2010**, *584*, 4121–4127. [CrossRef] [PubMed]
63. Morgan, M.A.J.; Popova, I.K.; Vaidya, A.; Burg, J.M.; Marunde, M.R.; Rendleman, E.J.; Dumar, Z.J.; Watson, R.; Meiners, M.J.; Howard, S.A.; et al. A Trivalent Nucleosome Interaction by PHIP/BRWD2 Is Disrupted in Neurodevelopmental Disorders and Cancer. *Genes Dev.* **2021**, *35*, 1642–1656. [CrossRef] [PubMed]
64. Webster, E.; Cho, M.T.; Alexander, N.; Desai, S.; Naidu, S.; Bekheirnia, M.R.; Lewis, A.; Retterer, K.; Juusola, J.; Chung, W.K. De Novo PHIP-Predicted Deleterious Variants Are Associated with Developmental Delay, Intellectual Disability, Obesity, and Dysmorphic Features. *Cold Spring Harb. Mol. Case Stud.* **2016**, *2*, a001172. [CrossRef] [PubMed]
65. Dietrich, J.; Lovell, S.; Veatch, O.J.; Butler, M.G. PHIP Gene Variants with Protein Modeling, Interactions, and Clinical Phenotypes. *Am. J. Med. Genet. Part A* **2022**, *188*, 579–589. [CrossRef] [PubMed]
66. Ferdinand, P.; Roffe, C. Hypoxia after Stroke: A Review of Experimental and Clinical Evidence. *Exp. Transl. Stroke Med.* **2016**, *8*, 9. [CrossRef] [PubMed]
67. Zhao, H.; Li, F.; Huang, Y.; Zhang, S.; Li, L.; Yang, Z.; Wang, R.; Tao, Z.; Han, Z.; Fan, J.; et al. Prognostic Significance of Plasma IL-2 and SIL-2Rα in Patients with First-Ever Ischaemic Stroke. *J. Neuroinflamm.* **2020**, *17*, 237. [CrossRef] [PubMed]
68. Lasek-Bal, A.; Jedrzejowska-Szypulka, H.; Student, S.; Warsz-Wianecka, A.; Zareba, K.; Puz, P.; Bal, W.; Pawletko, K.; Lewin-Kowalik, J. The Importance of Selected Markers of Inflammation and Blood-Brain Barrier Damage for Short-Term Ischemic Stroke Prognosis. *J. Physiol. Pharmacol.* **2019**, *70*, 209–217. [CrossRef]
69. Villa-González, M.; Martín-López, G.; Pérez-Álvarez, M.J. Dysregulation of MTOR Signaling after Brain Ischemia. *Int. J. Mol. Sci.* **2022**, *23*, 2814. [CrossRef]
70. Cuartero, M.I.; García-Culebras, A.; Torres-López, C.; Medina, V.; Fraga, E.; Vázquez-Reyes, S.; Jareño-Flores, T.; García-Segura, J.M.; Lizasoain, I.; Moro, M.Á. Post-Stroke Neurogenesis: Friend or Foe? *Front. Cell Dev. Biol.* **2021**, *9*, 613. [CrossRef]
71. Zhu, Z.; Ge, M.; Li, C.; Yu, L.; Gu, Y.; Hu, Y.; Cao, Z. Effects of P38 MAPK Signaling Pathway on Cognitive Function and Recovery of Neuronal Function after Hypoxic-Ischemic Brain Injury in Newborn Rats. *J. Clin. Neurosci.* **2020**, *78*, 365–370. [CrossRef]
72. Ahmed, H.A.; Ishrat, T.; Pillai, B.; Fouda, A.Y.; Sayed, M.A.; Eldahshan, W.; Waller, J.L.; Ergul, A.; Fagan, S.C. RAS Modulation Prevents Progressive Cognitive Impairment after Experimental Stroke: A Randomized, Blinded Preclinical Trial. *J. Neuroinflamm.* **2018**, *15*, 229. [CrossRef]
73. Almeida, A.; Sánchez-Morán, I.; Rodríguez, C. Mitochondrial–Nuclear P53 Trafficking Controls Neuronal Susceptibility in Stroke. *IUBMB Life* **2021**, *73*, 582–591. [CrossRef]
74. Sil, S.; Periyasamy, P.; Thangaraj, A.; Chivero, E.T.; Buch, S. PDGF/PDGFR Axis in the Neural Systems. *Mol. Aspects Med.* **2018**, *62*, 63–74. [CrossRef]
75. Gulati, A. Endothelin Receptors, Mitochondria and Neurogenesis in Cerebral Ischemia. *Curr. Neuropharmacol.* **2016**, *14*, 619–626. [CrossRef]
76. Edwards, D.N.; Bix, G.J. The Inflammatory Response After Ischemic Stroke: Targeting B2 and B1 Integrins. *Front. Neurosci.* **2019**, *13*, 540. [CrossRef] [PubMed]
77. Hayakawa, K.; Seo, J.H.; Miyamoto, N.; Pham, L.-D.D.; Navaratna, D.; Lo, E.H.; Arai, K. Brain Angiogenesis After Stroke. In *Biochemical Basis and Therapeutic Implications of Angiogenesis*; Springer International Publishing: Cham, Switzerland, 2017; pp. 473–494.
78. Yeh, E.T.H.; Chang, H.M. Cancer and Clot: Between a Rock and a Hard Place. *J. Am. Coll. Cardiol.* **2017**, *70*, 939–941. [CrossRef] [PubMed]
79. Demers, M.; Wagner, D.D. NETosis: A New Factor in Tumor Progression and Cancer-Associated Thrombosis. *Semin. Thromb. Hemost.* **2014**, *40*, 277–283. [CrossRef] [PubMed]
80. Riedl, J.; Preusser, M.; Nazari, P.M.S.; Posch, F.; Panzer, S.; Marosi, C.; Birner, P.; Thaler, J.; Brostjan, C.; Lötsch, D.; et al. Podoplanin Expression in Primary Brain Tumors Induces Platelet Aggregation and Increases Risk of Venous Thromboembolism. *Blood* **2017**, *129*, 1831–1839. [CrossRef] [PubMed]
81. Subramanian, A.; Tamayo, P.; Mootha, V.K.; Mukherjee, S.; Ebert, B.L.; Gillette, M.A.; Paulovich, A.; Pomeroy, S.L.; Golub, T.R.; Lander, E.S.; et al. Gene Set Enrichment Analysis: A Knowledge-Based Approach for Interpreting Genome-Wide Expression Profiles. *Proc. Natl. Acad. Sci. USA* **2005**, *102*, 15545–15550. [CrossRef] [PubMed]
82. Liberzon, A.; Birger, C.; Thorvaldsdóttir, H.; Ghandi, M.; Mesirov, J.P.; Tamayo, P. The Molecular Signatures Database HALLMARK Gene Set Collection. *Cell Syst.* **2015**, *1*, 417–425. [CrossRef]

83. Livak, K.J.; Schmittgen, T.D. Analysis of Relative Gene Expression Data Using Real-Time Quantitative PCR and the 2−ΔΔCT Method. *Methods* **2001**, *25*, 402–408. [CrossRef] [PubMed]
84. Ru, Y.; Kechris, K.J.; Tabakoff, B.; Hoffman, P.; Radcliffe, R.A.; Bowler, R.; Mahaffey, S.; Rossi, S.; Calin, G.A.; Bemis, L.; et al. The MultiMiR R Package and Database: Integration of MicroRNA-Target Interactions along with Their Disease and Drug Associations. *Nucleic Acids Res.* **2014**, *42*, 133. [CrossRef]
85. Liberzon, A.; Subramanian, A.; Pinchback, R.; Thorvaldsdottir, H.; Tamayo, P.; Mesirov, J.P. Molecular Signatures Database (MSigDB) 3.0. *Bioinformatics* **2011**, *27*, 1739–1740. [CrossRef] [PubMed]
86. Ashburner, M.; Ball, C.A.; Blake, J.A.; Botstein, D.; Butler, H.; Cherry, J.M.; Davis, A.P.; Dolinski, K.; Dwight, S.S.; Eppig, J.T.; et al. Gene Ontology: Tool for the Unification of Biology. The Gene Ontology Consortium. *Nat. Genet.* **2000**, *25*, 25–29. [CrossRef] [PubMed]
87. Carbon, S.; Douglass, E.; Good, B.M.; Unni, D.R.; Harris, N.L.; Mungall, C.J.; Basu, S.; Chisholm, R.L.; Dodson, R.J.; Hartline, E.; et al. The Gene Ontology Resource: Enriching a GOld Mine. *Nucleic Acids Res.* **2021**, *49*, D325–D334. [CrossRef]
88. Mi, H.; Muruganujan, A.; Thomas, P.D. PANTHER in 2013: Modeling the Evolution of Gene Function, and Other Gene Attributes, in the Context of Phylogenetic Trees. *Nucleic Acids Res.* **2013**, *41*, D377–D386. [CrossRef]
89. Thomas, P.D.; Ebert, D.; Muruganujan, A.; Mushayahama, T.; Albou, L.; Mi, H. PANTHER: Making Genome-scale Phylogenetics Accessible to All. *Protein Sci.* **2022**, *31*, 8–22. [CrossRef] [PubMed]
90. Kanehisa, M.; Sato, Y.; Kawashima, M. KEGG Mapping Tools for Uncovering Hidden Features in Biological Data. *Protein Sci.* **2022**, *31*, 47–53. [CrossRef]
91. Kanehisa, M.; Sato, Y. KEGG Mapper for Inferring Cellular Functions from Protein Sequences. *Protein Sci.* **2020**, *29*, 28–35. [CrossRef]
92. Huang, D.W.; Sherman, B.T.; Lempicki, R.A. Bioinformatics Enrichment Tools: Paths toward the Comprehensive Functional Analysis of Large Gene Lists. *Nucleic Acids Res.* **2009**, *37*, 1–13. [CrossRef]
93. Wiebe, D.S.; Omelyanchuk, N.A.; Mukhin, A.M.; Grosse, I.; Lashin, S.A.; Zemlyanskaya, E.V.; Mironova, V.V. Fold-Change-Specific Enrichment Analysis (FSEA): Quantification of Transcriptional Response Magnitude for Functional Gene Groups. *Genes* **2020**, *11*, 434. [CrossRef]
94. Jain, A.; Tuteja, G. TissueEnrich: Tissue-Specific Gene Enrichment Analysis. *Bioinformatics* **2019**, *35*, 1966–1967. [CrossRef]
95. Xu, X.; Wells, A.B.; O'Brien, D.R.; Nehorai, A.; Dougherty, J.D. Cell Type-Specific Expression Analysis to Identify Putative Cellular Mechanisms for Neurogenetic Disorders. *J. Neurosci.* **2014**, *34*, 1420–1431. [CrossRef]
96. Dougherty, J.D.; Schmidt, E.F.; Nakajima, M.; Heintz, N. Analytical Approaches to RNA Profiling Data for the Identification of Genes Enriched in Specific Cells. *Nucleic Acids Res.* **2010**, *38*, 4218–4230. [CrossRef] [PubMed]
97. Miller, J.A.; Ding, S.-L.; Sunkin, S.M.; Smith, K.A.; Ng, L.; Szafer, A.; Ebbert, A.; Riley, Z.L.; Royall, J.J.; Aiona, K.; et al. Transcriptional Landscape of the Prenatal Human Brain. *Nature* **2014**, *508*, 199–206. [CrossRef] [PubMed]
98. Ge, S.X.; Jung, D.; Yao, R. ShinyGO: A Graphical Gene-Set Enrichment Tool for Animals and Plants. *Bioinformatics* **2020**, *36*, 2628–2629. [CrossRef] [PubMed]
99. Wells, A.; Kopp, N.; Xu, X.; O'Brien, D.R.; Yang, W.; Nehorai, A.; Adair-Kirk, T.L.; Kopan, R.; Dougherty, J.D. The Anatomical Distribution of Genetic Associations. *Nucleic Acids Res.* **2015**, *43*, 10804–10820. [CrossRef] [PubMed]

Disclaimer/Publisher's Note: The statements, opinions and data contained in all publications are solely those of the individual author(s) and contributor(s) and not of MDPI and/or the editor(s). MDPI and/or the editor(s) disclaim responsibility for any injury to people or property resulting from any ideas, methods, instructions or products referred to in the content.

Review
New Insights into Oxidative Stress and Inflammatory Response in Neurodegenerative Diseases

Eveljn Scarian [1], Camilla Viola [1,2], Francesca Dragoni [3,4], Rosalinda Di Gerlando [3,4], Bartolo Rizzo [4], Luca Diamanti [5], Stella Gagliardi [4,*], Matteo Bordoni [1,†] and Orietta Pansarasa [1,†]

1. Cellular Models and Neuroepigenetics Unit, IRCCS Mondino Foundation, Via Mondino 2, 27100 Pavia, Italy; eveljn.scarian@mondino.it (E.S.); camilla.viola@mondino.it (C.V.); matteo.bordoni@mondino.it (M.B.); orietta.pansarasa@mondino.it (O.P.)
2. Department of Brain and Behavioral Sciences, University of Pavia, Via Agostino Bassi 21, 27100 Pavia, Italy
3. Department of Biology and Biotechnology "L. Spallanzani", University of Pavia, Via Adolfo Ferrata, 9, 27100 Pavia, Italy; francesca.dragoni@mondino.it (F.D.); rosalinda.digerlando@mondino.it (R.D.G.)
4. Molecular Biology and Transcriptomics Unit, IRCCS Mondino Foundation, Via Mondino 2, 27100 Pavia, Italy; bartolo.rizzo@mondino.it
5. Neuroncology Unit, IRCCS Mondino Foundation, Via Mondino 2, 27100 Pavia, Italy; luca.diamanti@mondino.it
* Correspondence: stella.gagliardi@mondino.it; Tel.: +39-038-238-0248
† These authors contributed equally to this work.

Abstract: Oxidative stress (OS) and inflammation are two important and well-studied pathological hallmarks of neurodegenerative diseases (NDDs). Due to elevated oxygen consumption, the high presence of easily oxidizable polyunsaturated fatty acids and the weak antioxidant defenses, the brain is particularly vulnerable to oxidative injury. Uncertainty exists over whether these deficits contribute to the development of NDDs or are solely a consequence of neuronal degeneration. Furthermore, these two pathological hallmarks are linked, and it is known that OS can affect the inflammatory response. In this review, we will overview the last findings about these two pathways in the principal NDDs. Moreover, we will focus more in depth on amyotrophic lateral sclerosis (ALS) to understand how anti-inflammatory and antioxidants drugs have been used for the treatment of this still incurable motor neuron (MN) disease. Finally, we will analyze the principal past and actual clinical trials and the future perspectives in the study of these two pathological mechanisms.

Keywords: oxidative stress; neurodegenerative diseases; amyotrophic lateral sclerosis; reactive oxygen species; inflammation

1. Introduction

Neurodegenerative diseases (NDDs) are a group of age-related disorders, which cause the death of neural cells of specific types [1]. They are more common in the community as the average age of the population rises, becoming a serious worldwide diffuse health problem [2]. Annual incidence rates of NDDs are typically approximated at 10 to 15 per 100,000 people worldwide [3]. The diagnosis of NDDs is challenging because of the variety of clinical signs and symptoms and it is frequently only confirmed with a neuropathological investigation following the patient's passing [4]. Despite their various symptoms, due to the distinct cell types and areas of the nervous system affected, they all manifest in two forms, a familial form and a sporadic one, not correlated with a familial history of the disease [1]. They share many pathological processes, including dysfunctions in the autophagosomal, ubiquitin/proteasomal, and lysosomal systems, proteins misfolding, and their aggregation. Moreover, they are all characterized by oxidative stress (OS) and neuroinflammation [5–7]. In this review, we will focus on the most common NDDs, Alzheimer's disease (AD), Parkinson's disease (PD), Huntington's disease (HD), and amyotrophic lateral sclerosis (ALS), as well as on the role of OS and neuroinflammation in these diseases. Furthermore, we will dig deeper into ALS and the use of antioxidant and anti-inflammatory drugs in its therapy.

2. Oxidative Stress

The term OS was first formulated in 1985 [8] and refers to an imbalance between oxidants and antioxidants in a biological system, either because of the presence of elevated levels of reactive oxygen species (ROS) or due to a deficient function of the antioxidant system [6]. In a metabolic system there is a redox balance: physiological deviations from this balance are referred to as "oxidative eustress", whereas non-physiological deviations are defined as "oxidative distress" [9]. Although oxygen is essential for human life, because of its structure and the presence of two unpaired electrons, it has the tendency to form radicals, including ROS. ROS are a class of oxygen-derived reactive molecules with a short-term life and a high reactivity [6] and include superoxide anions (O^{2-}), hydroxyl radical (OH), hydrogen peroxide (H_2O_2), nitric oxide (NO), and lipid radicals [10]. ROS can have both an exogenous and an endogenous production. Exogenous sources include specific pharmaceuticals, ionizing radiations, and the metabolism of environmental chemicals, whereas endogenous sources are mitochondrial or non-mitochondrial ROS-developing enzymes [11]. In healthy cells, more than 90% of ROS are produced when an electron escapes from the electron transport chain in mitochondria and attaches to oxygen, whereas 10% of ROS are produced by enzymes, including dihydroorotate dehydrogenase, monoamine oxidase, and nicotinamide adenine dinucleotide phosphate oxidase [12,13]. Due to elevated oxygen consumption, in the brain, there is a high production of ROS, mainly due to electron transport chain complex 1, which contributes to the neurodegeneration of cells modulating important biomolecules, including DNA, RNA, proteins, lipids, and pathways, such as nucleic acid oxidation and lipid peroxidation [6]. Moreover, it was widely demonstrated that ROS can damage mitochondria affecting their proteins, lipids, and DNA, hampering their functions and leading to various diseases [14–16]. In complex organisms, such as humans, lipid and protein oxidation are more relevant than DNA oxidation, especially regarding NDDs, in which oxidized proteins acquire a toxic function and aggregate [13]. Also noteworthy is the nitrosative stress, which refers to combined biochemical reactions of NO and O^{2-}, with the production of peroxynitrite anions. Peroxynitrite anions, in turn, can lead to the nitration of proteins, lipids, and DNA, affecting the enzyme activity of mitochondria and finally causing cell death [17]. It was widely demonstrated that nitrosative stress is associated with OS, inasmuch that some ROS involved in OS act also in the formation and scavenging pathways of nitrogen species. The combination of both OS and nitrosative stress is involved in many different pathologies, including NDDs [18].

There are many different mechanisms, both enzymatic and non-enzymatic, involved in the protection of the organism from the effects of ROS. The principal enzymatic antioxidants include the following: catalase, which is involved in the conversion of H_2O_2 to water and oxygen, using manganese or iron as cofactors; superoxide dismutases, which convert reactive O^{2-} to less reactive H_2O_2 and oxygen; and glutathione peroxidase, which allows for the reduction of H_2O_2 and lipid peroxides. Besides that, non-enzymatic antioxidants include thioredoxin; glutathione; vitamins A, E, and C; flavonoids; proteins; and trace elements [19–21] (Figure 1).

Numerous studies pointed out that OS-induced damages are key factors in the aging process and, consequently, in the development of NDDs. Various mitochondrial DNA deletions and a decrease in the number of antioxidants have been found in elderly individuals [22–25]. For these reasons, it is evident that treatments using antioxidants are fundamental to act against OS in mitochondria. To maintain mitochondrial homeostasis, drugs should accumulate in the mitochondria and interact with their targets. Conventional antioxidants do not accumulate in disease mitochondria, but in recent years, mitochondria-targeted antioxidant (MTA) compounds have been developed [26,27]. These compounds are antioxidant molecules conjugated with a carrier, such as triphenylphosphonium (TPP), which allows for the transport of antioxidants through cellular membranes, thanks to its lipophilicity [28]. They act by interrupting the intramitochondrial cascade caused by OS and lead to apoptosis [27].

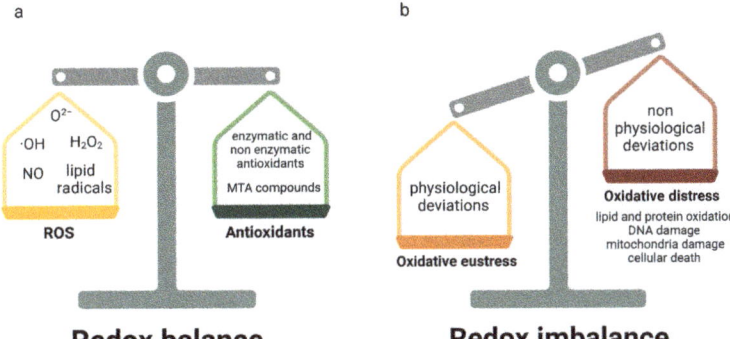

Figure 1. Redox balance and imbalance in organisms. (**a**) The redox balance in living organisms is maintained by the equilibrium between reactive oxygen species (ROS) levels and the action of antioxidants. O^{2-} = superoxide anions, OH = hydroxyl radical, H_2O_2 = hydrogen peroxide, NO = nitric oxide, MTA = mitochondria-targeted antioxidant. (**b**) Moreover, both physiological and non-physiological deviations in ROS levels could occur leading to oxidative eustress and oxidative distress, respectively. Oxidative distress causes lipid and protein oxidation, DNA damage, mitochondria damage and finally cellular death (figure created with Biorender.com accessed on 28 January 2024).

Different studies have demonstrated that the treatment using MTA compounds has beneficial effects against mitochondria OS. Among them, mitoquinone, resulted from the conjugation of a triphenylphosphonium carrier and a modified ubiquinone, is the most known, inasmuch as it acts in the scavenging of ROS in the mitochondria and remains active for a long time [29]. MitoVitE, derived from the conjugation of TPP and α-tocopherol, a type of vitamin E, acts by counteracting lipid peroxidation, protecting mitochondria and cells from OS and reducing apoptosis [29,30]. Finally, MitoTEMPO, composed of (2,2,6,6-Tetramethylpiperidin-1-yl)oxyl and TPP, acts by converting mitochondrial superoxide into water [31].

A valide alternative to TPP-targeting is the encapsulation of antioxidants in liposomes. Liposome-encapsulated antioxidants allow for the delivery of antioxidants, such as quercetin, N-acetyl-L-cysteine, and vitamin E, without altering their structures and bioactivity. They enter the cells via micropinocytosis, fusing with the mitochondrial membrane and releasing the antioxidants [26].

3. Neuroinflammation

Inflammation is the response of the immune system to adverse factors, including pathogens and toxic molecules. Normally, the inflammatory response acts as a defense mechanism to restore tissue homeostasis. When the tissue is injured, a chemical signaling cascade occurs, activating leukocyte chemotaxis at the site of injury. Leukocytes produce cytokines and induce the inflammatory response, characterized by swelling, heat, redness, pain, and a loss of tissue function [32,33]. It is a complex mechanism with the involvement of different cell types, including macrophages, monocytes, lymphocytes, and mast cells [34]. The inflammation resolution process occurs with a cessation of neutrophils' action and with a reduction in cytokines' gradient [32,35]. When immediate inflammatory responses to tissue injury are ineffective, chronic inflammation rises [36].

The term neuroinflammation refers to the inflammatory response in the brain and it is one of the main characteristics of NDDs. It could be defined as the inflammatory response to factors that cause a change in the homeostasis in the central nervous system

(CNS) [13]. It was widely demonstrated that the inflammatory response in the brain can cause cell injury and increase the blood–brain barrier permeability, leading to a decrease in its protective role [32]. In brain diseases characterized by inflammation, there is the activation of the brain's immune cells and microglia, which form the primary innate immunity of brain, with the consequent activation of inflammatory mediators, including cytokines, chemokines, secondary messengers, and ROS [37–39]. Moreover, microglia undergo cytoskeletal modifications and changes in receptors' expression, which allow for its migration toward sites of injury [40]. Curiously, CNS protection and host-organism benefits are the goals of microglial activation and of increased cytokine expression, which are also important for processes such as synaptic pruning and memory consolidation [41–45]. However, persistent, excessive, or amplified microglial activation can result in significant pathogenic alterations [40]. Moreover, it was observed that astrocytes play a critical role in the infiltration of CNS by leukocytes, represented mainly by lymphocytes and mononuclear phagocytes [46].

The inflammatory process is directly linked with OS. ROS can promote the expression of pro-inflammatory genes and, simultaneously, neuroinflammation can stimulate ROS production. In a physiological condition, in which redox balance occurs, the inflammatory response acts as a defense mechanism. On the contrary, under pathological conditions, the redox imbalance causes the activation of inflammatory mechanisms, leading to the secretion of pro-inflammatory molecules and of neoepitopes [46,47]. In parallel, pro-inflammatory cytokines, including interleukines (interleukin 1β and interleukin 6), interferons, and tumor necrosis factor, induce the generation of ROS in non-phagocytic cells, principally by the activation of NADPH oxidase (NOX) [46].

Both OS and inflammation are involved in NDDs' pathogenesis, causing common and different manifestations Their involvement is synthesized in Figure 2 and will be discussed in the next paragraphs.

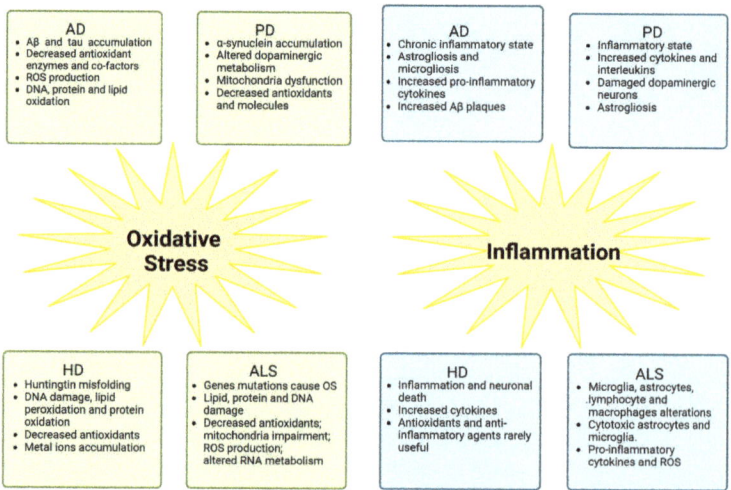

Figure 2. Clinical manifestations of OS and inflammation in four different neurodegenerative diseases (NDDs): Alzheimer's disease (AD), Parkinson's disease (PD), Huntington's disease (HD), and amyotrophic lateral sclerosis (ALS) (figure created with Biorender.com accessed on 28 January 2024).

4. Oxidative Stress and Inflammation in AD, PD, and HD

AD is the most common type of dementia and it is caused by the loss of cognitive and behavioral capacities, due to the death of neurons of the neocortex, enthorinal cortex, and hippocampus [48]. It is characterized by the accumulation of neurotoxic beta-amyloid (Aβ) oligomer peptides and of tau protein, which causes neuroinflammation, neurotransmitter imbalance, dendritic alterations, and synaptic impairments, all linked to the neurodegeneration [6]. Numerous studies have reported that OS induced by the accumulation of toxic Aβ peptides causes lipids, proteins, and DNA oxidation. Accumulation of Aβ plaques causes different damages, including the disruption of the electron transport chain via cytochrome oxidase inhibition, inevitably leading to OS [48–51]. Moreover, decreased levels of antioxidant enzymes were found in AD patients [52,53]. An important role of biometals, such as zinc, iron, and copper, was widely demonstrated in AD neurodegeneration, inasmuch as they have been frequently found in Aβ plaques. This causes a deficiency of such metals, important cofactors for antioxidant enzymes in brain cells [54–56]. Moreover, Cu^{2+} and Zn^{2+} can bind peptides causing a redox reaction and leading to the production of ROS [57].

Numerous clinical trials have focused on the association between AD and OS, studying the effects of fatty acid supplementation, with some beneficial effects, most of all in cognitive assessment [58–60]. For example, it was demonstrated that eicosapentaenoic and docosahexaenoic acids have antioxidant, anti-apoptotic, anti-inflammatory, and neurotrophic properties, enhancing nerve growth factor levels and improving cognitive function [60].

Various studies have demonstrated that AD is characterized by a chronic pro-inflammatory condition in the brain, including both astro- and microgliosis. Aβ-associated depositions cause an increase in pro-inflammatory cytokines' production by microglia, and, in turn, systemic inflammation enhances β-amyloid generation in the brain [61–63]. Moreover, it was recently demonstrated that cytokines produced by microglia, including interleukin 1α, tumor necrosis factor α, and complement component C1q, activate reactive astrocytes involved in neuronal death. Neuroinflammation might prime microglia for such activation [64].

PD is a NDD characterized by the loss of midbrain dopaminergic neurons of the *substantia nigra pars compacta*, causing a reduction of the dopaminergic input to basal ganglia and a hyperactivation of the cholinergic one. The aberrant activation of these pathways contributes to difficulties in memory and learning, and, above all, to the loss of control in motor functions [65].

OS and the overproduction of ROS are important factors involved in degeneration of dopaminergic neurons. The accumulation of ROS was associated with different mechanisms including the metabolism of dopamine itself, mitochondrial dysfunctions in neurons and neuroglia, inflammation, and increased levels of iron and calcium [13,66,67]. It was also observed that neurons of *substantia nigra* accumulate granules of neuromelanin, a pigment which can cause ROS production. Moreover, it was demonstrated that alterations in neuromelanin composition and density can cause α-synuclein aggregation and iron accumulation [68].

Additionally, PD mutations, including the ones on *DJ-1*, *PINK1*, *Parkin*, *SNCA*, and *LRRK2*, have numerous consequences on mitochondrial functions, causing an exacerbation of ROS production [69,70]. With regard to dopamine metabolism, this neurotransmitter is an unstable molecule that is prone to auto-oxidation to form quinones and free radicals. Numerous enzymes are involved in its metabolism and in its degradation by catalyzing its oxidative deamination. However, due to neuronal degeneration, there is an imbalance of these enzymes, which causes the production of ROS [69,70]. Moreover, two enzymes are involved in the defense against ROS, dopamine transporter and vesicular monoamine transporter 2. They both are involved in the uptake of free dopamine from synapses and in its packing into synaptic vesicles to be protected from oxidation. It was demonstrated that dopamine transporter concentration declines with age and that vesicular monoamine transporter 2 is inhibited by α-synuclein, the presynaptic neuronal protein which is found aggregated in PD [68]. Finally, it was proved that in PD patients' brains, there is a decreased concentration of important antioxidants, such as glutathione and vitamin E, and an alteration in the levels of calcium, iron, and lipids [71–76]. As for AD, also for PD, numerous clinical trials have been focused on OS in PD and have studied the deficiency of antioxidants in this pathology and how to ameliorate ROS-caused symptoms. For example, a still ongoing phase II clinical trial is evaluating the effect of the antioxidant N-acetyl cysteine on the dopaminergic function of PD patients [13].

The important role of neuroinflammation in PD was widely demonstrated, mainly due to the activation of microglia and astrocytes. Microglial cells would specifically harm dopaminergic neurons because they are more prevalent in the midbrain than in the other brain areas. It was proved that there was an abundant presence of reactive astrocytes and microglia and an increase in the complement component C1q in the *substantia nigra* of PD-affected subjects, suggesting PD-associated neuroinflammation [77–80]. Moreover, microglia-activated neuroinflammation mediators, such as cytokines and interleukins, have been detected in the cerebrospinal fluid (CSF) of PD patients [81]. Eventually, the fact that the human leukocyte antigen was found to be a risk factor for PD demonstrated that there is a possibility of a more general pro-inflammatory state in PD, not caused by neuronal loss, although it can worsen the neuroinflammation as well [82].

HD is an inherited NDD that occurs in young individuals. It is a protein-misfolding disease, where the huntingtin protein is mutated and causes an aberration in normal biological functions interacting with other proteins [83]. The mutant protein gains a toxic function leading to OS and inflammation. However, it is still not clear whether OS causes HD or it is a consequence of earlier events and the studies about this aspect are fewer than for other NDDs [84]. Oxidative damage in cells and tissues in HD models and patients has been reported. Lipid peroxidation, protein oxidation, and DNA damage have been linked to this pathology and to huntingtin mutation [85–90]. As for the other NDDs, an accumulation of metal ions, especially iron and copper, and a decrease in antioxidant concentrations have been found [91–95]. Moreover, mitochondrial dysfunctions have been detected in HD patients' brains [96,97]. It was recently demonstrated that the deregulation of HSF1, a transcriptional regulator of the heat shock response, contributes to mitochondrial dysregulation in HD, by impairing the peroxisome proliferator co-activator PGC-1α and its downstream targets such as the mitochondrial transcription factor TFAM and cytochrome c [97]. Neuronal death can activate inflammatory mechanisms, which in turn cause neurodegeneration leading to a vicious cycle [98]. Elevated levels of cytokines have been found in fluids of both animal models and HD patients [99–103]. Unfortunately, until now, anti-inflammatory and antioxidant agents have rarely achieved effectiveness in HD treatment [103].

5. Oxidative Stress and Inflammation in ALS

ALS is an NDD which affects the upper and lower motor neurons (MNs) of the cortex, brainstem, and spinal cord, causing the death of patients within three to five years after symptoms' onset. There are two types of ALS, a sporadic form and a familial one, which can be related to both mutations in specific genes and to epigenetic factors. Despite ALS principal symptoms being related to motor dysfunctions, patients often show signs of behavioral and cognitive impairment [1,104].

There are different factors involved in ALS onset and progression including the presence of OS. In fact, different studies reported OS hallmarks in ALS patients and animal models. Oxidative damage was found in lipids and proteins of post-mortem tissues, as well in plasma, urine, and CSF [105–109]. Moreover, it was demonstrated that nerve terminals are sensitive to ROS and to inflammation, amplifying the decline of neuromuscular junctions [110]. OS was often associated with gene mutations, especially in *SOD1*. *SOD1* catalyzes the conversion of O^{2-} into H_2O_2 and molecular oxygen, which are nontoxic for the cells. Specific *SOD1* mutations lead to a higher peroxidase activity and convert H_2O_2 to hydroxide, which inactivates the dismutase structure. Furthermore, O^{2-} leads to peroxynitrite production and finally to neuronal death [111]. It is obvious that mutations in this gene can cause serious problems in respiration and the metabolic activities of cells [112]. The gain of function of mutant *SOD1* and aberrant aggregation of this protein were associated with MNs' death in ALS patients. SOD1 protein aggregation contributes to dysfunction of the ubiquitin/proteasome system and interferes with mitophagy. In addition, mutant *SOD1* leads to impairment in the respiratory chain of mitochondria [113–115].

TARDBP encodes for the TDP-43 protein, involved in many different processes, including RNA transcription, maturation, transport, and translation. It also participates in intracellular stress management, taking part in the biogenesis and maintenance of stress granules. Mutation in *TARDBP* causes TDP-43 aggregation and cytoplasmic mislocalization, but TDP-43 inclusions were found also in non-mutated patients [111,116]. In turn, aggregated TDP43 causes a mitochondrial imbalance that increases OS [117–119]. It was found that OS induces conformation modifications in TDP-43, causing cysteine disulphide cross-linking or promoting lysine acetylation, leading to TDP-43 aggregation and its acquisition of an aberrant function [120,121]. Finally, mutated *TARDBP* decreases antioxidant expression [122,123], influencing the nuclear factor erythroid-2-related factor 2 (Nrf2) antioxidative pathway. TDP43 was also found in stress granules, structures formed in response to stress. In 2011, Dewey and co-authors demonstrated that both wild-type and mutant TDP-43 form stress granules, but mutant TDP-43 sets up larger ones and incorporates them earlier [123,124].

Other common ALS-associated gene mutations include the ones in *FUS* and in *C9ORF72*. *FUS* encodes for an RNA/DNA-binding protein and it is implicated in RNA metabolism and DNA repair. It was demonstrated that *FUS* deficits and mutations fail to repair OS-caused DNA damage due to nick ligation defects, eventually leading to MNs' death [125]. As for TDP-43, mutations in *FUS* cause mitochondria damage, a decrease in mitochondrial membrane potential and respiration, and a dysregulation in mitochondrial gene transcription [126,127]. In 2020, Tsai and co-authors demonstrated that in *FUS*-mutated cells, FUS protein associates with mitochondria and with mRNAs encoding mitochondrial respiratory chain components. This association causes mitochondrial networks' disorganization, impairment in aerobic respiration, and an increase in ROS production [126].

Finally, *C9ORF72* is the most commonly mutated gene in ALS patients. In 2016, Onesto and co-authors found that ROS production in *C9ORF72* mutated ALS patients' cells, causing hyperpolarization of mitochondrial membranes [128]. More recently, Birger and co-authors demonstrated that astrocytes carrying the *C9ORF72* expansion inhibit the production of antioxidant molecules, enhancing OS also in MNs [129]. Additionally, it was found that mutations in this gene increase O^{2-} levels and reduce mitochondrial potential and cell survival [130].

However, signs of OS, including protein and lipid peroxidation, were found in non-mutated ALS cases as well [131–133] and were associated with a decrease in antioxidant enzymes' activity and with a possible pro-oxidative state [134].

As for other NDDs, it is difficult to determine if oxidative damage is a primary cause or a secondary consequence of ALS. Moreover, it is very problematic to evaluate OS markers at an early stage of the disease, ruling out the possibility of evaluating if oxidative damage appears early or late in its course [133]. Nevertheless, animal models have brought some insights into this context. For example, in 2007, Kraft and co-authors obtained a mutant *SOD1* mouse and found an activation of nuclear Nrf2—an antioxidant response element during the disease course. The earliest activation occurred in distal muscles of mice and subsequently caused MN loss [135]. Vande Velde and co-authors arrived at the same conclusions in 2011. They found that mutant *SOD1* causes mitochondria disruption at an early pathogenic stage [136].

The exact oxidative mechanism in ALS is still to be determined, and the involvement of mitochondria in this process is not clear. Moreover, Edaravone, a drug approved in the USA for alleviating ALS symptoms, involved in lipid peroxides and hydroxyl radical elimination, is not particularly effective in disease treatment [137]. In 2019, Walczak and co-authors compared ALS patients and control subjects in terms of mitochondrial function and antioxidant enzymes, and they found a decreased expression in ALS patients' mitochondria complexes I, II, III, and IV proteins; in mitochondrial membrane potential; and in *SOD1* and catalase, both antioxidant enzymes [138]. In addition, ALS patients carrying mutations in *CHCHD10*, involved in ALS pathology and in mitochondrial cristae morphology maintenance, manifest fibroblasts with mitochondrial damage and mitochondrial network fragmentation [139].

With regard to oxidative DNA damage, 8-hydroxy 2 deoxyguanosine is the most abundant oxidative alteration in DNA, inasmuch as guanine has a low electron reduction potential [137]. Elevated levels of 8-hydroxy 2 deoxyguanosine were found in the motor cortex and spinal cord DNA of ALS patients [140,141]. Furthermore, signs of p53 activation, indicating the apoptosis process, were found in both ALS cellular models and in ALS patients [125,141–143]. Altered levels of antioxidant enzymes were found in ALS.

Apurinic/apyrimidinic endonuclease 1 is an enzyme involved in redox regulation and in DNA repair. Its concentration and localization were altered in both ALS patients and animal models [144–146]. In addition, alterations in the levels of 8-oxoguanine glycosylase, involved in the removal of oxidized guanine, were found in spinal MNs of both sporadic and mutated ALS cases [144,147].

OS can also bring about abnormalities in RNA metabolism, which in turn can cause OS. It was found that oxidative RNA modifications occur early in the disease progression and precede MN death. Proteins encoded by *TARDBP*, *FUS*, and *SOD1* are involved in miRNA processing and some miRNAs regulate the expression of genes involved in OS [137]. In 2017, Pegoraro and co-authors found an upregulation of both muscle-specific and inflammatory miRNAs in ALS patients compared to control subjects and this upregulation was associated with an earlier age of symptoms onset. Moreover, they found differential miRNA expressions in muscles from males and females, suggesting the influence of sexual hormones [148]. The expression of miR-388-3p, involved in both mitochondrial function and apoptosis, was found increased in *SOD1* mutant mice [149], while the expression of miR-34a, involved in OS regulation, was found decreased in both ALS patients and mouse models [150,151]. MiR-155, involved in inflammatory response and mitochondrial function, was found upregulated in skeletal muscles of ALS patients and in the spinal cord of *SOD1* mice [152–154].

Finally, hyperexcitability is a decisive characteristic of ALS, and it was detected before early clinical symptoms, with a strengthening which causes disruption in energy metabolism, mitochondrial disfunctions, and increased OS [155–157]. This altered neuronal excitability and the consequent manifestation of OS were associated with defects in ion channels, including sodium, potassium, calcium, and chloride ones, of neuronal and non-neuronal cells [158]. In fact, while most ALS patients do not manifest deleterious mutations in ion channel-associated genes, many studies reported alterations in channels in both mutated and non-mutated ALS subjects and animal models [158,159]. Already in 2006, Kaiser and co-authors demonstrated a reduction in potassium channels in SOD1^{G93A} mice leading inevitably to MN death. More recently, alterations in chloride channels were associated with muscle channelopathies, atrophy, and OS [160,161] and the decreased expression of calcium channels in the spinal MNs of SOD1^{G93A} mice was correlated with excess mitochondrial calcium and the production of ROS [162,163].

Noteworthy, Riluzole acts by blocking voltage-gated channels, especially sodium ones, allowing for the inhibition of glutamate release in presynaptic terminals and interfering with the excitatory transmission caused by this amino acid [164].

With regard to the inflammatory response, alterations in the immune system can cause an increase in neuroinflammation in ALS patients which has been associated with neuronal loss in both animal models and in humans [134]. Alterations were observed in all the cell types involved in inflammation, including microglia, astrocytes, lymphocytes, and macrophages. Activated microglia were found in both ALS patients and animal models, and they were correlated with MN deficits [165–167]. The loss of function of *C9ORF72* causes alterations in microglia, macrophages, and neuroinflammation [168]. In addition, different studies have demonstrated a defective lysosomal system with the accumulation of innate immune cells in *C9ORF72* mutated mice [169–171].

Many studies have demonstrated that microglia activation and their switch from a protective phenotype to a deleterious one can be mediated by the receptor P2X7, the inhibition of which may provide positive outcomes in ALS patients [172–175]. Furthermore, injured MNs induce microglia to acquire a cytotoxic phenotype with the consequent release of ROS and pro-inflammatory cytokines [176–179]. Among them, interleukin 6 was correlated with disease progression in ALS [180]. A more recent study tested a cohort of 53 ALS patients through positron emission tomography. Authors used [11C]-PBR28, a radiotracer that binds to a protein typically expressed in activated microglia, and found that glial activation is increased in the pathological brain region and is correlated with clinical measures [181].

Even mutated astrocytes are toxic to normal MNs, causing their death [182–184]. In 2017, Qian and co-authors demonstrated that both non-MNs and MNs degenerate after ALS astrocyte transplantation, suggesting that neural degeneration is not specific to MNs and that the astrocyte-mediated neuronal death occurs through a non-cell autonomous toxicity [185]. Moreover, ALS causes the loss of glutamate transporter on astrocytes, responsible for the uptake of excess glutamate from synaptic clefts. It was demonstrated that the inefficient glutamate uptake exacerbates MN degeneration [186,187]. As well as microglia, astrocytes exert toxic effects on MNs by secreting pro-inflammatory molecules, including NO, NOX2, prostaglandin E2, and leukotriene B4, or inducing necroptosis [188–191].

In addition to astrocytes and microglia, dysregulation in T lymphocytes and macrophages was observed in ALS patients and ALS animal models [192–197]. In 2020, Chiot and co-authors demonstrated that the replacement of macrophages in *SOD1* mice by more neurotrophic macrophages led to a decrease in macrophage and microglia activation. Moreover, they found that when the replacement occurs in pre-symptomatic stages, it causes a delay in disease onset, whereas when it occurs at the disease onset, it is able to increase mice survival [198].

6. ALS Therapeutic Approaches Related to OS and Inflammation

Several trials to find therapies for ALS have been conducted or are still on course, and some of them are related to **OS**. In this regard, one of two drugs approved in the USA for the treatment of ALS, Edaravone, acts as a **scavenger of ROS**, thus preventing OS propagation [199,200]. In a recent study, Ohta and co-authors demonstrated that in the CSF and plasma of ALS patients, there is a reduction in antioxidant capacities, measured using the OXY-adsorbent test, which is reversed by Edaravone treatment [201]. The other approved drug, Riluzole, blocks glutamatergic neurotransmission and inhibits glutamate release. Different studies have proved that it can also attenuate **OS** injuries in in vitro and in vivo ALS models [202,203]. However, the exact mechanism of action of Riluzole is still unknown.

Studies have been performed also on molecules which upregulate genes containing the antioxidant response element. Among them, sulforaphane activates the Nrf2/**antioxidant response** element pathway but did not show effects in ALS treatment [204,205]. A limitation in the use of sulforaphane could be that the combination of sulforaphane and antioxidants reduces the protective effects of sulforaphane itself, specifically in the induction of autophagy [206]. Moreover, further studies have pointed out possible side effects of sulforaphane, which can induce a lowering of the seizure threshold in mice [207] and can influence thyroid activity [208]. More recently, CuATSM, a positron emission tomography-imaging agent which is able to deliver copper to cells with altered mitochondria, has been proved to extend the survival and to delay ALS onset in SODG93A mice, acting on **OS response** [209,210]. However, it is not tolerated at a high dose in mice, causing toxicity signs including motor aberrations, weight loss, and low activity [190].

Studies have also focused on mitochondrial-targeting drugs, such as mitoquinone and Szeto-Schiller peptides, which act by **decreasing oxidative damage** and maintaining normal mitochondrial function [111,211]. Additionally, the p62-mediated mitophagy inducer was seen as a promoter of the quality control of mitochondria and an inducer of autophagy in damaged organelles, without evident adverse effects, acting as a potential ALS therapeutic molecule [212,213].

Other promising approaches to **reduce OS** are the use of phytochemicals, such as quercetin, which decreases ROS in *SOD1* mutated cells [214] but could, however, have possible nephrotoxic effects and interact with other drugs [215], and the use of cannabidiol or the target of cannabinoid receptors [216–218]. Finally, many studies have suggested the possibility to use **modifiers of OS-related molecules**, such as NOX inhibitors. NOX activity is unregulated in ALS patients and animal models, causing inflammation and glial activation. It was observed that the use of NOX inhibitors, such as perphenazine, thioridazine, and apocynin, reduces O^{2-} levels, increases the numbers of MNs, and extends the lifespan, but it could have also sedative effects [219,220].

Despite different approaches, finding a definitive drug is difficult, because the direct pathogenic mechanism of ALS is not clear. One promising option would be the design of **antioxidant therapies** also **associated with anti-inflammatory therapeutics** [110]. Multiple **anti-inflammatory compounds** have been tested and have been shown to be effective for ALS treatment, especially in animal models. Minocycline was tested on ALS animal models, demonstrating a high efficacy in reducing MN loss, extending mice survival, and suppressing microglia activation [221,222]. However, a phase III trial on 412 ALS patients revealed harmful effects, including gastrointestinal, respiratory, and neurological ones, without significant results on disease progression [223]. On the contrary, a recently concluded phase II trial on NP001, a regulator of macrophage activation, revealed the good tolerability of this compound, leading to the slowing of ALSFRS-R and vital capacity scores in a subgroup of treated patients [224,225]. The only side effect reported was higher infusion-related sensations of burning [225]. Better results were obtained with the use of masitinib, a tyrosine-kinase inhibitor, that is able to decrease aberrant glial cells, microgliosis, and MN degeneration in mice [226]. The clinical trial on ALS patients demonstrated a slowing in functional decline in patients and a prolonged survival by over two years, with the most common side effects including maculopapular rash and peripheral edema [227,228].

In the field of drug repurposing, Fingolimod, a modulator of sphingosine-1-phosphate receptor approved for the treatment of relapsing remitting multiple sclerosis, was tested on *SOD1* mutated mice and was observed to act on **inflammation**, having beneficial effects modulating microglia and innate immunity and reducing the levels of inducible NO synthase [229]. In a recent phase II trial, Fingolimod resulted as well tolerated by ALS patients and showed the possibility to reduce circulating lymphocytes, with no serious adverse events [230]. Moreover, it was demonstrated that Fingolimod acts also on **OS**, reducing the levels OS markers and increasing antioxidants, especially SOD [231,232]. A recent study by Yevgi and Demir tested the action of this drug on multiple sclerosis patients and demonstrated a reduction in the total OS after three months of treatment [233].

Other studies focused on the use of *immune modulatory drugs*. In a pilot trial of 2019, authors treated ALS patients with RNS60, an immune-modulatory agent, demonstrating its safety and tolerability, with common adverse effects including falls, headaches, nasopharyngitis, and contusions and no serious adverse effects [234]. More recently, a trial targeted T cells with a low dose of interleukine 2, demonstrating a high tolerability and an immunologically efficacy in ALS patients, with an increase in Treg levels. No serious adverse events were reported and the non-serious adverse effects were transient [235]. Moreover, numerous studies have focused on cell-based treatments, especially for the use of mesenchymal, embryonic, and neural progenitor cells [236,237].

Finally, it was demonstrated that the regular use of anti-hypertensive drugs could have a protective role against ALS incidence. Hypertension is one of the most common comorbidities in ALS and it was related to progression, incidence, and survival, mainly for the involvement of angiotensin 2 in ROS production. Angiotensin 2 is a potent stimulator of NAD(P)H oxidase, one of the major sources of ROS. ROS generated by NAD(P)H oxidase can induce the production of other ROS and could lead to inflammation [238–241]. In 2020, Pfeiffer and co-authors demonstrated that numerous hypertension drugs, including beta blockers, angiotensin-converting enzyme inhibitors, calcium channel blockers, diuretics, and angiotensin 2 receptor blockers, were correlated with a **lower risk of ALS** [242]. Moreover, it was demonstrated that the angiotensin system can be involved in different NDDs and that its blocking can be a new method for **neuroprotection** [243–245].

These studies demonstrated that many drugs tested are effective in animal models but not in clinical practice. This gap can be explained by the complexity of the ALS disease mechanism and by the fact that preclinical models could not completely recapitulate the disease processes which occur in humans [246.

The still ongoing clinical trials, testing the efficacy of the abovementioned drugs, are reported in Table 1.

Table 1. Ongoing clinical trials. List of the still ongoing clinical trials of the mentioned drugs (https://clinicaltrials.gov accessed on 29 January 2024).

Drug	Action Mechanism of the Drug	Name of the Trial	Clinical Trial ID	Clinical Trial Phase
Edaravone	Scavenger of ROS	Study to investigate the efficacy and safety of FAB122 (daily oral Edaravone) in patients with amyotrophic lateral sclerosis	NCT05178810	Phase III
		Radicava® (Edaravone) Findings in Biomarkers from ALS (REFINE-ALS)	NCT04259255	Phase IV
Riluzole	Glutamatergic neurotransmission blocking	Treatment combining riluzole and IFB-088 in bulbar amyotrophic lateral sclerosis (TRIALS protocol)	NCT05508074	Phase II
Cannabidiol and cannabinoids	OS reducing	Outcomes Mandate National Integration with Cannabis as Medicine (OMNI-Can)	NCT03944447	Phase II
		Safety and efficacy on spasticity symptoms of a cannabis sativa extract in motor neuron disease	NCT01776970	Phase II and phase III
		Efficacy of Cannabinoids in Amyotrophic Lateral Sclerosis or Motor Neurone Disease	NCT03690791	Phase III
		EMERALD TRIAL Open Label Extension Study (EMERALD-OLE)	NCT04997954	Phase IV
Masitinib	Anti-inflammatory compounds	Efficacy and Safety of Masitinib Versus Placebo in the Treatment of ALS Patients	NCT03127267	Phase III
RNS60	Immune modulatory drug	Nebulized RNS60 for the Treatment of Amyotrophic Lateral Sclerosis	NCT02988297	Phase II not yet recruiting
Stem cells	Immune system modulator	The Evaluation of the Effect of Mesenchymal Stem Cells on the Immune System of Patients with ALS (ALSTEM)	NCT04651855	Phase I and II
		Derivation of Induced Pluripotent Stem Cells from an Existing Collection of Human Somatic Cells	NCT00801333	Observational
		CNS10-NPC-GDNF Delivered to the Motor Cortex for ALS	NCT05306457	Phase I
		Neurologic Stem Cell Treatment Study (NEST)	NCT02795052	Interventional
		Development of iPS From Donated Somatic Cells of Patients with Neurological Diseases	NCT00874783	Interventional
Calcium channel blockers	ROS reducer	Rho Kinase Inhibitor in Amyotrophic Lateral Sclerosis (REAL)	NCT05218668	Phase II

7. Conclusive Remarks

OS and inflammation are important mechanisms involved in NDDs and, among them, in ALS pathology. They can be caused by external or internal triggers, such as chemicals and ROS-developing enzymes, respectively, but they always lead to pathological aberrations, including DNA and RNA damage, mitochondrial dysfunction, and cell death. Despite many studies focused on their role in neurological diseases, uncertainty still exists over whether they contribute to the development of NDDs or are solely a consequence of neuronal degeneration. This review summarized the recent findings on the involvement of these two pathological pathways in NDDs, with a specific focus on ALS. We highlighted that all the discussed NDDs, i.e., AD, PD, HD, and ALS, are characterized by an oxidative and inflammatory state which leads to similar pathological mechanisms, including cell damage, lipid and protein oxidation, DNA aberrations, and finally neuronal death. Moreover, we underlined how these two mechanisms are intrinsically correlated in a vicious cycle. The generation of ROS causes neuronal damage and the release of molecules that activate microglia and astrocytes. In turn, these cells release pro-inflammatory cytokines which cause inflammation and exacerbate neuronal injury.

Finally, we discussed some evidence of possible therapeutic approaches targeting OS and the inflammation pathway for the treatment of ALS. As for the other NDDs, many studies focused on the use of antioxidants and anti-inflammatory compounds for the treatment of this still incurable pathology, but few drugs, including NP001 and Fingolimod, have shown efficacy in humans especially for the multifactorial characteristic of these diseases. Although the finding of a definitive drug is difficult and there is a need for future studies, there are numerous clinical trials which will deepen the knowledge about these diseases and will elucidate the precise mechanisms underlining OS and the inflammatory response.

Author Contributions: Writing—original draft preparation: E.S.; writing—review and editing: E.S., M.B., C.V., F.D., R.D.G., B.R., S.G., L.D. and O.P.; conceptualization: E.S.; supervision: S.G., M.B. and O.P.; funding acquisition: O.P. and L.D.; project administration: M.B. and O.P. All authors have read and agreed to the published version of the manuscript.

Funding: This research was funded by the Italian Ministry of Health "Ricerca Corrente 2022–2024" granted to IRCCS Mondino Foundation.

Conflicts of Interest: The authors declare no conflicts of interest.

References

1. Pansarasa, O.; Garofalo, M.; Scarian, E.; Dragoni, F.; Garau, J.; Di Gerlando, R.; Diamanti, L.; Bordoni, M.; Gagliardi, S. Biomarkers in Human Peripheral Blood Mononuclear Cells: The State of the Art in Amyotrophic Lateral Sclerosis. *Int. J. Mol. Sci.* **2022**, *23*, 2580. [CrossRef]
2. Mayne, K.; White, J.A.; McMurran, C.E.; Rivera, F.J.; de la Fuente, A.G. Aging and Neurodegenerative Disease: Is the Adaptive Immune System a Friend or Foe? *Front. Aging Neurosci.* **2020**, *12*, 572090. [CrossRef]
3. Onohuean, H.; Akiyode, A.O.; Akiyode, O.; Igbinoba, S.I.; Alagbonsi, A.I. Epidemiology of neurodegenerative diseases in the East African region: A meta-analysis. *Front. Neurol.* **2022**, *13*, 1024004. [CrossRef]
4. Bruzova, M.; Rusina, R.; Stejskalova, Z.; Matej, R. Autopsy-diagnosed neurodegenerative dementia cases support the use of cerebrospinal fluid protein biomarkers in the diagnostic work-up. *Sci. Rep.* **2021**, *11*, 10837. [CrossRef]
5. Dugger, B.N.; Dickson, D.W. Pathology of Neurodegenerative Diseases. *Cold Spring Harb. Perspect. Biol.* **2017**, *9*, a028035. [CrossRef]
6. Singh, A.; Kukreti, R.; Saso, L.; Kukreti, S. Oxidative Stress: A Key Modulator in Neurodegenerative Diseases. *Molecules* **2019**, *24*, 1583. [CrossRef]
7. Kwon, H.S.; Koh, S.H. Neuroinflammation in neurodegenerative disorders: The roles of microglia and astrocytes. *Transl. Neurodegener.* **2020**, *9*, 42. [CrossRef]
8. Sies, H. *Oxidative Stress*; Academic Press: London, UK, 1985.
9. Sies, H. *Oxidative Stress: Eustress and Distress*, 1st ed.; Academic Press: London, UK, 2020.
10. Radi, R. Oxygen radicals, nitric oxide, and peroxynitrite: Redox pathways in molecular medicine. *Proc. Natl. Acad. Sci. USA* **2018**, *115*, 5839–5848. [CrossRef]
11. De Almeida, A.J.P.O.; de Oliveira, J.C.P.L.; da Silva Pontes, L.V.; de Souza Júnior, J.F.; Gonçalves, T.A.F.; Dantas, S.H.; de Almeida Feitosa, M.S.; Silva, A.O.; de Medeiros, I.A. ROS: Basic Concepts, Sources, Cellular Signaling, and its Implications in Aging Pathways. *Oxidative Med. Cell. Longev.* **2022**, *2022*, 1225578. [CrossRef]
12. Tirichen, H.; Yaigoub, H.; Xu, W.; Wu, C.; Li, R.; Li, Y. Mitochondrial Reactive Oxygen Species and Their Contribution in Chronic Kidney Disease Progression through Oxidative Stress. *Front. Physiol.* **2021**, *12*, 627837. [CrossRef]

13. Teleanu, D.M.; Niculescu, A.G.; Lungu, I.I.; Radu, C.I.; Vladâcenco, O.; Roza, E.; Costăchescu, B.; Grumezescu, A.M.; Teleanu, R.I. An Overview of Oxidative Stress, Neuroinflammation, and Neurodegenerative Diseases. *Int. J. Mol. Sci.* **2022**, *23*, 5938. [CrossRef]
14. Guo, C.; Sun, L.; Chen, X.; Zhang, D. Oxidative stress, mitochondrial damage and neurodegenerative diseases. *Neural Regen. Res.* **2013**, *8*, 2003–2014. [CrossRef]
15. Zorov, D.B.; Juhaszova, M.; Sollott, S.J. Mitochondrial reactive oxygen species (ROS) and ROS-induced ROS release. *Physiol. Rev.* **2014**, *94*, 909–950. [CrossRef]
16. Patergnani, S.; Bouhamida, E.; Leo, S.; Pinton, P.; Rimessi, A. Mitochondrial Oxidative Stress and "Mito-Inflammation": Actors in the Diseases. *Biomedicines* **2021**, *9*, 216. [CrossRef]
17. Wang, F.; Yuan, Q.; Chen, F.; Pang, J.; Pan, C.; Xu, F.; Chen, Y. Fundamental Mechanisms of the Cell Death Caused by Nitrosative Stress. *Front. Cell Dev. Biol.* **2021**, *9*, 742483. [CrossRef]
18. Cobb, C.A.; Cole, M.P. Oxidative and nitrative stress in neurodegeneration. *Neurobiol. Dis.* **2015**, *84*, 4–21. [CrossRef]
19. Kim, G.H.; Kim, J.E.; Rhie, S.J.; Yoon, S. The Role of Oxidative Stress in Neurodegenerative Diseases. *Exp. Neurobiol.* **2015**, *24*, 325–340. [CrossRef]
20. Niedzielska, E.; Smaga, I.; Gawlik, M.; Moniczewski, A.; Stankowicz, P.; Pera, J.; Filip, M. Oxidative Stress in Neurodegenerative Diseases. *Mol. Neurobiol.* **2016**, *53*, 4094–4125. [CrossRef]
21. Liu, Z.; Zhou, T.; Ziegler, A.C.; Dimitrion, P.; Zuo, L. Oxidative Stress in Neurodegenerative Diseases: From Molecular Mechanisms to Clinical Applications. *Oxidative Med. Cell. Longev.* **2017**, *2017*, 2525967. [CrossRef]
22. Imam, S.Z.; Karahalil, B.; Hogue, B.A.; Souza-Pinto, N.C.; Bohr, V.A. Mitochondrial and nuclear DNA-repair capacity of various brain regions in mouse is altered in an age-dependent manner. *Neurobiol. Aging* **2006**, *27*, 1129–1136. [CrossRef]
23. Tian, F.; Tong, T.J.; Zhang, Z.Y.; McNutt, M.A.; Liu, X.W. Age-dependent down-regulation of mitochondrial 8-oxoguanine DNA glycosylase in SAM-P/8 mouse brain and its effect on brain aging. *Rejuvenation Res.* **2009**, *12*, 209–215. [CrossRef]
24. Cui, H.; Kong, Y.; Zhang, H. Oxidative stress, mitochondrial dysfunction, and aging. *J. Signal Transduct.* **2012**, *2012*, 646354. [CrossRef]
25. Mikhed, Y.; Daiber, A.; Steven, S. Mitochondrial Oxidative Stress, Mitochondrial DNA Damage and Their Role in Age-Related Vascular Dysfunction. *Int. J. Mol. Sci.* **2015**, *16*, 15918–15953. [CrossRef]
26. Jiang, Q.; Yin, J.; Chen, J.; Ma, X.; Wu, M.; Liu, G.; Yao, K.; Tan, B.; Yin, Y. Mitochondria-Targeted Antioxidants: A Step towards Disease Treatment. *Oxidative Med. Cell. Longev.* **2020**, *2020*, 8837893. [CrossRef]
27. Fields, M.; Marcuzzi, A.; Gonelli, A.; Celeghini, C.; Maximova, N.; Rimondi, E. Mitochondria-Targeted Antioxidants, an Innovative Class of Antioxidant Compounds for Neurodegenerative Diseases: Perspectives and Limitations. *Int. J. Mol. Sci.* **2023**, *24*, 3739. [CrossRef]
28. Kulkarni, C.A.; Fink, B.D.; Gibbs, B.E.; Chheda, P.R.; Wu, M.; Sivitz, W.I.; Kerns, R.J. A Novel Triphenylphosphonium Carrier to Target Mitochondria without Uncoupling Oxidative Phosphorylation. *J. Med. Chem.* **2021**, *64*, 662–676. [CrossRef]
29. Zinovkin, R.A.; Zamyatnin, A.A. Mitochondria-Targeted Drugs. *Curr. Mol. Pharmacol.* **2019**, *12*, 202–214. [CrossRef]
30. Jauslin, M.L.; Meier, T.; Smith, R.A.; Murphy, M.P. Mitochondria-targeted antioxidants protect Friedreich Ataxia fibroblasts from endogenous oxidative stress more effectively than untargeted antioxidants. *FASEB J.* **2003**, *17*, 1972–1974. [CrossRef]
31. Hu, H.; Li, M. Mitochondria-targeted antioxidant mitotempo protects mitochondrial function against amyloid beta toxicity in primary cultured mouse neurons. *Biochem. Biophys. Res. Commun.* **2016**, *478*, 174–180. [CrossRef]
32. Chen, L.; Deng, H.; Cui, H.; Fang, J.; Zuo, Z.; Deng, J.; Li, Y.; Wang, X.; Zhao, L. Inflammatory responses and inflammation-associated diseases in organs. *Oncotarget* **2018**, *9*, 7204–7218. [CrossRef]
33. Bennett, J.M.; Reeves, G.; Billman, G.E.; Sturmberg, J.P. Inflammation-Nature's Way to Efficiently Respond to All Types of Challenges: Implications for Understanding and Managing "the Epidemic" of Chronic Diseases. *Front. Med.* **2018**, *5*, 316. [CrossRef]
34. Weavers, H.; Martin, P. The cell biology of inflammation: From common traits to remarkable immunological adaptations. *J. Cell Biol.* **2020**, *219*, e202004003. [CrossRef]
35. Serhan, C.N.; Savill, J. Resolution of inflammation: The beginning programs the end. *Nat. Immunol.* **2005**, *6*, 1191–1197. [CrossRef]
36. Furman, D.; Campisi, J.; Verdin, E.; Carrera-Bastos, P.; Targ, S.; Franceschi, C.; Ferrucci, L.; Gilroy, D.W.; Fasano, A.; Miller, G.W.; et al. Chronic inflammation in the etiology of disease across the life span. *Nat. Med.* **2019**, *25*, 1822–1832. [CrossRef]
37. Nelson, P.T.; Soma, L.A.; Lavi, E. Microglia in diseases of the central nervous system. *Ann. Med.* **2002**, *34*, 491–500. [CrossRef]
38. Block, M.L.; Zecca, L.; Hong, J.S. Microglia-mediated neurotoxicity: Uncovering the molecular mechanisms. *Nat. Rev. Neurosci.* **2007**, *8*, 57–69. [CrossRef]
39. Huang, X.; Hussain, B.; Chang, J. Peripheral inflammation and blood-brain barrier disruption: Effects and mechanisms. *CNS Neurosci. Ther.* **2021**, *27*, 36–47. [CrossRef]
40. DiSabato, D.J.; Quan, N.; Godbout, J.P. Neuroinflammation: The devil is in the details. *J. Neurochem.* **2016**, *139* (Suppl. S2), 136–153. [CrossRef]
41. Schafer, D.P.; Stevens, B. Phagocytic glial cells: Sculpting synaptic circuits in the developing nervous system. *Curr. Opin. Neurobiol.* **2013**, *23*, 1034–1040. [CrossRef]

42. Mottahedin, A.; Ardalan, M.; Chumak, T.; Riebe, I.; Ek, J.; Mallard, C. Effect of Neuroinflammation on Synaptic Organization and Function in the Developing Brain: Implications for Neurodevelopmental and Neurodegenerative Disorders. *Front. Cell. Neurosci.* **2017**, *11*, 190. [CrossRef]
43. Geloso, M.C.; D'Ambrosi, N. Microglial Pruning: Relevance for Synaptic Dysfunction in Multiple Sclerosis and Related Experimental Models. *Cells* **2021**, *10*, 686. [CrossRef]
44. Derecki, N.C.; Cardani, A.N.; Yang, C.H.; Quinnies, K.M.; Crihfield, A.; Lynch, K.R.; Kipnis, J. Regulation of learning and memory by meningeal immunity: A key role for IL-4. *J. Exp. Med.* **2010**, *207*, 1067–1080. [CrossRef]
45. Cornell, J.; Salinas, S.; Huang, H.Y.; Zhou, M. Microglia regulation of synaptic plasticity and learning and memory. *Neural. Regen. Res.* **2022**, *17*, 705–716. [CrossRef]
46. Solleiro-Villavicencio, H.; Rivas-Arancibia, S. Effect of Chronic Oxidative Stress on Neuroinflammatory Response Mediated by CD4. *Front. Cell. Neurosci.* **2018**, *12*, 114. [CrossRef]
47. Obrador, E.; Salvador, R.; López-Blanch, R.; Jihad-Jebbar, A.; Vallés, S.L.; Estrela, J.M. Oxidative Stress, Neuroinflammation and Mitochondria in the Pathophysiology of Amyotrophic Lateral Sclerosis. *Antioxidants* **2020**, *9*, 901. [CrossRef]
48. Kumar, A.; Sidhu, J.; Goyal, A.; Tsao, J. *Alzheimer Disease*; StatPearls Publishing: St. Petersburg, FL, USA, 2022; p. 29763097.
49. Swerdlow, R.H.; Burns, J.M.; Khan, S.M. The Alzheimer's disease mitochondrial cascade hypothesis. *J Alzheimers Dis.* **2010**, *20* (Suppl. S2), S265–S279. [CrossRef]
50. Picone, P.; Nuzzo, D.; Caruana, L.; Scafidi, V.; Di Carlo, M. Mitochondrial dysfunction: Different routes to Alzheimer's disease therapy. *Oxidative Med. Cell. Longev.* **2014**, *2014*, 780179. [CrossRef]
51. Tamagno, E.; Guglielmotto, M.; Vasciaveo, V.; Tabaton, M. Oxidative Stress and Beta Amyloid in Alzheimer's Disease. Which Comes First: The Chicken or the Egg? *Antioxidants* **2021**, *10*, 1479. [CrossRef]
52. Tofighi, N.; Asle-Rousta, M.; Rahnema, M.; Amini, R. Protective effect of alpha-linoleic acid on Aβ-induced oxidative stress, neuroinflammation, and memory impairment by alteration of α7 nAChR and NMDAR gene expression in the hippocampus of rats. *Neurotoxicology* **2021**, *85*, 245–253. [CrossRef]
53. Zhao, Y.; Zhao, B. Oxidative stress and the pathogenesis of Alzheimer's disease. *Oxidative Med. Cell. Longev.* **2013**, *2013*, 316523. [CrossRef]
54. Wang, X.; Wang, W.; Li, L.; Perry, G.; Lee, H.G.; Zhu, X. Oxidative stress and mitochondrial dysfunction in Alzheimer's disease. *Biochim. Biophys. Acta* **2014**, *1842*, 1240–1247. [CrossRef]
55. Cuajungco, M.P.; Fagét, K.Y. Zinc takes the center stage: Its paradoxical role in Alzheimer's disease. *Brain Res. Brain Res. Rev.* **2003**, *41*, 44–56. [PubMed]
56. Huang, X.; Moir, R.D.; Tanzi, R.E.; Bush, A.I.; Rogers, J.T. Redox-active metals, oxidative stress, and Alzheimer's disease pathology. *Ann. N. Y. Acad. Sci.* **2004**, *1012*, 153–163. [CrossRef] [PubMed]
57. Bagheri, S.; Squitti, R.; Haertlé, T.; Siotto, M.; Saboury, A.A. Role of Copper in the Onset of Alzheimer's Disease Compared to Other Metals. *Front. Aging Neurosci.* **2017**, *9*, 446. [CrossRef] [PubMed]
58. Cassidy, L.; Fernandez, F.; Johnson, J.B.; Naiker, M.; Owoola, A.G.; Broszczak, D.A. Oxidative stress in alzheimer's disease: A review on emergent natural polyphenolic therapeutics. *Complement. Ther. Med.* **2020**, *49*, 102294. [CrossRef]
59. Shinto, L.; Quinn, J.; Montine, T.; Dodge, H.H.; Woodward, W.; Baldauf-Wagner, S.; Waichunas, D.; Bumgarner, L.; Bourdette, D.; Silbert, L.; et al. A randomized placebo-controlled pilot trial of omega-3 fatty acids and alpha lipoic acid in Alzheimer's disease. *J. Alzheimers Dis.* **2014**, *38*, 111–120. [CrossRef]
60. Canhada, S.; Castro, K.; Perry, I.S.; Luft, V.C. Omega-3 fatty acids' supplementation in Alzheimer's disease: A systematic review. *Nutr. Neurosci.* **2018**, *21*, 529–538. [CrossRef]
61. Ajith, T.A. A Recent Update on the Effects of Omega-3 Fatty Acids in Alzheimer's Disease. *Curr. Clin. Pharmacol.* **2018**, *13*, 252–260. [CrossRef]
62. Kinney, J.W.; Bemiller, S.M.; Murtishaw, A.S.; Leisgang, A.M.; Salazar, A.M.; Lamb, B.T. Inflammation as a central mechanism in Alzheimer's disease. *Alzheimers Dement.* **2018**, *4*, 575–590. [CrossRef]
63. Newcombe, E.A.; Camats-Perna, J.; Silva, M.L.; Valmas, N.; Huat, T.J.; Medeiros, R. Inflammation: The link between comorbidities, genetics, and Alzheimer's disease. *J. Neuroinflamm.* **2018**, *15*, 276. [CrossRef]
64. Xie, J.; Van Hoecke, L.; Vandenbroucke, R.E. The Impact of Systemic Inflammation on Alzheimer's Disease Pathology. *Front. Immunol.* **2021**, *12*, 796867. [CrossRef] [PubMed]
65. Liddelow, S.A.; Guttenplan, K.A.; Clarke, L.E.; Bennett, F.C.; Bohlen, C.J.; Schirmer, L.; Bennett, M.L.; Münch, A.E.; Chung, W.S.; Peterson, T.C.; et al. Neurotoxic reactive astrocytes are induced by activated microglia. *Nature* **2017**, *541*, 481–487. [CrossRef]
66. Emamzadeh, F.N.; Surguchov, A. Parkinson's Disease: Biomarkers, Treatment, and Risk Factors. *Front. Neurosci.* **2018**, *12*, 612. [CrossRef]
67. Venkateshappa, C.; Harish, G.; Mythri, R.B.; Mahadevan, A.; Bharath, M.M.; Shankar, S.K. Increased oxidative damage and decreased antioxidant function in aging human substantia nigra compared to striatum: Implications for Parkinson's disease. *Neurochem. Res.* **2012**, *37*, 358–369. [CrossRef]
68. Kolodkin, A.N.; Sharma, R.P.; Colangelo, A.M.; Ignatenko, A.; Martorana, F.; Jennen, D.; Briedé, J.J.; Brady, N.; Barberis, M.; Mondeel, T.D.G.A.; et al. ROS networks: Designs, aging, Parkinson's disease and precision therapies. *npj Syst. Biol. Appl.* **2020**, *6*, 34. [CrossRef]

69. Trist, B.G.; Hare, D.J.; Double, K.L. Oxidative stress in the aging substantia nigra and the etiology of Parkinson's disease. *Aging Cell* **2019**, *18*, e13031. [CrossRef]
70. Dias, V.; Junn, E.; Mouradian, M.M. The role of oxidative stress in Parkinson's disease. *J. Parkinsons Dis.* **2013**, *3*, 461–491. [CrossRef]
71. Dorszewska, J.; Kowalska, M.; Prendecki, M.; Piekut, T.; Kozłowska, J.; Kozubski, W. Oxidative stress factors in Parkinson's disease. *Neural. Regen. Res.* **2021**, *16*, 1383–1391. [CrossRef]
72. Bjørklund, G.; Peana, M.; Maes, M.; Dadar, M.; Severin, B. The glutathione system in Parkinson's disease and its progression. *Neurosci. Biobehav. Rev.* **2021**, *120*, 470–478. [CrossRef]
73. Samavarchi Tehrani, S.; Sarfi, M.; Yousefi, T.; Ahmadi Ahangar, A.; Gholinia, H.; Mohseni Ahangar, R.; Maniati, M.; Saadat, P. Comparison of the calcium-related factors in Parkinson's disease patients with healthy individuals. *Caspian J. Intern. Med.* **2020**, *11*, 28–33. [CrossRef]
74. Chen, Q.; Chen, Y.; Zhang, Y.; Wang, F.; Yu, H.; Zhang, C.; Jiang, Z.; Luo, W. Iron deposition in Parkinson's disease by quantitative susceptibility mapping. *BMC Neurosci.* **2019**, *20*, 23. [CrossRef] [PubMed]
75. Xicoy, H.; Wieringa, B.; Martens, G.J.M. The Role of Lipids in Parkinson's Disease. *Cells* **2019**, *8*, 27. [CrossRef]
76. Fais, M.; Dore, A.; Galioto, M.; Galleri, G.; Crosio, C.; Iaccarino, C. Parkinson's Disease-Related Genes and Lipid Alteration. *Int. J. Mol. Sci.* **2021**, *22*, 7630. [CrossRef]
77. Filograna, R.; Beltramini, M.; Bubacco, L.; Bisaglia, M. Anti-Oxidants in Parkinson's Disease Therapy: A Critical Point of View. *Curr. Neuropharmacol.* **2016**, *14*, 260–271. [CrossRef] [PubMed]
78. McGeer, P.L.; McGeer, E.G. Glial reactions in Parkinson's disease. *Mov. Disord.* **2008**, *23*, 474–483. [CrossRef]
79. Joe, E.H.; Choi, D.J.; An, J.; Eun, J.H.; Jou, I.; Park, S. Astrocytes, Microglia, and Parkinson's Disease. *Exp. Neurobiol.* **2018**, *27*, 77–87. [CrossRef] [PubMed]
80. Depboylu, C.; Schorlemmer, K.; Klietz, M.; Oertel, W.H.; Weihe, E.; Höglinger, G.U.; Schäfer, M.K. Upregulation of microglial C1q expression has no effects on nigrostriatal dopaminergic injury in the MPTP mouse model of Parkinson disease. *J. Neuroimmunol.* **2011**, *236*, 39–46. [CrossRef]
81. Cho, K. Emerging Roles of Complement Protein C1q in Neurodegeneration. *Aging Dis.* **2019**, *10*, 652–663. [CrossRef]
82. Badanjak, K.; Fixemer, S.; Smajić, S.; Skupin, A.; Grünewald, A. The Contribution of Microglia to Neuroinflammation in Parkinson's Disease. *Int. J. Mol. Sci.* **2021**, *22*, 4676. [CrossRef]
83. Lai, T.T.; Kim, Y.J.; Ma, H.I.; Kim, Y.E. Evidence of Inflammation in Parkinson's Disease and Its Contribution to Synucleinopathy. *J. Mov. Disord.* **2022**, *15*, 1–14. [CrossRef]
84. McColgan, P.; Tabrizi, S.J. Huntington's disease: A clinical review. *Eur. J. Neurol.* **2018**, *25*, 24–34. [CrossRef]
85. Kumar, A.; Ratan, R.R. Oxidative Stress and Huntington's Disease: The Good, The Bad, and The Ugly. *J. Huntingt. Dis.* **2016**, *5*, 217–237. [CrossRef] [PubMed]
86. Lee, J.; Kosaras, B.; Del Signore, S.J.; Cormier, K.; McKee, A.; Ratan, R.R.; Kowall, N.W.; Ryu, H. Modulation of lipid peroxidation and mitochondrial function improves neuropathology in Huntington's disease mice. *Acta Neuropathol.* **2011**, *121*, 487–498. [CrossRef]
87. Peña-Bautista, C.; Vento, M.; Baquero, M.; Cháfer-Pericás, C. Lipid peroxidation in neurodegeneration. *Clin. Chim. Acta* **2019**, *497*, 178–188. [CrossRef] [PubMed]
88. Sorolla, M.A.; Rodríguez-Colman, M.J.; Vall-llaura, N.; Tamarit, J.; Ros, J.; Cabiscol, E. Protein oxidation in Huntington disease. *Biofactors* **2012**, *38*, 173–185. [CrossRef] [PubMed]
89. Maiuri, T.; Suart, C.E.; Hung, C.L.K.; Graham, K.J.; Barba Bazan, C.A.; Truant, R. DNA Damage Repair in Huntington's Disease and Other Neurodegenerative Diseases. *Neurotherapeutics* **2019**, *16*, 948–956. [CrossRef]
90. Askeland, G.; Dosoudilova, Z.; Rodinova, M.; Klempir, J.; Liskova, I.; Kuśnierczyk, A.; Bjørås, M.; Nesse, G.; Klungland, A.; Hansikova, H.; et al. Increased nuclear DNA damage precedes mitochondrial dysfunction in peripheral blood mononuclear cells from Huntington's disease patients. *Sci. Rep.* **2018**, *8*, 9817. [CrossRef]
91. Paul, B.D.; Snyder, S.H. Impaired Redox Signaling in Huntington's Disease: Therapeutic Implications. *Front. Mol. Neurosci.* **2019**, *12*, 68. [CrossRef]
92. Bartzokis, G.; Lu, P.H.; Tishler, T.A.; Fong, S.M.; Oluwadara, B.; Finn, J.P.; Huang, D.; Bordelon, Y.; Mintz, J.; Perlman, S. Myelin breakdown and iron changes in Huntington's disease: Pathogenesis and treatment implications. *Neurochem. Res.* **2007**, *32*, 1655–1664. [CrossRef]
93. Agrawal, S.; Fox, J.; Thyagarajan, B.; Fox, J.H. Brain mitochondrial iron accumulates in Huntington's disease, mediates mitochondrial dysfunction, and can be removed pharmacologically. *Free Radic. Biol. Med.* **2018**, *120*, 317–329. [CrossRef]
94. Pfalzer, A.C.; Yan, Y.; Kang, H.; Totten, M.; Silverman, J.; Bowman, A.B.; Erikson, K.; Claassen, D.O. Alterations in metal homeostasis occur prior to canonical markers in Huntington disease. *Sci. Rep.* **2022**, *12*, 10373. [CrossRef]
95. Johri, A.; Beal, M.F. Antioxidants in Huntington's disease. *Biochim. Biophys. Acta* **2012**, *1822*, 664–674. [CrossRef]
96. Essa, M.M.; Moghadas, M.; Ba-Omar, T.; Walid Qoronfleh, M.; Guillemin, G.J.; Manivasagam, T.; Justin-Thenmozhi, A.; Ray, B.; Bhat, A.; Chidambaram, S.B.; et al. Protective Effects of Antioxidants in Huntington's Disease: An Extensive Review. *Neurotox. Res.* **2019**, *35*, 739–774. [CrossRef]
97. Carmo, C.; Naia, L.; Lopes, C.; Rego, A.C. Mitochondrial Dysfunction in Huntington's Disease. *Adv. Exp. Med. Biol.* **2018**, *1049*, 59–83. [CrossRef] [PubMed]

98. Intihar, T.A.; Martinez, E.A.; Gomez-Pastor, R. Mitochondrial Dysfunction in Huntington's Disease; Interplay between HSF1, p53 and PGC-1α Transcription Factors. *Front. Cell. Neurosci.* **2019**, *13*, 103. [CrossRef] [PubMed]
99. Valadão, P.A.C.; Santos, K.B.S.; Ferreira E Vieira, T.H.; Macedo E Cordeiro, T.; Teixeira, A.L.; Guatimosim, C.; de Miranda, A.S. Inflammation in Huntington's disease: A few new twists on an old tale. *J. Neuroimmunol.* **2020**, *348*, 577380. [CrossRef] [PubMed]
100. Lin, C.L.; Wang, S.E.; Hsu, C.H.; Sheu, S.J.; Wu, C.H. Oral treatment with herbal formula B307 alleviates cardiac failure in aging R6/2 mice with Huntington's disease via suppressing oxidative stress, inflammation, and apoptosis. *Clin. Interv. Aging* **2015**, *10*, 1173–1187. [CrossRef] [PubMed]
101. Sánchez-López, F.; Tasset, I.; Agüera, E.; Feijóo, M.; Fernández-Bolaños, R.; Sánchez, F.M.; Ruiz, M.C.; Cruz, A.H.; Gascón, F.; Túnez, I. Oxidative stress and inflammation biomarkers in the blood of patients with Huntington's disease. *Neurol. Res.* **2012**, *34*, 721–724. [CrossRef]
102. Miller, J.R.; Träger, U.; Andre, R.; Tabrizi, S.J. Mutant Huntingtin Does Not Affect the Intrinsic Phenotype of Human Huntington's Disease T Lymphocytes. *PLoS ONE* **2015**, *10*, e0141793. [CrossRef]
103. Yang, H.M.; Yang, S.; Huang, S.S.; Tang, B.S.; Guo, J.F. Microglial Activation in the Pathogenesis of Huntington's Disease. *Front. Aging Neurosci.* **2017**, *9*, 193. [CrossRef]
104. Fatoba, O.; Ohtake, Y.; Itokazu, T.; Yamashita, T. Immunotherapies in Huntington's disease and α-Synucleinopathies. *Front. Immunol.* **2020**, *11*, 337. [CrossRef]
105. Scarian, E.; Fiamingo, G.; Diamanti, L.; Palmieri, I.; Gagliardi, S.; Pansarasa, O. The Role of VCP Mutations in the Spectrum of Amyotrophic Lateral Sclerosis-Frontotemporal Dementia. *Front. Neurol.* **2022**, *13*, 841394. [CrossRef]
106. Tam, O.H.; Rozhkov, N.V.; Shaw, R.; Kim, D.; Hubbard, I.; Fennessey, S.; Propp, N.; Fagegaltier, D.; Harris, B.T.; Ostrow, L.W.; et al. Postmortem Cortex Samples Identify Distinct Molecular Subtypes of ALS: Retrotransposon Activation, Oxidative Stress, and Activated Glia. *Cell Rep.* **2019**, *29*, 1164–1177.e1165. [CrossRef]
107. Ihara, Y.; Nobukuni, K.; Takata, H.; Hayabara, T. Oxidative stress and metal content in blood and cerebrospinal fluid of amyotrophic lateral sclerosis patients with and without a Cu, Zn-superoxide dismutase mutation. *Neurol. Res.* **2005**, *27*, 105–108. [CrossRef]
108. Calingasan, N.Y.; Chen, J.; Kiaei, M.; Beal, M.F. Beta-amyloid 42 accumulation in the lumbar spinal cord motor neurons of amyotrophic lateral sclerosis patients. *Neurobiol. Dis.* **2005**, *19*, 340–347. [CrossRef]
109. Simpson, E.P.; Henry, Y.K.; Henkel, J.S.; Smith, R.G.; Appel, S.H. Increased lipid peroxidation in sera of ALS patients: A potential biomarker of disease burden. *Neurology* **2004**, *62*, 1758–1765. [CrossRef] [PubMed]
110. D'Amico, E.; Factor-Litvak, P.; Santella, R.M.; Mitsumoto, H. Clinical perspective on oxidative stress in sporadic amyotrophic lateral sclerosis. *Free Radic. Biol. Med.* **2013**, *65*, 509–527. [CrossRef] [PubMed]
111. Pollari, E.; Goldsteins, G.; Bart, G.; Koistinaho, J.; Giniatullin, R. The role of oxidative stress in degeneration of the neuromuscular junction in amyotrophic lateral sclerosis. *Front. Cell Neurosci.* **2014**, *8*, 131. [CrossRef] [PubMed]
112. Motataianu, A.; Serban, G.; Barcutean, L.; Balasa, R. Oxidative Stress in Amyotrophic Lateral Sclerosis: Synergy of Genetic and Environmental Factors. *Int. J. Mol. Sci.* **2022**, *23*, 9339. [CrossRef] [PubMed]
113. Peggion, C.; Scalcon, V.; Massimino, M.L.; Nies, K.; Lopreiato, R.; Rigobello, M.P.; Bertoli, A. SOD1 in ALS: Taking Stock in Pathogenic Mechanisms and the Role of Glial and Muscle Cells. *Antioxidants* **2022**, *11*, 614. [CrossRef] [PubMed]
114. Kaur, S.J.; McKeown, S.R.; Rashid, S. Mutant SOD1 mediated pathogenesis of Amyotrophic Lateral Sclerosis. *Gene* **2016**, *577*, 109–118. [CrossRef] [PubMed]
115. Tak, Y.J.; Park, J.H.; Rhim, H.; Kang, S. ALS-Related Mutant SOD1 Aggregates Interfere with Mitophagy by Sequestering the Autophagy Receptor Optineurin. *Int. J. Mol. Sci.* **2020**, *21*, 7525. [CrossRef] [PubMed]
116. Ferri, A.; Cozzolino, M.; Crosio, C.; Nencini, M.; Casciati, A.; Gralla, E.B.; Rotilio, G.; Valentine, J.S.; Carrì, M.T. Familial ALS-superoxide dismutases associate with mitochondria and shift their redox potentials. *Proc. Natl. Acad. Sci. USA* **2006**, *103*, 13860–13865. [CrossRef] [PubMed]
117. Prasad, A.; Bharathi, V.; Sivalingam, V.; Girdhar, A.; Patel, B.K. Molecular Mechanisms of TDP-43 Misfolding and Pathology in Amyotrophic Lateral Sclerosis. *Front. Mol. Neurosci.* **2019**, *12*, 25. [CrossRef]
118. Zuo, X.; Zhou, J.; Li, Y.; Wu, K.; Chen, Z.; Luo, Z.; Zhang, X.; Liang, Y.; Esteban, M.A.; Zhou, Y.; et al. TDP-43 aggregation induced by oxidative stress causes global mitochondrial imbalance in ALS. *Nat. Struct. Mol. Biol.* **2021**, *28*, 132–142. [CrossRef] [PubMed]
119. Park, S.K.; Park, S.; Liebman, S.W. Respiration Enhances TDP-43 Toxicity, but TDP-43 Retains Some Toxicity in the Absence of Respiration. *J. Mol. Biol.* **2019**, *431*, 2050–2059. [CrossRef]
120. Gautam, M.; Jara, J.H.; Kocak, N.; Rylaarsdam, L.E.; Kim, K.D.; Bigio, E.H.; Hande Özdinler, P. Mitochondria, ER, and nuclear membrane defects reveal early mechanisms for upper motor neuron vulnerability with respect to TDP-43 pathology. *Acta Neuropathol.* **2019**, *137*, 47–69. [CrossRef]
121. Cohen, T.J.; Hwang, A.W.; Unger, T.; Trojanowski, J.Q.; Lee, V.M. Redox signalling directly regulates TDP-43 via cysteine oxidation and disulfide cross-linking. *EMBO J.* **2012**, *31*, 1241–1252. [CrossRef]
122. Cohen, T.J.; Hwang, A.W.; Restrepo, C.R.; Yuan, C.X.; Trojanowski, J.Q.; Lee, V.M. An acetylation switch controls TDP-43 function and aggregation propensity. *Nat. Commun.* **2015**, *6*, 5845. [CrossRef]
123. Tian, Y.P.; Che, F.Y.; Su, Q.P.; Lu, Y.C.; You, C.P.; Huang, L.M.; Wang, S.G.; Wang, L.; Yu, J.X. Effects of mutant TDP-43 on the Nrf2/ARE pathway and protein expression of MafK and JDP2 in NSC-34 cells. *Genet. Mol. Res.* **2017**, *16*, 4238. [CrossRef]

124. Moujalled, D.; Grubman, A.; Acevedo, K.; Yang, S.; Ke, Y.D.; Moujalled, D.M.; Duncan, C.; Caragounis, A.; Perera, N.D.; Turner, B.J.; et al. TDP-43 mutations causing amyotrophic lateral sclerosis are associated with altered expression of RNA-binding protein hnRNP K and affect the Nrf2 antioxidant pathway. *Hum. Mol. Genet.* **2017**, *26*, 1732–1746. [CrossRef]
125. Dewey, C.M.; Cenik, B.; Sephton, C.F.; Dries, D.R.; Mayer, P.; Good, S.K.; Johnson, B.A.; Herz, J.; Yu, G. TDP-43 is directed to stress granules by sorbitol, a novel physiological osmotic and oxidative stressor. *Mol. Cell. Biol.* **2011**, *31*, 1098–1108. [CrossRef]
126. Wang, H.; Guo, W.; Mitra, J.; Hegde, P.M.; Vandoorne, T.; Eckelmann, B.J.; Mitra, S.; Tomkinson, A.E.; Van Den Bosch, L.; Hegde, M.L. Mutant FUS causes DNA ligation defects to inhibit oxidative damage repair in Amyotrophic Lateral Sclerosis. *Nat. Commun.* **2018**, *9*, 3683. [CrossRef] [PubMed]
127. Tsai, Y.L.; Coady, T.H.; Lu, L.; Zheng, D.; Alland, I.; Tian, B.; Shneider, N.A.; Manley, J.L. ALS/FTD-associated protein FUS induces mitochondrial dysfunction by preferentially sequestering respiratory chain complex mRNAs. *Genes Dev.* **2020**, *34*, 785–805. [CrossRef] [PubMed]
128. Brunet, M.A.; Jacques, J.F.; Nassari, S.; Tyzack, G.E.; McGoldrick, P.; Zinman, L.; Jean, S.; Robertson, J.; Patani, R.; Roucou, X. The FUS gene is dual-coding with both proteins contributing to FUS-mediated toxicity. *EMBO Rep.* **2021**, *22*, e50640. [CrossRef] [PubMed]
129. Onesto, E.; Colombrita, C.; Gumina, V.; Borghi, M.O.; Dusi, S.; Doretti, A.; Fagiolari, G.; Invernizzi, F.; Moggio, M.; Tiranti, V.; et al. Gene-specific mitochondria dysfunctions in human TARDBP and C9ORF72 fibroblasts. *Acta Neuropathol. Commun.* **2016**, *4*, 47. [CrossRef]
130. Birger, A.; Ben-Dor, I.; Ottolenghi, M.; Turetsky, T.; Gil, Y.; Sweetat, S.; Perez, L.; Belzer, V.; Casden, N.; Steiner, D.; et al. Human iPSC-derived astrocytes from ALS patients with mutated C9ORF72 show increased oxidative stress and neurotoxicity. *EBioMedicine* **2019**, *50*, 274–289. [CrossRef]
131. Jiménez-Villegas, J.; Kirby, J.; Mata, V.; Cadenas, S.; Turner, M.R.; Malaspina, A.; Shaw, P.J.; Cuadrado, A.; Rojo, A.I. Dipeptide Repeat Pathology in C9orf72-ALS Is Associated with Redox, Mitochondrial and NRF2 Pathway Imbalance. *Antioxidants* **2022**, *11*, 1897. [CrossRef]
132. Ferrante, R.J.; Browne, S.E.; Shinobu, L.A.; Bowling, A.C.; Baik, M.J.; MacGarvey, U.; Kowall, N.W.; Brown, R.H.; Beal, M.F. Evidence of increased oxidative damage in both sporadic and familial amyotrophic lateral sclerosis. *J. Neurochem.* **1997**, *69*, 2064–2074. [CrossRef]
133. Shibata, N.; Nagai, R.; Uchida, K.; Horiuchi, S.; Yamada, S.; Hirano, A.; Kawaguchi, M.; Yamamoto, T.; Sasaki, S.; Kobayashi, M. Morphological evidence for lipid peroxidation and protein glycoxidation in spinal cords from sporadic amyotrophic lateral sclerosis patients. *Brain Res.* **2001**, *917*, 97–104. [CrossRef]
134. Cunha-Oliveira, T.; Montezinho, L.; Mendes, C.; Firuzi, O.; Saso, L.; Oliveira, P.J.; Silva, F.S.G. Oxidative Stress in Amyotrophic Lateral Sclerosis: Pathophysiology and Opportunities for Pharmacological Intervention. *Oxidative Med. Cell. Longev.* **2020**, *2020*, 5021694. [CrossRef]
135. Babu, G.N.; Kumar, A.; Chandra, R.; Puri, S.K.; Singh, R.L.; Kalita, J.; Misra, U.K. Oxidant-antioxidant imbalance in the erythrocytes of sporadic amyotrophic lateral sclerosis patients correlates with the progression of disease. *Neurochem. Int.* **2008**, *52*, 1284–1289. [CrossRef]
136. Kraft, A.D.; Resch, J.M.; Johnson, D.A.; Johnson, J.A. Activation of the Nrf2-ARE pathway in muscle and spinal cord during ALS-like pathology in mice expressing mutant SOD1. *Exp. Neurol.* **2007**, *207*, 107–117. [CrossRef]
137. Vande Velde, C.; McDonald, K.K.; Boukhedimi, Y.; McAlonis-Downes, M.; Lobsiger, C.S.; Bel Hadj, S.; Zandona, A.; Julien, J.P.; Shah, S.B.; Cleveland, D.W. Misfolded SOD1 associated with motor neuron mitochondria alters mitochondrial shape and distribution prior to clinical onset. *PLoS ONE* **2011**, *6*, e22031. [CrossRef]
138. Hosaka, T.; Hiroshi, T.; Akira, T. Biomolecular Modifications Linked to Oxidative Stress in Amyotrophic Lateral Sclerosis: Determining Promising Biomarkers Related to Oxidative Stress. *Processes* **2021**, *9*, 1667. [CrossRef]
139. Walczak, J.; Dębska-Vielhaber, G.; Vielhaber, S.; Szymański, J.; Charzyńska, A.; Duszyński, J.; Szczepanowska, J. Distinction of sporadic and familial forms of ALS based on mitochondrial characteristics. *FASEB J.* **2019**, *33*, 4388–4403. [CrossRef] [PubMed]
140. Anderson, C.J.; Bredvik, K.; Burstein, S.R.; Davis, C.; Meadows, S.M.; Dash, J.; Case, L.; Milner, T.A.; Kawamata, H.; Zuberi, A.; et al. ALS/FTD mutant CHCHD10 mice reveal a tissue-specific toxic gain-of-function and mitochondrial stress response. *Acta Neuropathol.* **2019**, *138*, 103–121. [CrossRef] [PubMed]
141. Shibata, N.; Nagai, R.; Miyata, S.; Jono, T.; Horiuchi, S.; Hirano, A.; Kato, S.; Sasaki, S.; Asayama, K.; Kobayashi, M. Nonoxidative protein glycation is implicated in familial amyotrophic lateral sclerosis with superoxide dismutase-1 mutation. *Acta Neuropathol.* **2000**, *100*, 275–284. [CrossRef] [PubMed]
142. Kim, B.W.; Jeong, Y.E.; Wong, M.; Martin, L.J. DNA damage accumulates and responses are engaged in human ALS brain and spinal motor neurons and DNA repair is activatable in iPSC-derived motor neurons with SOD1 mutations. *Acta Neuropathol. Commun.* **2020**, *8*, 7. [CrossRef] [PubMed]
143. Aguirre, N.; Beal, M.F.; Matson, W.R.; Bogdanov, M.B. Increased oxidative damage to DNA in an animal model of amyotrophic lateral sclerosis. *Free Radic. Res.* **2005**, *39*, 383–388. [CrossRef] [PubMed]
144. Barbosa, L.F.; Cerqueira, F.M.; Macedo, A.F.; Garcia, C.C.; Angeli, J.P.; Schumacher, R.I.; Sogayar, M.C.; Augusto, O.; Carrì, M.T.; Di Mascio, P.; et al. Increased SOD1 association with chromatin, DNA damage, p53 activation, and apoptosis in a cellular model of SOD1-linked ALS. *Biochim. Biophys. Acta* **2010**, *1802*, 462–471. [CrossRef]

145. Manabe, Y.; Warita, H.; Murakami, T.; Shiote, M.; Hayashi, T.; Nagano, I.; Shoji, M.; Abe, K. Early decrease of redox factor-1 in spinal motor neurons of presymptomatic transgenic mice with a mutant SOD1 gene. *Brain Res.* **2001**, *915*, 104–107. [CrossRef] [PubMed]
146. Shaikh, A.Y.; Martin, L.J. DNA base-excision repair enzyme apurinic/apyrimidinic endonuclease/redox factor-1 is increased and competent in the brain and spinal cord of individuals with amyotrophic lateral sclerosis. *Neuromol. Med.* **2002**, *2*, 47–60. [CrossRef]
147. Oliveira, T.T.; Coutinho, L.G.; de Oliveira, L.O.A.; Timoteo, A.R.S.; Farias, G.C.; Agnez-Lima, L.F. APE1/Ref-1 Role in Inflammation and Immune Response. *Front. Immunol.* **2022**, *13*, 793096. [CrossRef]
148. Kikuchi, H.; Furuta, A.; Nishioka, K.; Suzuki, S.O.; Nakabeppu, Y.; Iwaki, T. Impairment of mitochondrial DNA repair enzymes against accumulation of 8-oxo-guanine in the spinal motor neurons of amyotrophic lateral sclerosis. *Acta Neuropathol.* **2002**, *103*, 408–414. [CrossRef] [PubMed]
149. Pegoraro, V.; Merico, A.; Angelini, C. Micro-RNAs in ALS muscle: Differences in gender, age at onset and disease duration. *J. Neurol. Sci.* **2017**, *380*, 58–63. [CrossRef]
150. Li, C.; Wei, Q.; Gu, X.; Chen, Y.; Chen, X.; Cao, B.; Ou, R.; Shang, H. Decreased Glycogenolysis by miR-338-3p Promotes Regional Glycogen Accumulation Within the Spinal Cord of Amyotrophic Lateral Sclerosis Mice. *Front. Mol. Neurosci.* **2019**, *12*, 114. [CrossRef] [PubMed]
151. Rizzuti, M.; Filosa, G.; Melzi, V.; Calandriello, L.; Dioni, L.; Bollati, V.; Bresolin, N.; Comi, G.P.; Barabino, S.; Nizzardo, M.; et al. MicroRNA expression analysis identifies a subset of downregulated miRNAs in ALS motor neuron progenitors. *Sci. Rep.* **2018**, *8*, 10105. [CrossRef]
152. Zhou, F.; Zhang, C.; Guan, Y.; Chen, Y.; Lu, Q.; Jie, L.; Gao, H.; Du, H.; Zhang, H.; Liu, Y.; et al. Screening the expression characteristics of several miRNAs in G93A-SOD1 transgenic mouse: Altered expression of miRNA-124 is associated with astrocyte differentiation by targeting Sox2 and Sox9. *J. Neurochem.* **2018**, *145*, 51–67. [CrossRef]
153. Di Pietro, L.; Baranzini, M.; Berardinelli, M.G.; Lattanzi, W.; Monforte, M.; Tasca, G.; Conte, A.; Logroscino, G.; Michetti, F.; Ricci, E.; et al. Potential therapeutic targets for ALS: MIR206, MIR208b and MIR499 are modulated during disease progression in the skeletal muscle of patients. *Sci. Rep.* **2017**, *7*, 9538. [CrossRef]
154. Koval, E.D.; Shaner, C.; Zhang, P.; du Maine, X.; Fischer, K.; Tay, J.; Chau, B.N.; Wu, G.F.; Miller, T.M. Method for widespread microRNA-155 inhibition prolongs survival in ALS-model mice. *Hum. Mol. Genet.* **2013**, *22*, 4127–4135. [CrossRef]
155. Butovsky, O.; Jedrychowski, M.P.; Cialic, R.; Krasemann, S.; Murugaiyan, G.; Fanek, Z.; Greco, D.J.; Wu, P.M.; Doykan, C.E.; Kiner, O.; et al. Targeting miR-155 restores abnormal microglia and attenuates disease in SOD1 mice. *Ann. Neurol.* **2015**, *77*, 75–99. [CrossRef] [PubMed]
156. Vucic, S.; Kiernan, M.C. Cortical excitability testing distinguishes Kennedy's disease from amyotrophic lateral sclerosis. *Clin. Neurophysiol.* **2008**, *119*, 1088–1096. [CrossRef] [PubMed]
157. Bae, J.S.; Simon, N.G.; Menon, P.; Vucic, S.; Kiernan, M.C. The puzzling case of hyperexcitability in amyotrophic lateral sclerosis. *J. Clin. Neurol.* **2013**, *9*, 65–74. [CrossRef] [PubMed]
158. Shibuya, K.; Otani, R.; Suzuki, Y.I.; Kuwabara, S.; Kiernan, M.C. Neuronal Hyperexcitability and Free Radical Toxicity in Amyotrophic Lateral Sclerosis: Established and Future Targets. *Pharmaceuticals* **2022**, *15*, 433. [CrossRef] [PubMed]
159. Stringer, R.N.; Weiss, N. Pathophysiology of ion channels in amyotrophic lateral sclerosis. *Mol. Brain* **2023**, *16*, 82. [CrossRef] [PubMed]
160. Kaiser, M.; Maletzki, I.; Hülsmann, S.; Holtmann, B.; Schulz-Schaeffer, W.; Kirchhoff, F.; Bähr, M.; Neusch, C. Progressive loss of a glial potassium channel (KCNJ10) in the spinal cord of the SOD1 (G93A) transgenic mouse model of amyotrophic lateral sclerosis. *J. Neurochem.* **2006**, *99*, 900–912. [CrossRef] [PubMed]
161. Tarantino, N.; Canfora, I.; Camerino, G.M.; Pierno, S. Therapeutic Targets in Amyotrophic Lateral Sclerosis: Focus on Ion Channels and Skeletal Muscle. *Cells* **2022**, *11*, 415. [CrossRef]
162. Camerino, G.M.; Fonzino, A.; Conte, E.; De Bellis, M.; Mele, A.; Liantonio, A.; Tricarico, D.; Tarantino, N.; Dobrowolny, G.; Musarò, A.; et al. Elucidating the Contribution of Skeletal Muscle Ion Channels to Amyotrophic Lateral Sclerosis in search of new therapeutic options. *Sci. Rep.* **2019**, *9*, 3185. [CrossRef]
163. Jaiswal, M.K. Calcium, mitochondria, and the pathogenesis of ALS: The good, the bad, and the ugly. *Front. Cell. Neurosci.* **2013**, *7*, 199. [CrossRef]
164. Anzilotti, S.; Brancaccio, P.; Simeone, G.; Valsecchi, V.; Vinciguerra, A.; Secondo, A.; Petrozziello, T.; Guida, N.; Sirabella, R.; Cuomo, O.; et al. Preconditioning, induced by sub-toxic dose of the neurotoxin L-BMAA, delays ALS progression in mice and prevents Na^+/Ca^{2+} exchanger 3 downregulation. *Cell Death Dis.* **2018**, *9*, 206. [CrossRef]
165. Liu, J.; Wang, F. Role of Neuroinflammation in Amyotrophic Lateral Sclerosis: Cellular Mechanisms and Therapeutic Implications. *Front. Immunol.* **2017**, *8*, 1005. [CrossRef]
166. Corcia, P.; Tauber, C.; Vercoullie, J.; Arlicot, N.; Prunier, C.; Praline, J.; Nicolas, G.; Venel, Y.; Hommet, C.; Baulieu, J.L.; et al. Molecular imaging of microglial activation in amyotrophic lateral sclerosis. *PLoS ONE* **2012**, *7*, e52941. [CrossRef]
167. Turner, M.R.; Cagnin, A.; Turkheimer, F.E.; Miller, C.C.; Shaw, C.E.; Brooks, D.J.; Leigh, P.N.; Banati, R.B. Evidence of widespread cerebral microglial activation in amyotrophic lateral sclerosis: An [^{11}C](R)-PK11195 positron emission tomography study. *Neurobiol. Dis.* **2004**, *15*, 601–609. [CrossRef]

168. Boillée, S.; Yamanaka, K.; Lobsiger, C.S.; Copeland, N.G.; Jenkins, N.A.; Kassiotis, G.; Kollias, G.; Cleveland, D.W. Onset and progression in inherited ALS determined by motor neurons and microglia. *Science* **2006**, *312*, 1389–1392. [CrossRef] [PubMed]
169. O'Rourke, J.G.; Bogdanik, L.; Yáñez, A.; Lall, D.; Wolf, A.J.; Muhammad, A.K.; Ho, R.; Carmona, S.; Vit, J.P.; Zarrow, J.; et al. C9orf72 is required for proper macrophage and microglial function in mice. *Science* **2016**, *351*, 1324–1329. [CrossRef] [PubMed]
170. Atanasio, A.; Decman, V.; White, D.; Ramos, M.; Ikiz, B.; Lee, H.C.; Siao, C.J.; Brydges, S.; LaRosa, E.; Bai, Y.; et al. C9orf72 ablation causes immune dysregulation characterized by leukocyte expansion, autoantibody production, and glomerulonephropathy in mice. *Sci. Rep.* **2016**, *6*, 23204. [CrossRef] [PubMed]
171. Sullivan, P.M.; Zhou, X.; Robins, A.M.; Paushter, D.H.; Kim, D.; Smolka, M.B.; Hu, F. The ALS/FTLD associated protein C9orf72 associates with SMCR8 and WDR41 to regulate the autophagy-lysosome pathway. *Acta Neuropathol. Commun.* **2016**, *4*, 51. [CrossRef] [PubMed]
172. Yiangou, Y.; Facer, P.; Durrenberger, P.; Chessell, I.P.; Naylor, A.; Bountra, C.; Banati, R.R.; Anand, P. COX-2, CB_2 and P2X7-immunoreactivities are increased in activated microglial cells/macrophages of multiple sclerosis and amyotrophic lateral sclerosis spinal cord. *BMC Neurol.* **2006**, *6*, 12. [CrossRef] [PubMed]
173. D'Ambrosi, N.; Finocchi, P.; Apolloni, S.; Cozzolino, M.; Ferri, A.; Padovano, V.; Pietrini, G.; Carrì, M.T.; Volonté, C. The proinflammatory action of microglial P2 receptors is enhanced in SOD1 models for amyotrophic lateral sclerosis. *J. Immunol.* **2009**, *183*, 4648–4656. [CrossRef] [PubMed]
174. Apolloni, S.; Parisi, C.; Pesaresi, M.G.; Rossi, S.; Carrì, M.T.; Cozzolino, M.; Volonté, C.; D'Ambrosi, N. The NADPH oxidase pathway is dysregulated by the P2X7 receptor in the SOD1-G93A microglia model of amyotrophic lateral sclerosis. *J. Immunol.* **2013**, *190*, 5187–5195. [CrossRef]
175. Apolloni, S.; Amadio, S.; Parisi, C.; Matteucci, A.; Potenza, R.L.; Armida, M.; Popoli, P.; D'Ambrosi, N.; Volonté, C. Spinal cord pathology is ameliorated by P2X7 antagonism in a SOD1-mutant mouse model of amyotrophic lateral sclerosis. *Dis. Model Mech.* **2014**, *7*, 1101–1109. [CrossRef]
176. Blasco, H.; Corcia, P.; Pradat, P.F.; Bocca, C.; Gordon, P.H.; Veyrat-Durebex, C.; Mavel, S.; Nadal-Desbarats, L.; Moreau, C.; Devos, D.; et al. Metabolomics in cerebrospinal fluid of patients with amyotrophic lateral sclerosis: An untargeted approach via high-resolution mass spectrometry. *J. Proteome Res.* **2013**, *12*, 3746–3754. [CrossRef]
177. Liao, B.; Zhao, W.; Beers, D.R.; Henkel, J.S.; Appel, S.H. Transformation from a neuroprotective to a neurotoxic microglial phenotype in a mouse model of ALS. *Exp. Neurol.* **2012**, *237*, 147–152. [CrossRef] [PubMed]
178. Moreno-Martinez, L.; Calvo, A.C.; Muñoz, M.J.; Osta, R. Are Circulating Cytokines Reliable Biomarkers for Amyotrophic Lateral Sclerosis? *Int. J. Mol. Sci.* **2019**, *20*, 2759. [CrossRef] [PubMed]
179. Tortelli, R.; Zecca, C.; Piccininni, M.; Benmahemed, S.; Dell'Abate, M.T.; Barulli, M.R.; Capozzo, R.; Battista, P.; Logroscino, G. Plasma Inflammatory Cytokines Are Elevated in ALS. *Front. Neurol.* **2020**, *11*, 552295. [CrossRef] [PubMed]
180. Lu, C.H.; Allen, K.; Oei, F.; Leoni, E.; Kuhle, J.; Tree, T.; Fratta, P.; Sharma, N.; Sidle, K.; Howard, R.; et al. Systemic inflammatory response and neuromuscular involvement in amyotrophic lateral sclerosis. *Neurol. Neuroimmunol. Neuroinflamm.* **2016**, *3*, e244. [CrossRef] [PubMed]
181. Alshikho, M.J.; Zürcher, N.R.; Loggia, M.L.; Cernasov, P.; Reynolds, B.; Pijanowski, O.; Chonde, D.B.; Izquierdo Garcia, D.; Mainero, C.; Catana, C.; et al. Integrated magnetic resonance imaging and [^{11}C]-PBR28 positron emission tomographic imaging in amyotrophic lateral sclerosis. *Ann. Neurol.* **2018**, *83*, 1186–1197. [CrossRef] [PubMed]
182. Nagai, M.; Re, D.B.; Nagata, T.; Chalazonitis, A.; Jessell, T.M.; Wichterle, H.; Przedborski, S. Astrocytes expressing ALS-linked mutated SOD1 release factors selectively toxic to motor neurons. *Nat. Neurosci.* **2007**, *10*, 615–622. [CrossRef] [PubMed]
183. Di Giorgio, F.P.; Carrasco, M.A.; Siao, M.C.; Maniatis, T.; Eggan, K. Non-cell autonomous effect of glia on motor neurons in an embryonic stem cell-based ALS model. *Nat. Neurosci.* **2007**, *10*, 608–614. [CrossRef] [PubMed]
184. Papadeas, S.T.; Kraig, S.E.; O'Banion, C.; Lepore, A.C.; Maragakis, N.J. Astrocytes carrying the superoxide dismutase 1 (SOD1^{G93A}) mutation induce wild-type motor neuron degeneration in vivo. *Proc. Natl. Acad. Sci. USA* **2011**, *108*, 17803–17808. [CrossRef] [PubMed]
185. Qian, K.; Huang, H.; Peterson, A.; Hu, B.; Maragakis, N.J.; Ming, G.L.; Chen, H.; Zhang, S.C. Sporadic ALS Astrocytes Induce Neuronal Degeneration In Vivo. *Stem Cell Rep.* **2017**, *8*, 843–855. [CrossRef] [PubMed]
186. Howland, D.S.; Liu, J.; She, Y.; Goad, B.; Maragakis, N.J.; Kim, B.; Erickson, J.; Kulik, J.; DeVito, L.; Psaltis, G.; et al. Focal loss of the glutamate transporter EAAT2 in a transgenic rat model of SOD1 mutant-mediated amyotrophic lateral sclerosis (ALS). *Proc. Natl. Acad. Sci. USA* **2002**, *99*, 1604–1609. [CrossRef] [PubMed]
187. Pardo, A.C.; Wong, V.; Benson, L.M.; Dykes, M.; Tanaka, K.; Rothstein, J.D.; Maragakis, N.J. Loss of the astrocyte glutamate transporter GLT1 modifies disease in SOD1^{G93A} mice. *Exp. Neurol.* **2006**, *201*, 120–130. [CrossRef] [PubMed]
188. Hensley, K.; Abdel-Moaty, H.; Hunter, J.; Mhatre, M.; Mou, S.; Nguyen, K.; Potapova, T.; Pye, Q.N.; Qi, M.; Rice, H.; et al. Primary glia expressing the G93A-SOD1 mutation present a neuroinflammatory phenotype and provide a cellular system for studies of glial inflammation. *J. Neuroinflamm.* **2006**, *3*, 2. [CrossRef]
189. Marchetto, M.C.; Muotri, A.R.; Mu, Y.; Smith, A.M.; Cezar, G.G.; Gage, F.H. Non-cell-autonomous effect of human SOD1 G37R astrocytes on motor neurons derived from human embryonic stem cells. *Cell Stem Cell* **2008**, *3*, 649–657. [CrossRef]
190. Re, D.B.; Le Verche, V.; Yu, C.; Amoroso, M.W.; Politi, K.A.; Phani, S.; Ikiz, B.; Hoffmann, L.; Koolen, M.; Nagata, T.; et al. Necroptosis drives motor neuron death in models of both sporadic and familial ALS. *Neuron* **2014**, *81*, 1001–1008. [CrossRef]

191. Ito, Y.; Ofengeim, D.; Najafov, A.; Das, S.; Saberi, S.; Li, Y.; Hitomi, J.; Zhu, H.; Chen, H.; Mayo, L.; et al. RIPK1 mediates axonal degeneration by promoting inflammation and necroptosis in ALS. *Science* **2016**, *353*, 603–608. [CrossRef]
192. Bowerman, M.; Vincent, T.; Scamps, F.; Perrin, F.E.; Camu, W.; Raoul, C. Neuroimmunity dynamics and the development of therapeutic strategies for amyotrophic lateral sclerosis. *Front. Cell. Neurosci.* **2013**, *7*, 214. [CrossRef] [PubMed]
193. Beers, D.R.; Zhao, W.; Wang, J.; Zhang, X.; Wen, S.; Neal, D.; Thonhoff, J.R.; Alsuliman, A.S.; Shpall, E.J.; Rezvani, K.; et al. ALS patients' regulatory T lymphocytes are dysfunctional, and correlate with disease progression rate and severity. *JCI Insight* **2017**, *2*, e89530. [CrossRef] [PubMed]
194. Zondler, L.; Müller, K.; Khalaji, S.; Bliederhäuser, C.; Ruf, W.P.; Grozdanov, V.; Thiemann, M.; Fundel-Clemes, K.; Freischmidt, A.; Holzmann, K.; et al. Peripheral monocytes are functionally altered and invade the CNS in ALS patients. *Acta Neuropathol.* **2016**, *132*, 391–411. [CrossRef]
195. Murdock, B.J.; Bender, D.E.; Kashlan, S.R.; Figueroa-Romero, C.; Backus, C.; Callaghan, B.C.; Goutman, S.A.; Feldman, E.L. Increased ratio of circulating neutrophils to monocytes in amyotrophic lateral sclerosis. *Neurol Neuroimmunol. Neuroinflamm.* **2016**, *3*, e242. [CrossRef]
196. Van Dyke, J.M.; Smit-Oistad, I.M.; Macrander, C.; Krakora, D.; Meyer, M.G.; Suzuki, M. Macrophage-mediated inflammation and glial response in the skeletal muscle of a rat model of familial amyotrophic lateral sclerosis (ALS). *Exp. Neurol.* **2016**, *277*, 275–282. [CrossRef]
197. Du, Y.; Zhao, W.; Thonhoff, J.R.; Wang, J.; Wen, S.; Appel, S.H. Increased activation ability of monocytes from ALS patients. *Exp. Neurol.* **2020**, *328*, 113259. [CrossRef] [PubMed]
198. Chiot, A.; Zaïdi, S.; Iltis, C.; Ribon, M.; Berriat, F.; Schiaffino, L.; Jolly, A.; de la Grange, P.; Mallat, M.; Bohl, D.; et al. Modifying macrophages at the periphery has the capacity to change microglial reactivity and to extend ALS survival. *Nat. Neurosci.* **2020**, *23*, 1339–1351. [CrossRef] [PubMed]
199. Nagase, M.; Yamamoto, Y.; Miyazaki, Y.; Yoshino, H. Increased oxidative stress in patients with amyotrophic lateral sclerosis and the effect of edaravone administration. *Redox Rep.* **2016**, *21*, 104–112. [CrossRef] [PubMed]
200. Cha, S.J.; Kim, K. Effects of the Edaravone, a Drug Approved for the Treatment of Amyotrophic Lateral Sclerosis, on Mitochondrial Function and Neuroprotection. *Antioxidants* **2022**, *11*, 195. [CrossRef] [PubMed]
201. Ohta, Y.; Yamashita, T.; Nomura, E.; Hishikawa, N.; Ikegami, K.; Osakada, Y.; Matsumoto, N.; Kawahara, Y.; Yunoki, T.; Takahashi, Y.; et al. Improvement of a decreased anti-oxidative activity by edaravone in amyotrophic lateral sclerosis patients. *J. Neurol. Sci.* **2020**, *415*, 116906. [CrossRef] [PubMed]
202. Noh, K.M.; Hwang, J.Y.; Shin, H.C.; Koh, J.Y. A novel neuroprotective mechanism of riluzole: Direct inhibition of protein kinase C. *Neurobiol. Dis.* **2000**, *7*, 375–383. [CrossRef] [PubMed]
203. Sala, G.; Arosio, A.; Conti, E.; Beretta, S.; Lunetta, C.; Riva, N.; Ferrarese, C.; Tremolizzo, L. Riluzole Selective Antioxidant Effects in Cell Models Expressing Amyotrophic Lateral Sclerosis Endophenotypes. *Clin. Psychopharmacol. Neurosci.* **2019**, *17*, 438–442. [CrossRef] [PubMed]
204. Tarozzi, A.; Angeloni, C.; Malaguti, M.; Morroni, F.; Hrelia, S.; Hrelia, P. Sulforaphane as a potential protective phytochemical against neurodegenerative diseases. *Oxidative Med. Cell. Longev.* **2013**, *2013*, 415078. [CrossRef]
205. Santín-Márquez, R.; Alarcón-Aguilar, A.; López-Diazguerrero, N.E.; Chondrogianni, N.; Königsberg, M. Sulforaphane—Role in aging and neurodegeneration. *Geroscience* **2019**, *41*, 655–670. [CrossRef]
206. Jo, C.; Kim, S.; Cho, S.J.; Choi, K.J.; Yun, S.M.; Koh, Y.H.; Johnson, G.V.; Park, S.I. Sulforaphane induces autophagy through ERK activation in neuronal cells. *FEBS Lett.* **2014**, *588*, 3081–3088. [CrossRef]
207. Socała, K.; Nieoczym, D.; Kowalczuk-Vasilev, E.; Wyska, E.; Wlaź, P. Increased seizure susceptibility and other toxicity symptoms following acute sulforaphane treatment in mice. *Toxicol. Appl. Pharmacol.* **2017**, *326*, 43–53. [CrossRef]
208. Ziros, P.G.; Habeos, I.G.; Chartoumpekis, D.V.; Ntalampyra, E.; Somm, E.; Renaud, C.O.; Bongiovanni, M.; Trougakos, I.P.; Yamamoto, M.; Kensler, T.W.; et al. NFE2-Related Transcription Factor 2 Coordinates Antioxidant Defense with Thyroglobulin Production and Iodination in the Thyroid Gland. *Thyroid* **2018**, *28*, 780–798. [CrossRef] [PubMed]
209. Williams, J.R.; Trias, E.; Beilby, P.R.; Lopez, N.I.; Labut, E.M.; Bradford, C.S.; Roberts, B.R.; McAllum, E.J.; Crouch, P.J.; Rhoads, T.W.; et al. Copper delivery to the CNS by CuATSM effectively treats motor neuron disease in SOD^{G93A} mice co-expressing the Copper-Chaperone-for-SOD. *Neurobiol. Dis.* **2016**, *89*, 1–9. [CrossRef] [PubMed]
210. Lum, J.S.; Brown, M.L.; Farrawell, N.E.; McAlary, L.; Ly, D.; Chisholm, C.G.; Snow, J.; Vine, K.L.; Karl, T.; Kreilaus, F.; et al. CuATSM improves motor function and extends survival but is not tolerated at a high dose in SOD1. *Sci. Rep.* **2021**, *11*, 19392. [CrossRef]
211. Miquel, E.; Cassina, A.; Martínez-Palma, L.; Souza, J.M.; Bolatto, C.; Rodríguez-Bottero, S.; Logan, A.; Smith, R.A.; Murphy, M.P.; Barbeito, L.; et al. Neuroprotective effects of the mitochondria-targeted antioxidant MitoQ in a model of inherited amyotrophic lateral sclerosis. *Free Radic. Biol. Med.* **2014**, *70*, 204–213. [CrossRef] [PubMed]
212. East, D.A.; Fagiani, F.; Crosby, J.; Georgakopoulos, N.D.; Bertrand, H.; Schaap, M.; Fowkes, A.; Wells, G.; Campanella, M. PMI: A $\Delta\Psi m$ independent pharmacological regulator of mitophagy. *Chem. Biol.* **2014**, *21*, 1585–1596. [CrossRef] [PubMed]
213. Deng, Z.; Lim, J.; Wang, Q.; Purtell, K.; Wu, S.; Palomo, G.M.; Tan, H.; Manfredi, G.; Zhao, Y.; Peng, J.; et al. ALS-FTLD-linked mutations of SQSTM1/p62 disrupt selective autophagy and NFE2L2/NRF2 anti-oxidative stress pathway. *Autophagy* **2020**, *16*, 917–931. [CrossRef]

214. Said Ahmed, M.; Hung, W.Y.; Zu, J.S.; Hockberger, P.; Siddique, T. Increased reactive oxygen species in familial amyotrophic lateral sclerosis with mutations in SOD1. *J. Neurol. Sci.* **2000**, *176*, 88–94. [CrossRef]
215. Andres, S.; Pevny, S.; Ziegenhagen, R.; Bakhiya, N.; Schäfer, B.; Hirsch-Ernst, K.I.; Lampen, A. Safety Aspects of the Use of Quercetin as a Dietary Supplement. *Mol. Nutr. Food Res.* **2018**, *62*, 1700447. [CrossRef]
216. Moreno-Martet, M.; Espejo-Porras, F.; Fernández-Ruiz, J.; de Lago, E. Changes in endocannabinoid receptors and enzymes in the spinal cord of SOD1^{G93A} transgenic mice and evaluation of a Sativex®-like combination of phytocannabinoids: Interest for future therapies in amyotrophic lateral sclerosis. *CNS Neurosci. Ther.* **2014**, *20*, 809–815. [CrossRef]
217. Espejo-Porras, F.; García-Toscano, L.; Rodríguez-Cueto, C.; Santos-García, I.; de Lago, E.; Fernandez-Ruiz, J. Targeting glial cannabinoid CB$_2$ receptors to delay the progression of the pathological phenotype in TDP-43 (A315T) transgenic mice, a model of amyotrophic lateral sclerosis. *Br. J. Pharmacol.* **2019**, *176*, 1585–1600. [CrossRef] [PubMed]
218. Rodríguez-Cueto, C.; García-Toscano, L.; Santos-García, I.; Gómez-Almería, M.; Gonzalo-Consuegra, C.; Espejo-Porras, F.; Fernández-Ruiz, J.; de Lago, E. Targeting the CB$_2$ receptor and other endocannabinoid elements to delay disease progression in amyotrophic lateral sclerosis. *Br. J. Pharmacol.* **2021**, *178*, 1373–1387. [CrossRef] [PubMed]
219. Harraz, M.M.; Marden, J.J.; Zhou, W.; Zhang, Y.; Williams, A.; Sharov, V.S.; Nelson, K.; Luo, M.; Paulson, H.; Schöneich, C.; et al. SOD1 mutations disrupt redox-sensitive Rac regulation of NADPH oxidase in a familial ALS model. *J. Clin. Investig.* **2008**, *118*, 659–670. [CrossRef] [PubMed]
220. Seredenina, T.; Nayernia, Z.; Sorce, S.; Maghzal, G.J.; Filippova, A.; Ling, S.C.; Basset, O.; Plastre, O.; Daali, Y.; Rushing, E.J.; et al. Evaluation of NADPH oxidases as drug targets in a mouse model of familial amyotrophic lateral sclerosis. *Free Radic. Biol. Med.* **2016**, *97*, 95–108. [CrossRef]
221. Van Den Bosch, L.; Tilkin, P.; Lemmens, G.; Robberecht, W. Minocycline delays disease onset and mortality in a transgenic model of ALS. *Neuroreport* **2002**, *13*, 1067–1070. [CrossRef]
222. Yong, V.W.; Wells, J.; Giuliani, F.; Casha, S.; Power, C.; Metz, L.M. The promise of minocycline in neurology. *Lancet Neurol.* **2004**, *3*, 744–751. [CrossRef]
223. Gordon, P.H.; Moore, D.H.; Miller, R.G.; Florence, J.M.; Verheijde, J.L.; Doorish, C.; Hilton, J.F.; Spitalny, G.M.; MacArthur, R.B.; Mitsumoto, H.; et al. Efficacy of minocycline in patients with amyotrophic lateral sclerosis: A phase III randomised trial. *Lancet Neurol.* **2007**, *6*, 1045–1053. [CrossRef]
224. Miller, R.G.; Block, G.; Katz, J.S.; Barohn, R.J.; Gopalakrishnan, V.; Cudkowicz, M.; Zhang, J.R.; McGrath, M.S.; Ludington, E.; Appel, S.H.; et al. Randomized phase 2 trial of NP001-a novel immune regulator: Safety and early efficacy in ALS. *Neurol. Neuroinmunol. Neuroinflamm.* **2015**, *2*, e100. [CrossRef]
225. Miller, R.G.; Zhang, R.; Bracci, P.M.; Azhir, A.; Barohn, R.; Bedlack, R.; Benatar, M.; Berry, J.D.; Cudkowicz, M.; Kasarskis, E.J.; et al. Phase 2B randomized controlled trial of NP001 in amyotrophic lateral sclerosis: Pre-specified and post hoc analyses. *Muscle Nerve* **2022**, *66*, 39–49. [CrossRef]
226. Trias, E.; Ibarburu, S.; Barreto-Núñez, R.; Babdor, J.; Maciel, T.T.; Guillo, M.; Gros, L.; Dubreuil, P.; Díaz-Amarilla, P.; Cassina, P.; et al. Post-paralysis tyrosine kinase inhibition with masitinib abrogates neuroinflammation and slows disease progression in inherited amyotrophic lateral sclerosis. *J. Neuroinflamm.* **2016**, *13*, 177. [CrossRef]
227. Mora, J.S.; Genge, A.; Chio, A.; Estol, C.J.; Chaverri, D.; Hernández, M.; Marín, S.; Mascias, J.; Rodriguez, G.E.; Povedano, M.; et al. Masitinib as an add-on therapy to riluzole in patients with amyotrophic lateral sclerosis: A randomized clinical trial. *Amyotroph. Lateral Scler. Front. Degener.* **2020**, *21*, 5–14. [CrossRef] [PubMed]
228. Mora, J.S.; Bradley, W.G.; Chaverri, D.; Hernández-Barral, M.; Mascias, J.; Gamez, J.; Gargiulo-Monachelli, G.M.; Moussy, A.; Mansfield, C.D.; Hermine, O.; et al. Long-term survival analysis of masitinib in amyotrophic lateral sclerosis. *Ther. Adv. Neurol. Disord.* **2021**, *14*, 17562864211030365. [CrossRef]
229. Potenza, R.L.; De Simone, R.; Armida, M.; Mazziotti, V.; Pèzzola, A.; Popoli, P.; Minghetti, L. Fingolimod: A Disease-Modifier Drug in a Mouse Model of Amyotrophic Lateral Sclerosis. *Neurotherapeutics* **2016**, *13*, 918–927. [CrossRef]
230. Berry, J.D.; Paganoni, S.; Atassi, N.; Macklin, E.A.; Goyal, N.; Rivner, M.; Simpson, E.; Appel, S.; Grasso, D.L.; Mejia, N.I.; et al. Phase IIa trial of fingolimod for amyotrophic lateral sclerosis demonstrates acceptable acute safety and tolerability. *Muscle Nerve* **2017**, *56*, 1077–1084. [CrossRef] [PubMed]
231. Adamczyk, B.; Koziarska, D.; Kasperczyk, S.; Adamczyk-Sowa, M. Are antioxidant parameters in serum altered in patients with relapsing-remitting multiple sclerosis treated with II-line immunomodulatory therapy? *Free Radic. Res.* **2018**, *52*, 1083–1093. [CrossRef] [PubMed]
232. Adamczyk, B.; Wawrzyniak, S.; Kasperczyk, S.; Adamczyk-Sowa, M. The Evaluation of Oxidative Stress Parameters in Serum Patients with Relapsing-Remitting Multiple Sclerosis Treated with II-Line Immunomodulatory Therapy. *Oxidative Med. Cell. Longev.* **2017**, *2017*, 9625806. [CrossRef]
233. Yevgi, R.; Demir, R. Oxidative stress activity of fingolimod in multiple sclerosis. *Clin. Neurol. Neurosurg.* **2021**, *202*, 106500. [CrossRef]
234. Paganoni, S.; Alshikho, M.J.; Luppino, S.; Chan, J.; Pothier, L.; Schoenfeld, D.; Andres, P.L.; Babu, S.; Zürcher, N.R.; Loggia, M.L.; et al. A pilot trial of RNS60 in amyotrophic lateral sclerosis. *Muscle Nerve* **2019**, *59*, 303–308. [CrossRef]
235. Camu, W.; Mickunas, M.; Veyrune, J.L.; Payan, C.; Garlanda, C.; Locati, M.; Juntas-Morales, R.; Pageot, N.; Malaspina, A.; Andreasson, U.; et al. Repeated 5-day cycles of low dose aldesleukin in amyotrophic lateral sclerosis (IMODALS): A phase 2a randomised, double-blind, placebo-controlled trial. *EBioMedicine* **2020**, *59*, 102844. [CrossRef]

236. Czarzasta, J.; Habich, A.; Siwek, T.; Czapliński, A.; Maksymowicz, W.; Wojtkiewicz, J. Stem cells for ALS: An overview of possible therapeutic approaches. *Int. J. Dev. Neurosci.* **2017**, *57*, 46–55. [CrossRef]
237. Glass, J.D.; Hertzberg, V.S.; Boulis, N.M.; Riley, J.; Federici, T.; Polak, M.; Bordeau, J.; Fournier, C.; Johe, K.; Hazel, T.; et al. Transplantation of spinal cord-derived neural stem cells for ALS: Analysis of phase 1 and 2 trials. *Neurology* **2016**, *87*, 392–400. [CrossRef] [PubMed]
238. Moreau, C.; Brunaud-Danel, V.; Dallongeville, J.; Duhamel, A.; Laurier-Grymonprez, L.; de Reuck, J.; Wiart, A.C.; Perez, T.; Richard, F.; Amouyel, P.; et al. Modifying effect of arterial hypertension on amyotrophic lateral sclerosis. *Amyotroph. Lateral Scler.* **2012**, *13*, 194–201. [CrossRef]
239. Lian, L.; Liu, M.; Cui, L.; Guan, Y.; Liu, T.; Cui, B.; Zhang, K.; Tai, H.; Shen, D. Environmental risk factors and amyotrophic lateral sclerosis (ALS): A case-control study of ALS in China. *J. Clin. Neurosci.* **2019**, *66*, 12–18. [CrossRef] [PubMed]
240. Hu, N.; Ji, H. Medications on hypertension, hyperlipidemia, diabetes, and risk of amyotrophic lateral sclerosis: A systematic review and meta-analysis. *Neurol. Sci.* **2022**, *43*, 5189–5199. [CrossRef] [PubMed]
241. Wen, H.; Gwathmey, J.K.; Xie, L.H. Oxidative stress-mediated effects of angiotensin II in the cardiovascular system. *World J. Hypertens.* **2012**, *23*, 34–44. [CrossRef]
242. Pfeiffer, R.M.; Mayer, B.; Kuncl, R.W.; Check, D.P.; Cahoon, E.K.; Rivera, D.R.; Freedman, D.M. Identifying potential targets for prevention and treatment of amyotrophic lateral sclerosis based on a screen of medicare prescription drugs. *Amyotroph. Lateral Scler. Front. Degener.* **2020**, *21*, 235–245. [CrossRef]
243. De Morais, S.D.B.; Shanks, J.; Zucker, I.H. Integrative Physiological Aspects of Brain RAS in Hypertension. *Curr. Hypertens. Rep.* **2018**, *20*, 10. [CrossRef]
244. Abiodun, O.A.; Ola, M.S. Role of brain renin angiotensin system in neurodegeneration: An update. *Saudi J. Biol. Sci.* **2020**, *27*, 905–912. [CrossRef] [PubMed]
245. Petrov, D.; Mansfield, C.; Moussy, A.; Hermine, O. ALS Clinical Trials Review: 20 Years of Failure. Are We Any Closer to Registering a New Treatment? *Front. Aging Neurosci.* **2017**, *9*, 68. [CrossRef] [PubMed]

Disclaimer/Publisher's Note: The statements, opinions and data contained in all publications are solely those of the individual author(s) and contributor(s) and not of MDPI and/or the editor(s). MDPI and/or the editor(s) disclaim responsibility for any injury to people or property resulting from any ideas, methods, instructions or products referred to in the content.

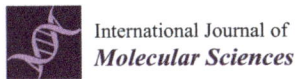 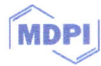

Article

CD163-Mediated Small-Vessel Injury in Alzheimer's Disease: An Exploration from Neuroimaging to Transcriptomics

Yuewei Chen [1,2,3,†], Peiwen Lu [1,3,†], Shengju Wu [4], Jie Yang [1,2,3], Wanwan Liu [1,‡] for the Alzheimer's Disease Neuroimaging Initiative, Zhijun Zhang [4,*] and Qun Xu [1,2,3,*]

1. Health Management Center, Renji Hospital of Medical School, Shanghai Jiao Tong University, Shanghai 200127, China; chenyuewei_js@163.com (Y.C.); lupeiwen0803@163.com (P.L.); liuwanwan@renji.com (W.L.)
2. Department of Neurology, Renji Hospital of Medical School, Shanghai Jiao Tong University, Shanghai 200127, China
3. Renji-UNSW CHeBA (Centre for Healthy Brain Ageing of University of New South Wales) Neurocognitive Center, Renji Hospital of Medical School, Shanghai Jiao Tong University, Shanghai 200127, China
4. School of Biomedical Engineering, Shanghai Jiao Tong University, Shanghai 200030, China
* Correspondence: zhangzj@sjtu.edu.cn (Z.Z.); xuqun@renji.com (Q.X.)
† These authors contributed equally to this work.
‡ Data used in preparation of this article were obtained from the Alzheimer's Disease Neuroimaging Initiative (ADNI) database (https://adni.loni.usc.edu/). As such, the investigators within the ADNI contributed to the design and implementation of ADNI and/or provided data but did not participate in analysis or writing of this report. A complete listing of ADNI investigators can be found at: http://adni.loni.usc.edu/wp-content/uploads/how_to_apply/ADNI_Acknowledgement_List.pdf.

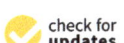

Citation: Chen, Y.; Lu, P.; Wu, S.; Yang, J.; Liu, W., for the Alzheimer's Disease Neuroimaging Initiative; Zhang, Z.; Xu, Q. CD163-Mediated Small-Vessel Injury in Alzheimer's Disease: An Exploration from Neuroimaging to Transcriptomics. *Int. J. Mol. Sci.* **2024**, *25*, 2293. https://doi.org/10.3390/ijms25042293

Academic Editor: Nicoletta Marchesi

Received: 10 January 2024
Revised: 10 February 2024
Accepted: 11 February 2024
Published: 14 February 2024

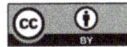

Copyright: © 2024 by the authors. Licensee MDPI, Basel, Switzerland. This article is an open access article distributed under the terms and conditions of the Creative Commons Attribution (CC BY) license (https://creativecommons.org/licenses/by/4.0/).

Abstract: Patients with Alzheimer's disease (AD) often present with imaging features indicative of small-vessel injury, among which, white-matter hyperintensities (WMHs) are the most prevalent. However, the underlying mechanism of the association between AD and small-vessel injury is still obscure. The aim of this study is to investigate the mechanism of small-vessel injury in AD. Differential gene expression analyses were conducted to identify the genes related to WMHs separately in mild cognitive impairment (MCI) and cognitively normal (CN) subjects from the ADNI database. The WMH-related genes identified in patients with MCI were considered to be associated with small-vessel injury in early AD. Functional enrichment analyses and a protein–protein interaction (PPI) network were performed to explore the pathway and hub genes related to the mechanism of small-vessel injury in MCI. Subsequently, the Boruta algorithm and support vector machine recursive feature elimination (SVM-RFE) algorithm were performed to identify feature-selection genes. Finally, the mechanism of small-vessel injury was analyzed in MCI from the immunological perspectives; the relationship of feature-selection genes with various immune cells and neuroimaging indices were also explored. Furthermore, 5×FAD mice were used to demonstrate the genes related to small-vessel injury. The results of the logistic regression analyses suggested that WMHs significantly contributed to MCI, the early stage of AD. A total of 276 genes were determined as WMH-related genes in patients with MCI, while 203 WMH-related genes were obtained in CN patients. Among them, only 15 genes overlapped and were thus identified as the crosstalk genes. By employing the Boruta and SVM-RFE algorithms, CD163, ALDH3B1, MIR22HG, DTX2, FOLR2, ALDH2, and ZNF23 were recognized as the feature-selection genes linked to small-vessel injury in MCI. After considering the results from the PPI network, CD163 was finally determined as the critical WMH-related gene in MCI. The expression of CD163 was correlated with fractional anisotropy (FA) values in regions that are vulnerable to small-vessel injury in AD. The immunostaining and RT-qPCR results from the verifying experiments demonstrated that the indicators of small-vessel injury presented in the cortical tissue of 5×FAD mice and related to the upregulation of CD163 expression. CD163 may be the most pivotal candidates related to small-vessel injury in early AD.

Keywords: CD163; Alzheimer's disease; white-matter hyperintensities; mild cognitive impairment; transcriptome

1. Introduction

Alzheimer's disease (AD) and cerebral small-vessel disease (CSVD) rank as the predominant causes of dementia [1]. Recent data prognosticates that, by 2050, the prevalence of dementia will triple worldwide. Notably, this estimate increases threefold when considering a biological definition of AD, rather than relying on clinical criteria [2]. AD, a neurodegenerative disorder, manifests through the abnormal accumulation of amyloid beta (Aβ) plaques and neurofibrillary tangles (NFTs), along with progressive neuronal loss, culminating in brain atrophy, cognitive decline, and behavioral disturbances [3]. The continuum of AD, stretching over a period of 15–25 years, can be present without any overt symptoms via a stage of mild cognitive impairment (MCI) leading up to dementia [2]. The stage of MCI is always considered as early AD, which is a critical period for disease modification. In addition, CSVD, encompassing white-matter lesions (WML), an enlarged perivascular space (EPVS), cortical superficial siderosis, lacunes, and cerebral microbleeds [4], plays a pivotal role not only in the direct etiology of vascular dementia but is also prominently encountered within AD brains [5,6]. The two-hit vascular hypothesis for AD proposes that primary damage to the brain microcirculation (hit one) initiates a non-amyloidogenic pathway leading to Aβ accumulation (hit two). These peptides, in turn, exert vasculotoxic and neurotoxic effects [7].

White-matter hyperintensities (WMH) have traditionally been viewed as one of the most prevalent neuroimaging features of small-vessel injury, especially for CSVD. Many neuroimaging studies have shown a relationship between AD pathologies and WMH [8,9]. For instance, a recent study emphasized the clinical relevance of WMHs in AD, especially posterior WMHs, and most notably, splenium of the corpus callosum (S-CC) WMH [10]. Another study pointed that posterior WMHs might be related to degenerative mechanisms secondary to AD pathology, while anterior WMH could be associated with both CSVD and degenerative mechanisms [11], indicating that the pathological mechanism of small-vessel injury in AD may be different from that in sporadic CSVD. Compared with traditional structural MRI sequences, indices extracted from diffusion tensor imaging (DTI) more sensitively detected white-matter microstructure damages due to small-vessel injury [12–14].

Recently, bioinformatics approaches have been developed to explore the underlying mechanisms of diseases. Feature-selection algorithms, including the Boruta algorithm and support vector machine recursive feature elimination (SVM-RFE) algorithm, have already been applied in transcriptomic, proteomic, and metabolomic analyses for targeted substance screening [15–18]. However, there have been few studies on the mechanisms of small-vessel injury in AD based on these technologies. Therefore, the primary objective of this study is to investigate the distinct mechanism of small-vessel injury in AD, by utilizing neuroimaging with transcriptome analysis, immunological explorations, and further experimental verification.

AD datasets sourced from the ADNI database were employed for comprehensive systemic analysis. First, logistic regression models were constructed to evaluate the contributions of WMH and cerebral atrophy in distinct stages of AD. Second, transcript-level differential analysis was conducted to obtain DEGs. Third, hub genes were identified using maximal clique centrality (MCC) and the molecular complex detection (MCODE). Fourth, the Boruta algorithm and SVM-RFE algorithm were used to obtain feature-selection genes. Machine Learning models were then employed to verify the robustness of these feature-selection genes. Fifth, the correlation analyses between feature-selection genes, the abundance of infiltrating immune cells, and neuroimaging features were subsequently conducted to illustrate the small-vessel injury during early AD from immunological perspectives and establish connections in multidimensional data. Finally, the results were further validated through cellular and animal experiments. The detailed analytic workflow chart is shown in Figure 1.

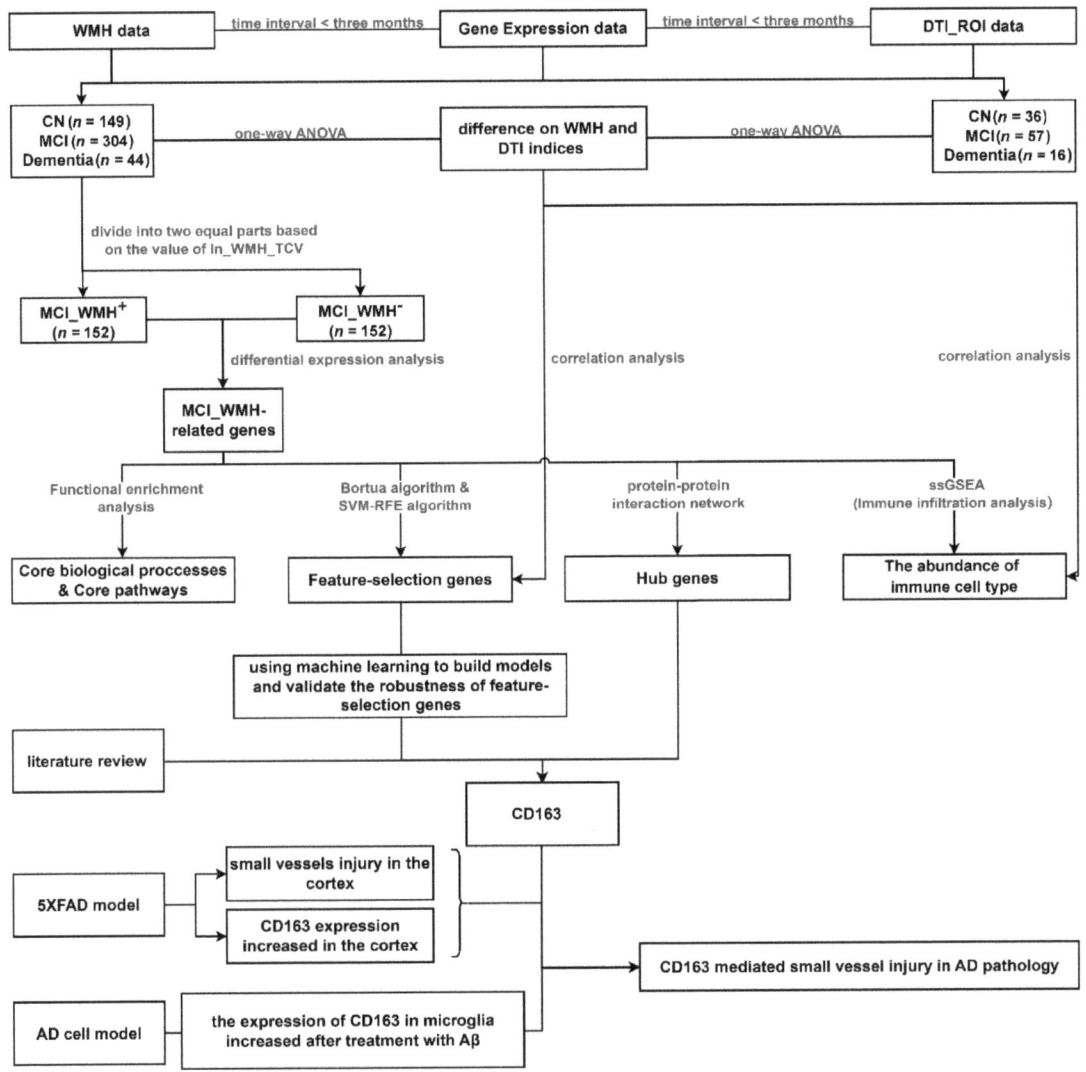

Figure 1. The study workflow chart. Abbreviations: WMH, white-matter hyperintensities; DTI_ROI, diffusion tensor imaging region of interest; CN, cognitively normal; MCI, mild cognitive impairment; AD, Alzheimer's disease; ln_WMH_TCV, natural logarithm of standardized white-matter hyperintensities (WMH) to total cerebrum cranial volume (TCV); MCI_WMH+, mild cognitive impairment with severe white-matter hyperintensities, whose values of ' ln_WMH_TCV' were above the median; MCI_WMH−, mild cognitive impairment with no or mild white-matter hyperintensities, whose values of ' ln_WMH_TCV' were below the median.

2. Results

2.1. WMH and Cerebral Atrophy Both Contributed to Early Stage of Alzheimer's Disease

Demographic characteristics, neuropsychological tests, and neuroimaging findings of the different cognitive groups are shown in Table 1. Standardized total cerebrum brain volume to total cerebrum cranial volume (TCB_TCV) and standardized segmented total hippocampi volume to TCV (T_hippo_TCV) significantly decreased sequentially in cognitively normal (CN) patients, MCI, AD (all $p < 0.05$). Meanwhile, indicators of WMH did not exhibit significant differences among the groups (all $p > 0.05$). Differences in DTI indices, including fractional anisotropy (FA), and mean, axial, and radial diffusivity (MD, AxD, RD) values, were observed among the three groups, especially for the following fiber bundles: tapetum, bilateral splenium of the corpus callosum, bilateral fornix, posterior thalamic radiation_left, fornix (cres)/Stria terminalis_left (FDR-adjusted $p < 0.05$). These were consistent with the vulnerable regions reported in previous studies [14] and may be associated with AD pathology (Figure 2A,B, Table S1).

Table 1. Demographic characteristics, neuropsychological tests, and neuroimaging indices.

	CN (n = 149)	MCI (n = 304)	Dementia (n = 44)	p
Demographic characteristics				
Male, n (%)	68 (45.60%)	163 (53.60%)	25 (56.80%)	0.090
Age, mean (SD)	73.45 (5.99) [b]	71.46 (7.42) [ac]	75.23 (9.20) [b]	0.001
Education, mean (SD)	16.68 (2.53) [c]	16.10 (2.64)	15.50 (2.71) [a]	0.013
APOEε4 carriers, n (%)	105/38/6 (70.50%/25.50%/4.00%) [bc]	175/106/23 (57.60%/34.90%/7.60%) [ac]	11/26/7 (25.00%/59.10%/15.90%) [ab]	<0.001
Neuropsychological tests				
MMSE, mean (SD)	29.03 (1.21) [bc]	28.11 (1.62) [ac]	22.52 (3.04) [ab]	<0.001
FAQ, mean (SD)	0.16 (0.60) [bc]	2.44 (3.56) [ac]	13.57 (7.20) [ab]	<0.001
MoCA, mean (SD)	25.72 (2.16) [bc]	23.52 (3.07) [ac]	17.19 (4.93) [ab]	<0.001
CDRSB, mean (SD)	0.03 (0.14) [bc]	1.38 (0.86) [ac]	4.64 (1.77) [ab]	<0.001
Neuroimaging				
ln_WMH_TCV, mean (SD)	−1.34 (1.16)	×1.23 (1.20)	−0.99 (1.10)	0.209
TCB_TCV, mean (SD)	77.71 (2.52) [c]	77.56 (3.02) [c]	74.26 (2.39) [ab]	<0.001
T_hippo_TCV, mean (SD)	0.56 (0.05) [bc]	0.54 (0.07) [ac]	0.46 (0.07) [ab]	<0.001

The χ2-test for gender and APOEε4, and one-way ANOVA were performed to assess group comparison for other indices, and Bonferroni correction for homoscedasticity and Tamhane's T2 test for heteroscedasticity were carried out; $p < 0.05$ was considered to be statistically significant. a: Significantly different from NC; b: Significantly different from MCI; c: Significantly different from dementia. Abbreviations: CN, cognitively normal; MCI, mild cognitive impairment; SD, standard deviation; MMSE, mini mental state examination; FAQ, functional activities questionnaire; MoCA, Montreal cognitive assessment; CDRSB, clinical dementia rating scale sum of boxes; ln_WMH_TCV, natural logarithm of standardized white-matter hyperintensities (WMH) to total cerebrum cranial volume (TCV); TCB_TCV, standardized total cerebrum brain volume (TCB) to total cerebrum cranial volume (TCV); T_hippo_TCV, standardized segmented total hippocampi volume (T_hippo) to total cerebrum cranial volume (TCV).

Multivariate logistic regression models revealed that TCB_TCV was associated with both MCI and dementia (all $p < 0.05$), while the natural logarithm of standardized WMH to TCV (ln_WMH_TCV) was only related to MCI ($p < 0.05$). Joint diagnostic effectiveness for TCB_TCV and ln_WMH_TCV in MCI yielded an area under the curve (AUC) value of 0.682 (TCB_TCV: OR = 0.882 (0.804~0.966) $p < 0.01$; ln_WMH_TCV, OR = 1.278 (1.053~1.559) $p < 0.05$) (Table 2, Figure 2C).

2.2. Differentially Expressed Genes (DEGs) and Functional Enrichment Analysis of WMH-Related Genes in MCI

Demographic characteristics, neuropsychological tests, and neuroimaging indices for either CN patients or those with MCI stratified by the median of ln_WMH_TCV are shown in Table S2. WMH+ indicates where the values of 'ln_WMH_TCV' were above the median, while WMH− indicates values below the median. A total of 109 upregulated DEGs and 94 downregulated DEGs were identified in the CN_WMH+ group, while 112 upregulated DEGs and 164 downregulated DEGs were identified in the MCI_WMH+ group (Figure 3A,B). Only 15 genes overlapped between the CN_WMH+ and MCI_WMH+ groups (Figure 3C). These results suggested that the mechanism of small-vessel injury in patients with MCI (due to AD pathology) differed from that in CN patients.

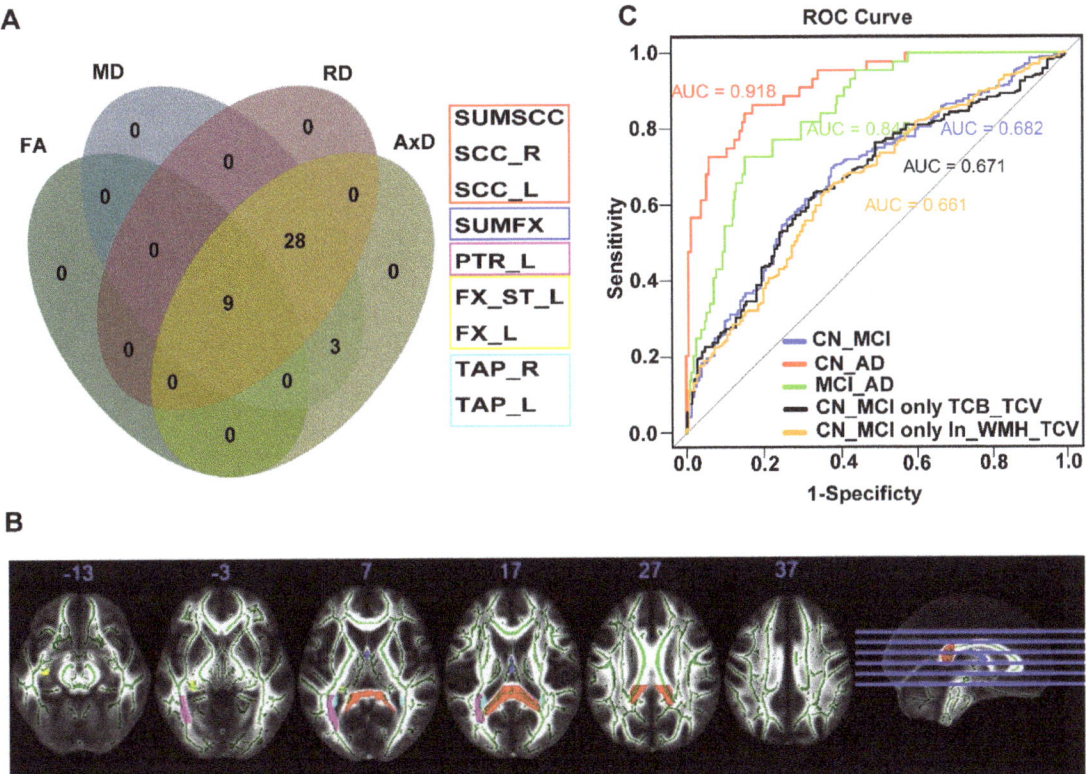

Figure 2. The difference among CN, MCI, and dementia in DTI indices and the prediction accuracy of ln_WMH_TCV and TCB_TCV in predicting AD progression: (**A**) The intersection of difference in FA, MD, RD, and AxD indices were considered the most fragile fiber bundles; (**B**) The predictive effectiveness of cerebral atrophy and small-vessel injury at different stages of AD diagnosis; (**C**) different cross-sectional views of the fragile fiber bundles. Red: bilateral splenium of the corpus callosum (SUMSCC, SCC_R, SCC_L), blue: bilateral fornix (SUMFX), violet: posterior thalamic radiation_left (PTR_L), yellow: fornix (cres)/stria terminalis_left (FX_ST_L, FX_L), cyan: tapetum (TAP_R, TAP_L). Abbreviations: FA, fractional anisotropy; MD, mean diffusivity; RD, radial diffusivity; AxD, axial diffusivity, TAP_R, tapetum right; TAP_L, tapetum left; SUMSCC, bilateral splenium of the corpus callosum; SUMFX, bilateral fornix; SCC_R, splenium of corpus callosum right; SCC_L, splenium of corpus callosum left; PTR_L, posterior thalamic radiation left; FX_ST_L, fornix (cres)/stria terminalis left; FX_L, fornix left; CN, cognitively normal; MCI, mild cognitive impairment; AD, Alzheimer's disease; ROC, receiver operating characteristic; AUC, area under the curve; TCB_TCV, standardized total cerebrum brain volume (TCB) to total cerebrum cranial volume (TCV); ln_WMH_TCV, natural logarithm of standardized white-matter hyperintensities (WMH) to total cerebrum cranial volume (TCV).

The results of the gene set enrichment analysis (GSEA) of the Kyoto Encyclopedia of Genes and Genomes (KEGG) pathways further revealed that the WMH-related genes in MCI were mainly enriched in pathways related to infection, immunity, and metabolism, including "lysosomes", "phagosomes", "neutrophil extracellular trap formation", "Influenza A" and "retinol metabolism" (Figure 3D,E). GSEA of gene ontology (GO) yielded similar outcomes as well (Supplementary Figure S1).

Table 2. Logistic regression analysis of diagnosis during AD continuum.

	Odds Ratio (95% CI)	p	C-Statistics
CN vs. MCI [1]			
ln_WMH_TCV	1.262 (1.041–1.537)	0.019	0.6614
CN vs. MCI [2]			
TCB_TCV	0.887 (0.809–0.970)	0.010	0.671
CN vs. MCI [3]			
ln_WMH_TCV	1.278 (1.053–1.559)	0.014	0.682
TCB_TCV	0.882 (0.804–0.966)	0.007	
CN vs. Dementia [4]			
ln_WMH_TCV	1.322 (0.874–2.083)	0.202	0.918
TCB_TCV	0.505 (0.385–0.634)	<0.001	
MCI vs. Dementia [5]			
ln_WMH_TCV	1.081 (0.759–1.548)	0.668	0.845
TCB_TCV	0.657 (0.554–0.768)	<0.001	

Model [1] and [2] only included ln_WMH_TCV or TCB_TCV for univariate logistic regression analysis, Model [3], [4], and [5] included two dependent variables, ln_WMH_TCV and TCB_TCV, for multivariate logistic regression. All logistic regression models were adjusted for age, gender, APOEε4, and education. Abbreviations: 95% CI, 95% confidence interval; C-statistics, concordance statistic; CN, cognitively normal; MCI, mild cognitive impairment; ln_WMH_TCV, natural logarithm of standardized white-matter hyperintensities (WMH) to total cerebrum cranial volume (TCV); TCB_TCV, standardized total cerebrum brain volume (TCB) to total cerebrum Cranial Volume (TCV).

2.3. PPI Network Construction of WMH-Related Genes in MCI

Based on the STRING results, a PPI network of WMH-related genes was constructed using 269 nodes and 285 edges in MCI (Figure 4A). A total of 19 genes and 30 genes were identified as being closely related genes using the MCODE (Figure 4B–D) and cyto-Hubba plugins (MCC) (Figure 4E), respectively. Interestingly, there were 15 hub genes that overlapped in both hub genes selection processes (Figure 4F).

2.4. Feature-Selection Genes from WMH-Related Genes in MCI

Based on the MCI_WMH-related gene set, 15 feature-selection genes were selected using the Boruta algorithm (ALDH2, MAST2, TCN2, CD163, ALDH3B1, CCDC170, ZNF23, MIR22HG, CCR6, NLRP3, PNPLA8, FOLR2, DTX2, EPHX1, PLEK) and 22 feature-selection genes were selected using the SVM-RFE algorithm. The results of feature-selection genes based on the Boruta and SVM-RFE algorithms are shown in Figure 5A,B. A total of seven variables were selected by both algorithms (Figure 5C), namely CD163, ALDH3B1, MIR22HG, DTX2, FOLR2, and ALDH2, ZNF23. Using the above feature-selection genes, seven machine learning models were established to predict the degree of WMH in the MCI group. The receiver operating characteristic (ROC) curve of each model showed predictive effectiveness, represented by the AUC value (Figure 5D). The gradient boosting machine (GBM) (AUC = 0.741) was the best model for predicting the degree of WMH in MCI groups, followed by random forest (RF) (AUC = 0.727) and k-nearest neighbors (KNN) (AUC = 0.705). The predictive effectiveness of seven machine learning methods in the training set is illustrated in Supplementary Figure S2. In summary, these seven genes were identified as the feature-selection genes and demonstrated their potential as biomarkers for predicting the degree of small-vessel injury in patients with MCI. From the expression values of boxplots, CD163, FOLR2, ALDH3B1, DTX2, and ALDH2 were highly expressed in the MCI group with severe small-vessel injury (Figure 5E).

2.5. Immune Landscape and Feature-Selection-Genes Correlation Analysis

The boxplot of infiltrating immune cell types revealed that the abundances of regulatory T cells, macrophages, monocytes, natural killer T cells, myeloid-derived suppressor cells, central memory CD8 T cells, and immature dendritic cells were much more increased in the MCI_WMH+ group than in the MCI_WMH– group, whereas the activated B cells were significantly reduced (Figure 6A). The correlation between feature-selection gene expression and the abundance of infiltrating immune cell types showed that most immunocytes positively connected with the seven feature-selection genes (Figure 6B). These results implied that the inflammatory components play an essential role in small-vessel injury in MCI, and most feature-selection genes are primarily associated with the positive regulation of immune function.

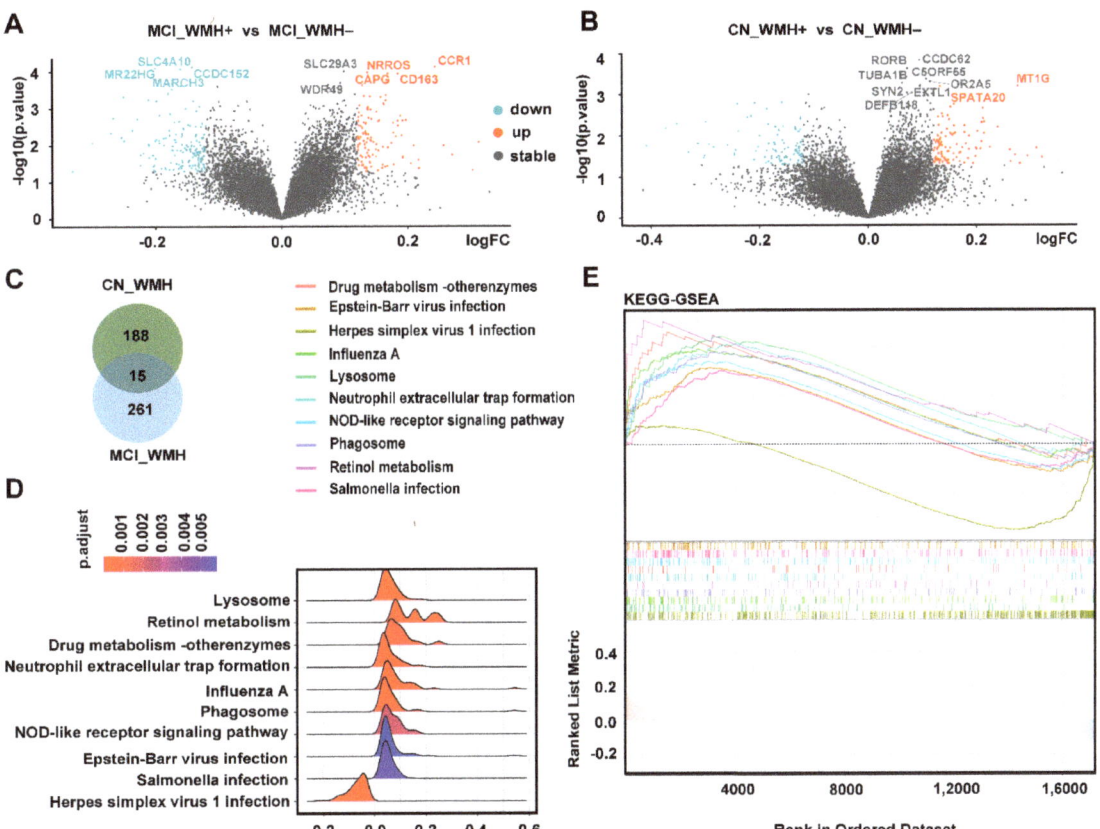

Figure 3. Identification of DEGs and functional enrichment analysis: (**A**) Volcano plot of DEGs constructed using the fold-change values (0.12) and p-value (0.05); red-orange color dots represent genes upregulated in MCI_WMH+, gray dots represent genes not differing significantly between MCI_WMH+ and MCI_WMH−, and cyan dots represent genes downregulated in MCI_WMH+. (**B**) Volcano plot of DEGs constructed using the fold-change values (0.12) and p-value (0.05); red-orange color dots represent genes upregulated in CN_WMH+ group, gray dots represent genes not differing significantly between CN_WMH+ and CN_WMH− groups, and cyan dots represent genes downregulated in CN_WMH+ group. (**C**) Venn plot. Only fifteen genes shared between WMH-related genes in CN patients and those with MCI. (**D**,**E**) The results of GSEA analysis of KEGG in MCI_WMH+ samples. Abbreviations: MCI_WMH+, mild cognitive impairment with severe white-matter hyperintensities; MCI_WMH−, mild cognitive impairment with no or mild white-matter hyperintensities; CN_WMH+, cognitively normal with severe white-matter hyperintensities; CN_WMH−, cognitively normal with no or mild white-matter hyperintensities; KEGG_GSEA, gene set enrichment analysis (GSEA) of Kyoto Encyclopedia of Genes and Genomes (KEGG) pathways; DEGs, differentially expressed genes.

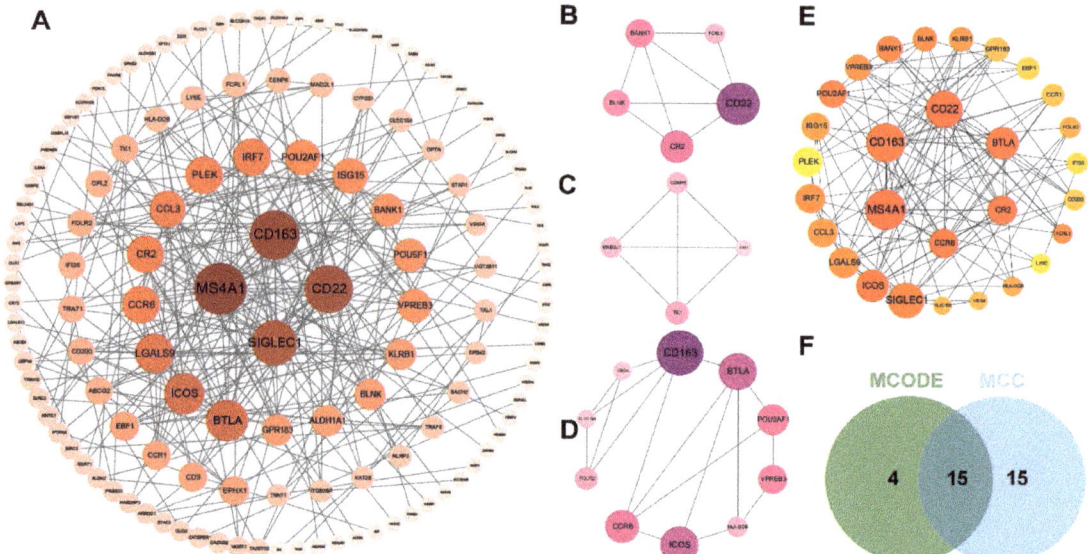

Figure 4. Screening of closely related genes and hub genes of WMH-related genes in MCI group using cytoHubba and MCODE plugins: (**A**) Macroscopic display of PPI networks for all DEGs of WMH-related genes in MCI group, with a redder color indicating a higher degree score; the gene nodes in the topological characteristics of this PPI network were ranked in descending order of degree value (**B–D**), with a deeper purple color indicating a higher score. The top three modules' genes are filtered by MCODE; (**E**) A redder color indicates a higher score and a yellower color indicates a lower score. The hub genes are filtered by the MCC for the top 30 genes; (**F**) Venn plot the common genes are both filtered by MCODE and MCC. Abbreviations: MCODE, molecular complex detection; MCC, maximal clique centrality.

The feature-selection genes, especially CD163 and FOLR2, exhibited significant correlations with FA values. This correlation was related to the fragility of small vessels in specific brain regions, with a tendency towards the left side, including left posterior thalamic radiation and the left fornix, considered as posterior WMHs (Figure 6C, Table S3).

Based on the results of PPI and machine learning, CD163 and FOLR2 were determined as the key WMH-related genes of MCI (Figure 6D). The significant correlations of either CD163 or FOLR2 with ln_WMH_TCV are shown in Figure 6E.

2.6. AD Pathology Resulted in Small-Vessel Injury and Elevated CD163 Expression

To further validate the alterations in the expression of CD163 following small-vessel injury in the context of AD pathology, we performed experiments using 6-month-old 5×FAD mice. Immunofluorescence results revealed the existence of cortical EPVS, which is an important indicator of small-vessel injury (Figure 7A–E). Real-time quantitative polymerase chain reaction (RT-qPCR) results from cortical tissues exhibited the upregulation of CD163 expression (Figure 7F). RT-qPCR analysis of rat primary microglia showed that CD163 expression increased after Aβ treatment (Figure 7G,H). This suggested that AD pathologies, especially Aβ plaques, may contribute to small-vessel injury and upregulate the expression of CD163.

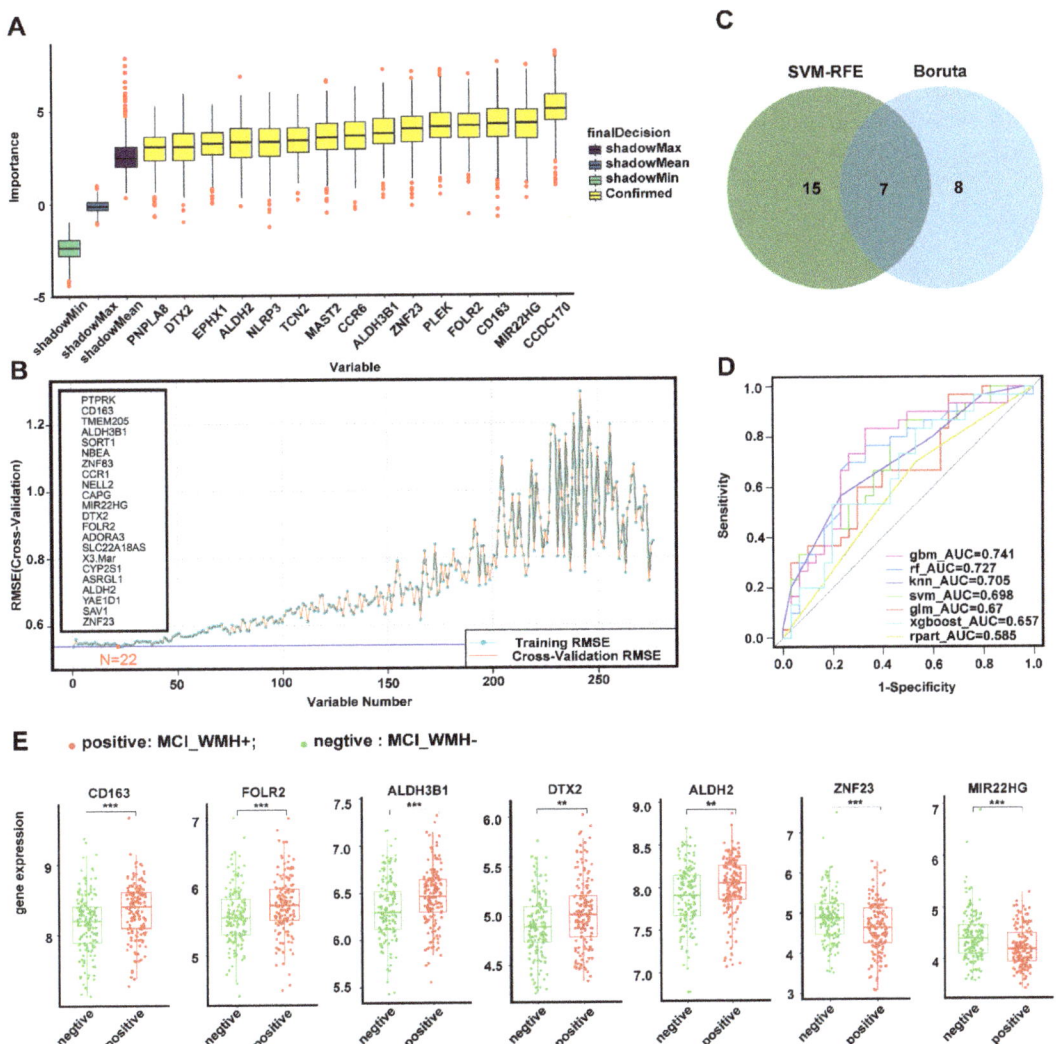

Figure 5. Screening feature-selection genes from DEGs between mild and severe small-vessel injury in MCI group: (**A**) 15 feature-selection genes were screened by Boruta algorithm; (**B**) 22 feature-selected genes were screened by SVM-RFE algorithm; (**C**) Venn plot, seven variables including CD163, FOLR2, ALDH3B1, DTX2, ALDH2, ZNF23, and MIR22HG intersected by Boruta and SVM-RFE algorithms; (**D**) the ROC curve of seven machine learning models, and the AUC value represents the model predictive effectiveness in testing set; (**E**) the expression level of feature-selection genes CD163, FOLR2, ALDH3B1, DTX2, ALDH2, ZNF23, and MIR22HG in the MCI between mild and severe small-vessel injury. CD163, p-value = 1.2×10^{-4}; FOLR2, p-value = 6.4×10^{-4}; ALDH3B1, p-value = 4.7×10^{-4}; DTX2, p-value = 1.8×10^{-3}; ALDH2, p-value = 3×10^{-3}; ZNF23, p-value = 5.1×10^{-4}; MIR22HG, p-value = 8.6×10^{-5}. ** $p < 0.01$; *** $p < 0.001$. Abbreviations: SVM-RFE, support vector machine recursive feature elimination; RMSE, root mean square error; AUC, area under the curve; gbm, gradient boosting machine; rf, random forest; KNN, k-nearest neighbors; SVM, support vector machine; GLM, generalized linear model; XGboost, extreme gradient boosting; rpart, recursive partition tree.

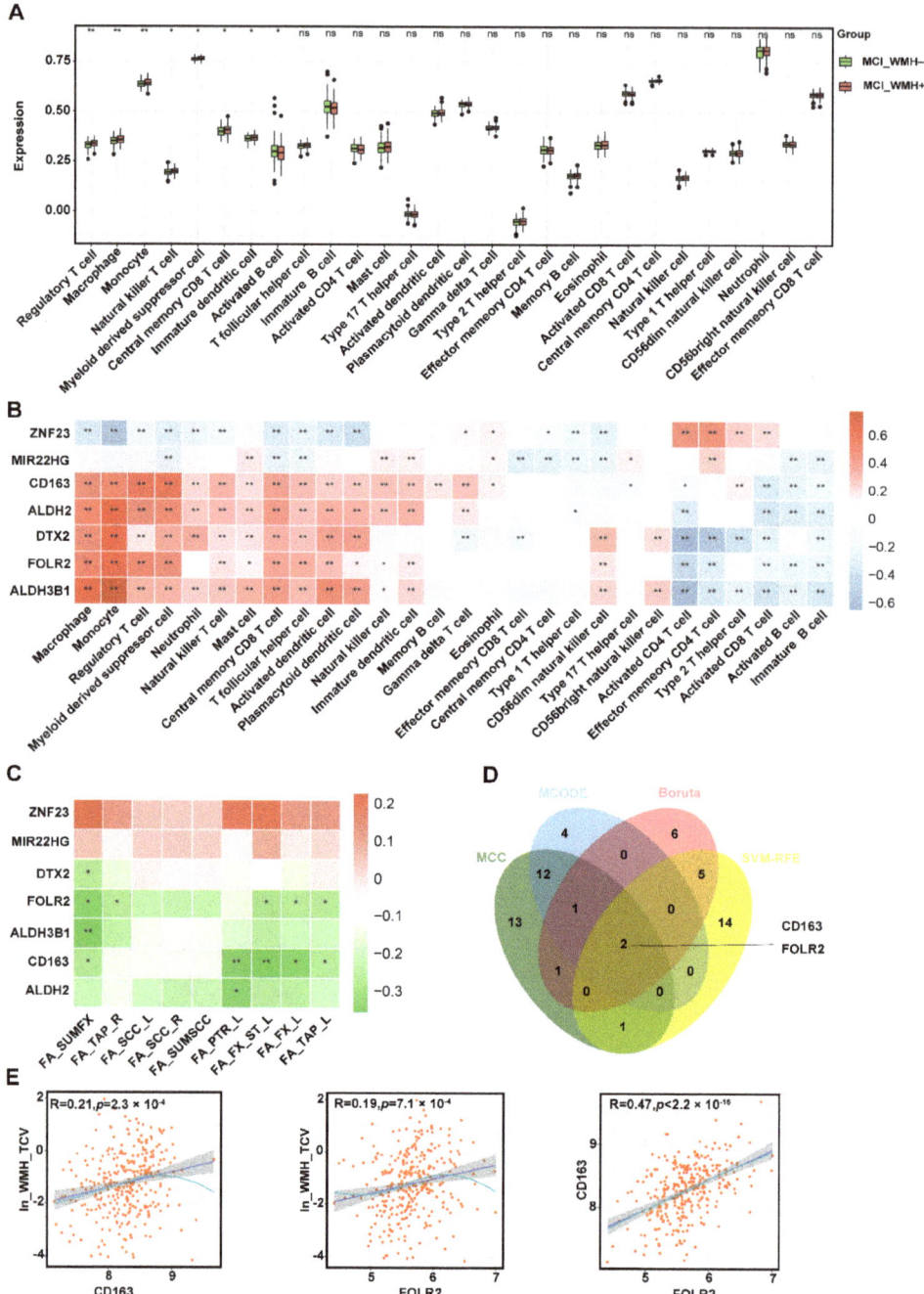

Figure 6. Alterations in the abundance of immune cells in MCI group with severe small-vessel injury (MCI_WMH+) and correlation analysis between hub genes with the abundance of immune cell and FA values: (**A**) Estimated proportions of 28 immune cell types between two groups in MCI group; (**B**) Correlation analysis of hub genes with different immune cell types; (**C**) Correlation analysis of hub genes with differential brain-area FA values; (**D**) Venn plot, two genes (CD163 and

FOLR2) intersected by Feature-selection algorithms and PPI. (**E**) The correlation between CD163, FOLR2, and ln_WMH_TCV. * $p < 0.05$; ** $p < 0.01$. Abbreviations: FA, fractional anisotropy; SUMFX, bilateral fornix; TAP_R, tapetum right; SCC_L, splenium of corpus callosum left; SCC_R, splenium of corpus callosum right; SUMSCC, bilateral splenium of the corpus callosum; PTR_L, posterior thalamic radiation left; FX_ST_L, fornix (cres)/stria terminalis left; FX_L, fornix left; TAP_L, tapetum left; ln_WMH_TCV, natural logarithm of standardized white-matter hyperintensities (WMH) to total cerebrum cranial volume (TCV).

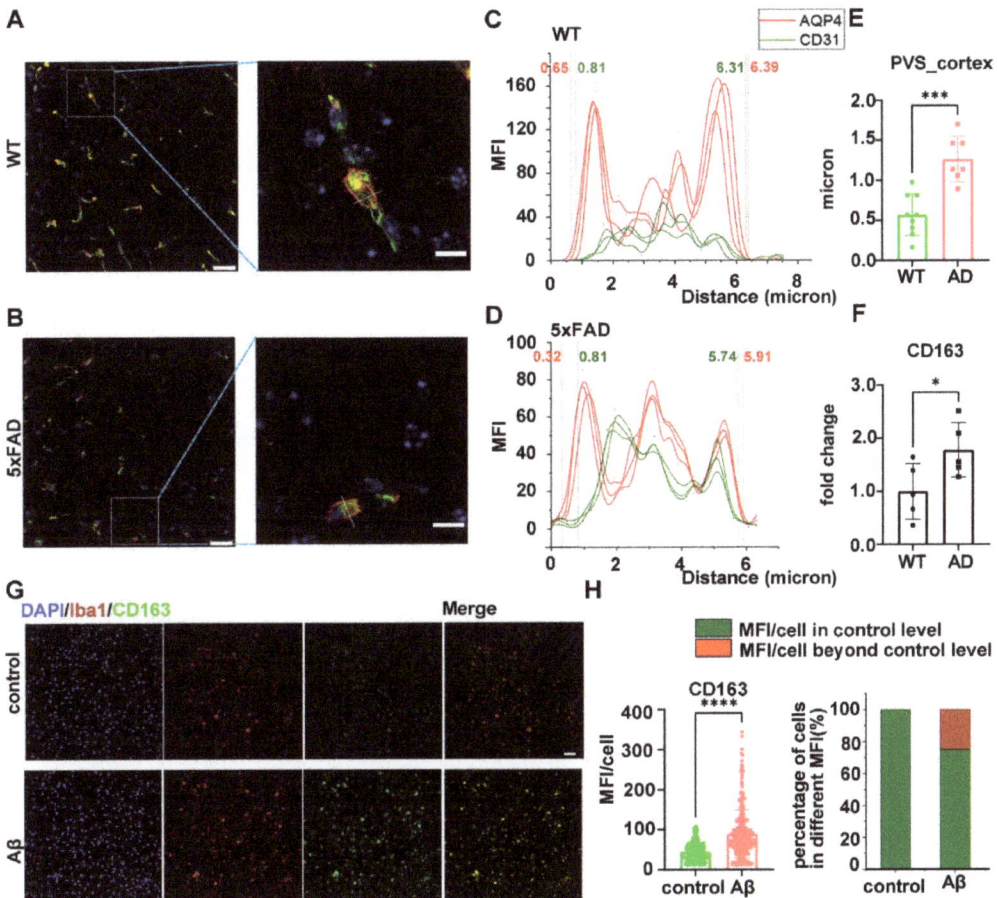

Figure 7. AD pathology leads to small-vessel injury and elevates CD163 expression. Immunofluorescence staining results of (**A**) 5×FAD cerebral cortex (left scale bar = 25 um; right scale bar = 10 um) and (**B**) WT cerebral cortex, green: CD31; red: AQP4; magenta: Aβ; blue: DAPI. (**C–E**) Calculation of the width of the perivascular spaces and the comparation between WT and 5×FAD. (**F**) rt-qPCR results from cortical tissues exhibited an upregulation of CD163 expression in 5×FAD mice. (**G**) Immunofluorescence staining: control vs. Aβ-treated rat primary microglia (scale bar = 50 um), green: CD163; red: iba-1; blue: DAPI. (**H**) Immunofluorescence staining results of CD163 showing the MFI and the percentage of cells in different MFIs. * $p < 0.05$; *** $p < 0.001$; **** $p < 0.0001$. Abbreviations: MFI, mean fluorescence intensity; Aβ, amyloid beta.

3. Discussion

There has been limited research centered around transcriptomic strategies on the mechanisms of small-vessel injury in AD. Through comprehensive analyses of clinical data, reviews of the relevant literature, and the verification experiments, our study suggested a distinct mechanism of small-vessel injury in early-stage AD.

From both clinical and neuroimaging perspectives, although WMHs did not show significant differences among the three groups, sensitive DTI indices, such as FA values, identified vulnerable regions associated with small-vessel injury in the AD continuum. We also identified that WMHs, an indicator of small-vessel injury associated with the diagnosis of early-stage AD, and TCB, which represents cerebral atrophy, can associated with the entire course of AD. Small-vessel injury played a potential role in the initial phases of the disease, whereas degenerative factors predominated in all stages of the disease [19,20]. These results also provide evidence to support the "two-hit vascular hypothesis" of AD etiology [21].

After bioinformatics analyses, we found that the gene expression of small-vessel injury in patients with MCI were quite different from that in CN patients. Increasing evidence shows that WMHs may predict the probability for diagnosing MCI [19,22], and the period of MCI is a crucial period for disease intervention within the AD continuum. This intrigues us and we subsequently wish to focus on small-vessel injury in the context of MCI. Seven feature-selection genes (CD163, FOLR2, ALDH3B1, MIR22HG, DTX2, ALDH2, and ZNF23), out of 276 WMH-related genes in MCI, were selected by the Boruta algorithm and the SVM-RFE algorithm and further validated as the predictable biomarkers of WMH through seven machine learning risk prediction models. Notably, they were highly correlated with the immune cells, as well as the immune-related pathway, indicating a potential role through immune-related biological pathways in the development of small-vessel injury in early AD. Finally, CD163 and FOLR2 were identified as the pivotal genes.

CD163, a glycoprotein within class B of the scavenger receptor cysteine-rich superfamily, primarily participates in iron metabolism, inflammation, and immune responses. Traditionally, its expression was thought to be restricted to perivascular and meningeal macrophages (Supplementary Figure S3) [23,24]. However, CD163 is also expressed in the microglia in various nervous system diseases, such as AD, Parkinson's disease (PD), HIV-encephalitis, multiple sclerosis, and head injury tissue [24–27]. Notably, CD163 exhibits heightened expression in AD, particularly in the frontal and occipital cortices, with co-localization with Aβ; in addition, it was found at a higher density around compromised blood vessels [24,28]. Our experimental results also reveal the presence of small-vessel injury in the cortex of 5×FAD mice, accompanied by an elevated expression of CD163. Additionally, exposure to Aβ induces the increase in CD163 expression in primary microglial cells. Research on human coronary artery plaques has demonstrated that the presence of CD163$^+$ macrophages were associated with increased expression of endothelial vascular cell adhesion molecule (VCAM), angiogenesis, inflammatory cell recruitment, and high microvascular permeability through the CD163/HIF1α/VEGF-A pathway [29].

Increased CD163 expression was found in the MCI_WMH+ group by our analysis. Therefore, it is reasonable to hypothesize that early hypoperfusion may hinder Aβ clearance, thereby promoting Aβ deposition and upregulating CD163 expression. This upregulation of CD163 expression, driven by the CD163/HIF1α/VEGF pathway, initiates non-functional angiogenesis, chronic inflammatory cell recruitment, and heightened vascular permeability, and exacerbates Aβ deposition. These processes create a detrimental feedback loop, ultimately resulting in development of the MCI stage. Certainly, these hypotheses need further validation by modulating the expression of CD163 in microglial cells to investigate its impact on the blood-brain barrier (BBB).

The GO annotations for FOLR2, which encode a member of the folate receptor (FOLR) family, include folic acid binding and folic acid transmembrane transporter activity. Folate deficiency is associated with cerebrovascular diseases, neurological diseases, and mood disorders [30]. Given the reported protection exerted by folic acid against oxidative stress, resulting from exposure to amyloid beta [31], the observed upregulation of folate receptors and folate binding could represent a response to the increased intracellular vitamin need. Therefore, lower circulating serum folate may be attributable to increased folate binding in peripheral tissues such as via fibroblasts [32]. In addition, the upregulation of FOLR2 may contribute to an unfavorable vascular phenotypic switch induced by obesity [33]. However, limited evidence exists on the relationship between this gene and cerebral blood vessels, especially small vessels.

It is noteworthy that CD163 and FOLR2 serve as frequently observed biomarkers of M2 macrophages [34–37], which are well-known for their anti-inflammatory properties [38]. Our investigation also revealed a positive correlation between the expression of CD163 and FOLR2, suggesting an upregulation of anti-inflammatory macrophages in patients with MCI with pronounced cerebral small-vessel injury. An increased abundance of anti-inflammatory macrophages may signify a compensatory response to an elevated immune milieu within the organism. Furthermore, this finding aligns with the heightened macrophage abundance revealed by immune infiltration analysis.

However, ALDH2 and ALDH3B1 are both members of the aldehyde dehydrogenase (ALDH) protein family, critical for detoxifying aldehydes. ALDH2, a nuclear gene, is transported and functions in the mitochondrial matrix. Elevated blood ALDH2 expression may indicate a protective response to toxic aldehydes in mitochondria [39]. ALDH2 mRNA expression was significantly higher in late-onset AD than in controls and increased with age in wildtype mice [40]. ALDH3B1 also protects cells from oxidative stress [41] and may have protective roles in various brain diseases including epilepsy [42].

DTX2 is a member of the DELTEX (DTX) family of E3 ubiquitin ligases (comprising five members: DTX1, DTX2, DTX3, DTX3L, and DTX4) in mammals and it is closely related to cell growth, differentiation, apoptosis, signal transduction, and some diseases, including tumors [43,44]. MIR22HG, a well-studied lncRNA, functions as a master regulator in diverse malignancies, playing a critical role in various aspects of carcinogenesis, including proliferation, apoptosis, invasion, and metastasis [45]. ZNF23 induces apoptosis in human ovarian cancer cells [46]. However, these three genes have been the subject of limited research in regard to the nervous system.

There are several limitations of this study that are worthy of mentioning. Firstly, brain MRI and gene expression data were available only in the subsamples, primarily due to limited access. Notably, there is a lack of databases containing comprehensive neuroimaging and gene expression data for the AD continuum. To compensate for this limitation, we randomly divided the dataset into a training set (20%) and a testing set (80%), employing as many as seven machine learning algorithms to create ROC curves and verify the robustness of these feature-selection genes. The predictive effectiveness of the GBM, RF, and KNN algorithms had accuracies exceeding 0.7, confirming the robustness of our results. In addition, we are in the process of constructing an independent AD-cohort dataset to further evaluate the generalizability of these feature-selection genes.

Secondly, we have only validated the coexistence of small-vessel injury and elevated CD163 expression in the context of AD pathology. More systematic experiments, including the modulation of CD163 expression in microglia, are required to investigate its impact and the underlying mechanisms of small-vessel injury in the future. Despite the insufficient evidence from the literature reviews regarding the association between FOLR2 and small-vessel injury, this represents one of the research directions that requires further experimental validation.

Finally, some cells and molecules from the central nervous system (CNS) can traverse the BBB and enter the peripheral blood, which provide insights for the state of the CNS, especially in disease research and monitoring. It is essential to acknowledge that peripheral changes cannot directly and fully reveal the pathological and physiological changes in the brain, which is an inherent limitation when studying central diseases through peripheral approaches.

4. Materials and Methods

4.1. Description of ADNI Subjects in the Study, Dataset Acquisition, and Data Preprocessing

Brain imaging and gene expression data were obtained from the ADNI database (http://adni.loni.usc.edu; accessed on 3 July 2023), a large dataset established in 2003 to measure the progression of healthy and cognitively impaired participants with brain scans, biological markers, and neuropsychological assessments [47]. Peripheral blood samples were collected and the Affymetrix Human Genome U219 Array (Affymetrix, Santa Clara, CA, USA) was utilized for expression profiling. Tabulation of gene expression profiles from blood RNA and all quality control and normalizations were conducted by ADNI before inclusion in the dataset.

Diagnosis, age, gender, education, cognitive test scores, and the most recent imaging data, including WMH as well as DTI indices extracted from MRI, were obtained from ADNI. Using the conversion between VISCODE and VISCODE2, the intervals between MRI, diagnosis, and blood sample collection were controlled so as to not exceed three months.

TCB and WMH were adopted to represent the severity of cerebral atrophy and small-vessel injuries [48–50]. For analytical purposes, Both TCB and WMH were standardized by TCV and subsequently multiplied by 100. WMH_TCV was a natural logarithm transformed to mitigate the impact of left skewness distributions (Supplementary Figure S4).

Logistic regression models were utilized to estimate the odds ratios (ORs) and 95% confidence intervals (CIs) for AD stages associated with cerebral atrophy and small-vessel injury. Age, gender, education level, and APOE mutation were adjusted before regression and correlation analysis.

4.2. MRI Analysis

DTI indices including FA, MD, AxD, and the RD of white matter, were sourced from the ADNI database under the same screening criteria as previously described. The GRETNA toolbox [51] was used to perform a one-way ANOVA on the DTI data of the three groups (CN, MCI, dementia), controlling for age, gender, and education level, and corrected for false discovery rate (FDR). Referring to the "JHU ICBM-DTI-81 White-Matter Labels" fiber bundles label, differential fiber bundles were extracted by employing FMRIB's Software Library (FSL) [52,53] and subsequently visualized using the MRIcron toolbox.

4.3. Differential Gene Expression Analysis

To identify WMH-related genes both in the CN and MCI groups, each group was separately stratified into two subgroups. These subgroups, denoted as the WMH+ and WMH− groups, were distinguished based on the median ln_WMH_TCV. This categorization allowed a comprehensive exploration of WMH-related genetic factors within and between the CN and MCI groups. Differential gene expression analysis between WMH- and WMH+ groups with MCI was undertaken using the *limma* package in R (v4.2) [54]. $|\log2(\text{fold change})| > 0.12$, and $p < 0.05$ were considered as screening thresholds to obtain DEGs. Volcano plots of DEGs were plotted using *ggplot2* in R.

4.4. Enrichment Analysis

Functional enrichment analysis was carried out using three domains of gene ontology (GO), including biological process (BP), cellular component (CC), and molecular function (MF). KEGG pathway analysis was adopted to identify the pathways of biological molecular interaction. GSEA, utilizing annotations from both GO and KEGG, was executed with the *clusterProfiler* R package [55]. Visualization of the results was achieved using *gseaplot2*, with significance set at a threshold of $p < 0.05$.

4.5. Protein–Protein Interactions (PPIs)

All of the DEGs were imported into the STRING online database (https://cn.string-db.org/; accessed on 12 October 2023), a functional protein association network, assembling all known and predicted proteins. The PPI network interactions file with medium confidence scores $\geq$ 0.4 was downloaded. The MCC plugin [56] and MCODE plugin in Cytoscape were used for further analysis of the interaction network and hub genes. The criteria of MCODE were set as degree cutoff = 2, node score cutoff = 0.2, k-core = 2, and max depth = 100. And the top subnetworks were shown using the MCODE plugin. Subsequently, MCODE analysis was performed and the top three modules in each DEG's upregulated and downregulated PPI network were obtained. The hub genes were filtered by the MCC plugin for the top 30 genes.

4.6. Identification and Validation of Feature-Selection Genes Using Machine Learning

The dataset's DEGs were subjected to feature selection using the Boruta algorithm [57] and the SVM-RFE algorithm. Following the execution of these algorithms, we determined the feature-selection genes by identifying the intersection of the selected features, and subsequently integrated them into the machine learning model. Seven machine learning algorithms were used to build models, namely the generalized linear model (GLM), gradient boosting machine (GBM), K-nearest neighbors (KNN), random forest (RF), extreme gradient boosting (XGBoost), support vector machine (SVM), and recursive partition tree (RPART). The data of 304 patients with MCI were randomly divided into the training set (80%) and testing set (20%) according to the ratio of 8:2. In order to assess the robustness of the model, we employed tenfold cross-validation on the training set and repeated it three times. On the training set, seven machine learning algorithms were used to build the models, and the testing set was used to test the effectiveness of the model. The model with the maximum AUC value of the receiver ROC was evaluated as the best model. The R packages used included *Boruta*, *caret*, *e1071*, *pROC*, *XGboost*, and *dplyr*.

4.7. Immune Cell Infiltration

The relative abundances of 28 infiltrating immune cells in the ADNI dataset were quantified using the ssGSEA algorithm. Boxplots were drawn to demonstrate the differential abundances of the 28 infiltrating immune cells.

4.8. The Correlation Analyses of Feature-Selection Genes

Spearman correlations were calculated for the abundances of 28 infiltrating immune cells and FA values, which represent specific fiber bundles susceptible to microvascular damage in the MCI group, with feature-selection genes, followed by visualization using the *pheatmap* package.

4.9. Animal and Cell Experiments
4.9.1. Animal and Cell Model of Alzheimer's Disease

Animal experiments were approved by the Animal Ethics and Experimentation Committee of Shanghai Jiao Tong University, Shanghai, China, and carried out according to the Guide for the Care and Use of Laboratory Animals: Reporting of In Vivo Experiments (ARRIVE) guidelines [58]. Five-month-old $5 \times$FAD and WT mice were purchased from Aniphe Biolaboratory Inc. (n = 5). The mice had free access to food and water ad libitum. Mice were sacrificed one month later (m = 6 month); left brain tissues were obtained for immunofluorescence (IF) staining and right brain tissues for RT-qPCR analysis.

Primary mixed glial cells were prepared from the frontal cortices of grouped male and female post-natal day 2 Sprague Dawley rats from the same litter, purchased from Beijing Vital River Laboratory Animal Technology Co., Ltd. In brief, cerebral cortices were cleaned from all meninges, digested in trypsin, and dissociated into a single-cell suspension by trituration through syringes. The cells were plated onto a Poly-D-lysine 75T bottle and grown in Dulbecco's modified Eagle's media (DMEM) supplemented with 10% inactivated fetal bovine serum (FBS) and 1% antibiotics (P/S, penicillin/streptomycin; NCM). The next day, cells were washed with DMEM to remove debris, and the media were changed twice per week. After 10 days, loosely attached microglia were removed from underlying astrocytes by shaking the bottle at 180 RPM for 30 min at 37 °C. Cells were collected, replated onto dishes in the original culture medium, and allowed to adhere overnight. The next day, the media were replaced with new media. Primary microglia were treated with 5uM Aβ_{1-42} (GL Biochem Ltd., Shanghai, China) for 18 h to construct a cell model of Alzheimer's disease.

4.9.2. IF Staining

Brain tissues were fixed with 4% paraformaldehyde (PFA) for 10 min. For IF staining, the tissue slices were permeabilized with 0.1% Triton X-100 for 10 min, blocked with 1% BSA for 1 h at 37 °C, and then incubated with antibodies against AQP4 (Servicebio, Wuhan, China, GB12529, 1:200), CD31 (R&D, AF3628, 1:200), and Aβ (Abcam, ab201060, 1:200) at 4 °C overnight. The next day, tissue slices were incubated with fluorescent secondary antibodies for 1 h at room temperature. The nuclei were stained with DAPI Fluoromount-G™ (Yeasen, Shanghai, China, 36308ES20) for 10 min prior to imaging.

After the same pre-treatment as before, the cell slides were incubated with antibodies against CD163 (ProteinTech Group, Chicago, IL, USA, Cat No: 16646-1-AP, 1:400) and iba-1 (WAKO, 011-27991) and the next steps are also consistent with the above. Representative regions and cells were selected and photographed.

4.9.3. RNA Extraction and RT-qPCR

RNA was extracted from the cerebral cortex tissues using NGzol reagent (Invitrogen, Waltham, MA, USA, 15596018) and reverse-transcribed to cDNA using the Hifair® II 1st Strand cDNA Synthesis Kit (Yeasen Biotechnology, Shanghai, China, 11119ES60). Primer sequences were obtained from PrimerBank (https://pga.mgh.harvard.edu/primerbank; accessed on 20 October 2023) and synthesized at Synbio Technologies (Suzhou, China) (Table 3). RT-qPCR was performed using the Hieff® qPCR SYBR Green Master Mix (High Rox Plus; Yeasen Biotechnology, 11203ES03) on a 7900HT Fast real-time PCR System. PCR amplification was conducted in triplicate for each sample, and the expression of target genes was normalized to GAPDH. Relative expression was determined using the $2^{-\Delta\Delta Ct}$ method.

Table 3. The RT-PCR primer.

Gene	Primer
CD163 (mouse)	CD163-F AATCACATCATGGCACAGGTCACC CD163-R TCGTCGCTTCAGAGTCCACAGG
GADPH (mouse)	GAPDH-F GGCAAATTCAACGGCACAGTCAAG GAPDH-R TCGCTCCTGGAAGATGGTGATGG

4.10. Statistical Analysis

Differences between two groups were assessed using the Student's t-test. For comparisons involving three groups, in the analysis of normally distributed continuous variables, group characteristics were compared using a one-way analysis of variance (ANOVA), followed by a Bonferroni multiple-comparison post-hoc test. In cases where the assumption of equal variance was violated, Tamhane's T2 test was applied [59]. The Kruskal-Wallis test for continuous variables with skewed distribution and the chi-square test for categorical variables were also used. All clinical statistical analyses were performed using IBM SPSS Statistics (version 26.0), and experimental data analyses were performed using GraphPad Prism 9 (GraphPad Software Inc., La Jolla, CA, USA). A two-tailed p-value of <0.05 was considered statistically significant.

5. Conclusions

Utilizing the ADNI database and combining the comprehensive reports showed that CD163 is related to small-vessel injury in AD patients. Subsequent validation studies revealed a potential correlation between CD163 and small-vessel injury in the cortical tissue of 5×FAD mice. Additionally, we conducted an analysis of the correlation among the expression levels of feature-selection genes, the abundance of infiltrating immune cells, and DTI indices in brain regions affected by small-vessel injury. These insights may contribute to an enhanced comprehension of the pathological mechanisms of MCI, specifically in relation to small-vessel injury. Furthermore, we suggest that high-risk individuals take measures aimed at preventing microvascular damage, including the control of vascular risk factors such as hypertension, diabetes, hyperlipidemia, etc., as well as the promotion of healthy lifestyles, especially limiting alcohol consumption and embracing an anti-inflammatory dietary regimen.

In conclusion, this research may serve as a predictive tool for estimating the conversion probability from being CN to having MCI and provide novel insights into the physiological mechanisms of early AD with small-vessel injury.

Supplementary Materials: The following supporting information can be downloaded at: https://www.mdpi.com/article/10.3390/ijms25042293/s1.

Author Contributions: Q.X. and Z.Z. conceived the project, designed the experiments, and revised the manuscript. Y.C. and P.L. cleaned, collected, and analyzed the data, and drafted the manuscript and figures. S.W. constructed animal and cell experiments. S.W., J.Y. and W.L. advised on experimental design and data analysis. Q.X. and Z.Z. administrated the project and provided the funding. All authors have read and agreed to the published version of the manuscript.

Funding: This study was supported by grants from the Shanghai Science and Technology Committee Project (Natural Science Funding; No. 23ZR1439200), the National Key R&D Program of China (2022YFA1603604 [ZZ]), and the National Natural Science Foundation of China (82271320 [ZZ]).

Institutional Review Board Statement: Animal experiments were conducted in accordance with the Animal Research: Reporting of In Vivo Experiments (ARRIVE) guidelines and received approval from the Institutional Animal Care and Use Committee of Shanghai Jiao Tong University, Shanghai, China (Project identification code: 20220309, date of approval: 1 March 2022).

Informed Consent Statement: Not applicable.

Data Availability Statement: All data is available from ADNI (https://adni.loni.usc.edu/).

Acknowledgments: Data collection and sharing for this project was funded by the Alzheimer's Disease Neuroimaging Initiative (ADNI) (National Institutes of Health Grant U01 AG024904) and DOD ADNI (Department of Defense award number W81XWH-12-2-0012). The ADNI is funded by the National Institute on Aging, the National Institute of Biomedical Imaging and Bioengineering, and through generous contributions from the following: AbbVie, Alzheimer's Association; Alzheimer's Drug Discovery Foundation; Araclon Biotech; BioClinica, Inc.; Biogen; Bristol-Myers Squibb Company; CereSpir, Inc.; Cogstate; Eisai Inc.; Elan Pharmaceuticals, Inc.; Eli Lilly and Company; EuroImmun; F. Hoffmann-La Roche Ltd. and its affiliated company Genentech, Inc.; Fujirebio; GE Healthcare; IXICO Ltd.; Janssen Alzheimer Immunotherapy Research & Development, LLC.; Johnson & Johnson Pharmaceutical Research & Development LLC.; Lumosity; Lundbeck; Merck & Co., Inc.; Meso Scale Diagnostics, LLC.; NeuroRx Research; Neurotrack Technologies; Novartis Pharmaceuticals Corporation; Pfizer Inc.; Piramal Imaging; Servier; Takeda Pharmaceutical Company; and Transition Therapeutics. The Canadian Institutes of Health Research provides funds to support ADNI clinical sites in Canada. Private sector contributions are facilitated by the Foundation for the National Institutes of Health (www.fnih.org). The grantee organization is the Northern California Institute for Research and Education, and the study was coordinated by the Alzheimer's Therapeutic Research Institute at the University of Southern California. ADNI data are disseminated by the Laboratory for Neuro Imaging at the University of Southern California.

Conflicts of Interest: The authors declare no conflicts of interest.

References

1. Jia, L.; Du, Y.; Chu, L.; Zhang, Z.; Li, F.; Lyu, D.; Li, Y.; Li, Y.; Zhu, M.; Jiao, H.; et al. Prevalence, risk factors, and management of dementia and mild cognitive impairment in adults aged 60 years or older in China: A cross-sectional study. *Lancet Public Health* **2020**, *5*, e661–e671. [CrossRef] [PubMed]
2. Scheltens, P.; De Strooper, B.; Kivipelto, M.; Holstege, H.; Chételat, G.; Teunissen, C.E.; Cummings, J.; van der Flier, W.M. Alzheimer's disease. *Lancet* **2021**, *397*, 1577–1590. [CrossRef] [PubMed]
3. Vinters, H.V. Emerging concepts in Alzheimer's disease. *Annu. Rev. Pathol.* **2015**, *10*, 291–319. [CrossRef]
4. Wardlaw, J.M.; Smith, E.E.; Biessels, G.J.; Cordonnier, C.; Fazekas, F.; Frayne, R.; Lindley, R.I.; O'Brien, J.T.; Barkhof, F.; Benavente, O.R.; et al. Neuroimaging standards for research into small vessel disease and its contribution to ageing and neurodegeneration. *Lancet Neurol.* **2013**, *12*, 822–838. [CrossRef] [PubMed]
5. Yoshita, M.; Fletcher, E.; Harvey, D.; Ortega, M.; Martinez, O.; Mungas, D.M.; Reed, B.R.; DeCarli, C.S. Extent and distribution of white matter hyperintensities in normal aging, MCI, and AD. *Neurology* **2006**, *67*, 2192–2198. [CrossRef] [PubMed]
6. Gertje, E.C.; van Westen, D.; Panizo, C.; Mattsson-Carlgren, N.; Hansson, O. Association of Enlarged Perivascular Spaces and Measures of Small Vessel and Alzheimer Disease. *Neurology* **2021**, *96*, e193–e202. [CrossRef] [PubMed]
7. Zlokovic, B.V. Neurovascular pathways to neurodegeneration in Alzheimer's disease and other disorders. *Nat. Rev. Neurosci.* **2011**, *12*, 723–738. [CrossRef] [PubMed]
8. Graff-Radford, J.; Arenaza-Urquijo, E.M.; Knopman, D.S.; Schwarz, C.G.; Brown, R.D.; Rabinstein, A.A.; Gunter, J.L.; Senjem, M.L.; Przybelski, S.A.; Lesnick, T.; et al. White matter hyperintensities: Relationship to amyloid and tau burden. *Brain* **2019**, *142*, 2483–2491. [CrossRef]
9. Ottoy, J.; Ozzoude, M.; Zukotynski, K.; Adamo, S.; Scott, C.; Gaudet, V.; Ramirez, J.; Swardfager, W.; Cogo-Moreira, H.; Lam, B.; et al. Vascular burden and cognition: Mediating roles of neurodegeneration and amyloid PET. *Alzheimer's Dement.* **2022**, *19*, 1503–1517. [CrossRef]
10. Garnier-Crussard, A.; Bougacha, S.; Wirth, M.; Dautricourt, S.; Sherif, S.; Landeau, B.; Gonneaud, J.; De Flores, R.; de la Sayette, V.; Vivien, D.; et al. White matter hyperintensity topography in Alzheimer's disease and links to cognition. *Alzheimer's Dement.* **2021**, *18*, 422–433. [CrossRef]
11. McAleese, K.E.; Miah, M.; Graham, S.; Hadfield, G.M.; Walker, L.; Johnson, M.; Colloby, S.J.; Thomas, A.J.; DeCarli, C.; Koss, D.; et al. Frontal white matter lesions in Alzheimer's disease are associated with both small vessel disease and AD-associated cortical pathology. *Acta Neuropathol.* **2021**, *142*, 937–950. [CrossRef] [PubMed]
12. Alexander, A.L.; Lee, J.E.; Lazar, M.; Field, A.S. Diffusion tensor imaging of the brain. *Neurotherapeutics* **2007**, *4*, 316–329. [CrossRef] [PubMed]
13. Zhuo, Y.; Fang, F.; Lu, L.; Li, T.; Lian, J.; Xiong, Y.; Kong, D.; Li, K. White matter impairment in type 2 diabetes mellitus with and without microvascular disease. *Neuroimage Clin.* **2019**, *24*, 101945. [CrossRef] [PubMed]
14. Nir, T.M.; Jahanshad, N.; Villalon-Reina, J.E.; Toga, A.W.; Jack, C.R.; Weiner, M.W.; Thompson, P.M.; Alzheimer's Disease Neuroimaging, I. Effectiveness of regional DTI measures in distinguishing Alzheimer's disease, MCI, and normal aging. *Neuroimage Clin.* **2013**, *3*, 180–195. [CrossRef] [PubMed]
15. Yang, Q.; Li, B.; Chen, S.; Tang, J.; Li, Y.; Li, Y.; Zhang, S.; Shi, C.; Zhang, Y.; Mou, M.; et al. MMEASE: Online meta-analysis of metabolomic data by enhanced metabolite annotation, marker selection and enrichment analysis. *J. Proteom.* **2021**, *232*, 104023. [CrossRef]
16. Li, F.; Zhou, Y.; Zhang, Y.; Yin, J.; Qiu, Y.; Gao, J.; Zhu, F. POSREG: Proteomic signature discovered by simultaneously optimizing its reproducibility and generalizability. *Brief. Bioinform.* **2022**, *23*, bbac040. [CrossRef] [PubMed]
17. Fu, J.; Zhang, Y.; Liu, J.; Lian, X.; Tang, J.; Zhu, F. Pharmacometabonomics: Data processing and statistical analysis. *Brief. Bioinform.* **2021**, *22*, bbab138. [CrossRef] [PubMed]
18. Yang, Y.; Cao, Y.; Han, X.; Ma, X.; Li, R.; Wang, R.; Xiao, L.; Xie, L. Revealing EXPH5 as a potential diagnostic gene biomarker of the late stage of COPD based on machine learning analysis. *Comput. Biol. Med.* **2023**, *154*, 106621. [CrossRef]
19. Cheng, Z.Z.; Gao, F.; Lv, X.Y.; Wang, Q.; Wu, Y.; Sun, B.L.; Shen, Y. Features of Cerebral Small Vessel Disease Contributes to the Differential Diagnosis of Alzheimer's Disease. *J. Alzheimers Dis.* **2023**, *91*, 795–804. [CrossRef]
20. Apatiga-Perez, R.; Soto-Rojas, L.O.; Campa-Cordoba, B.B.; Luna-Viramontes, N.I.; Cuevas, E.; Villanueva-Fierro, I.; Ontiveros-Torres, M.A.; Bravo-Munoz, M.; Flores-Rodriguez, P.; Garces-Ramirez, L.; et al. Neurovascular dysfunction and vascular amyloid accumulation as early events in Alzheimer's disease. *Metab. Brain Dis.* **2022**, *37*, 39–50. [CrossRef]
21. Eisenmenger, L.B.; Peret, A.; Famakin, B.M.; Spahic, A.; Roberts, G.S.; Bockholt, J.H.; Johnson, K.M.; Paulsen, J.S. Vascular contributions to Alzheimer's disease. *Transl. Res.* **2023**, *254*, 41–53. [CrossRef] [PubMed]
22. Groechel, R.C.; Tripodis, Y.; Alosco, M.L.; Mez, J.; Qiao Qiu, W.; Goldstein, L.; Budson, A.E.; Kowall, N.W.; Shaw, L.M.; Weiner, M.; et al. Biomarkers of Alzheimer's disease in Black and/or African American Alzheimer's Disease Neuroimaging Initiative (ADNI) participants. *Neurobiol. Aging* **2023**, *131*, 144–152. [CrossRef] [PubMed]
23. Kristiansen, M.; Graversen, J.H.; Jacobsen, C.; Sonne, O.; Hoffman, H.J.; Law, S.K.; Moestrup, S.K. Identification of the haemoglobin scavenger receptor. *Nature* **2001**, *409*, 198–201. [CrossRef] [PubMed]
24. Pey, P.; Pearce, R.K.; Kalaitzakis, M.E.; Griffin, W.S.; Gentleman, S.M. Phenotypic profile of alternative activation marker CD163 is different in Alzheimer's and Parkinson's disease. *Acta Neuropathol. Commun.* **2014**, *2*, 21. [CrossRef] [PubMed]

25. Nguyen, A.T.; Wang, K.; Hu, G.; Wang, X.; Miao, Z.; Azevedo, J.A.; Suh, E.; Van Deerlin, V.M.; Choi, D.; Roeder, K.; et al. APOE and TREM2 regulate amyloid-responsive microglia in Alzheimer's disease. *Acta Neuropathol.* **2020**, *140*, 477–493. [CrossRef]
26. Nissen, S.K.; Shrivastava, K.; Schulte, C.; Otzen, D.E.; Goldeck, D.; Berg, D.; Moller, H.J.; Maetzler, W.; Romero-Ramos, M. Alterations in Blood Monocyte Functions in Parkinson's Disease. *Mov. Disord.* **2019**, *34*, 1711–1721. [CrossRef] [PubMed]
27. Zhu, M.; Hou, T.; Jia, L.; Tan, Q.; Qiu, Y.; Du, Y.; Alzheimer's Disease Neuroimaging, I. Development and validation of a 13-gene signature associated with immune function for the detection of Alzheimer's disease. *Neurobiol. Aging* **2023**, *125*, 62–73. [CrossRef] [PubMed]
28. Yang, A.C.; Vest, R.T.; Kern, F.; Lee, D.P.; Agam, M.; Maat, C.A.; Losada, P.M.; Chen, M.B.; Schaum, N.; Khoury, N.; et al. A human brain vascular atlas reveals diverse mediators of Alzheimer's risk. *Nature* **2022**, *603*, 885–892. [CrossRef]
29. Guo, L.; Akahori, H.; Harari, E.; Smith, S.L.; Polavarapu, R.; Karmali, V.; Otsuka, F.; Gannon, R.L.; Braumann, R.E.; Dickinson, M.H.; et al. CD163+ macrophages promote angiogenesis and vascular permeability accompanied by inflammation in atherosclerosis. *J. Clin. Invest.* **2018**, *128*, 1106–1124. [CrossRef]
30. D'Anci, K.E.; Rosenberg, I.H. Folate and brain function in the elderly. *Curr. Opin. Clin. Nutr. Metab. Care* **2004**, *7*, 659–664. [CrossRef]
31. Dhitavat, S.; Ortiz, D.; Rogers, E.; Rivera, E.; Shea, T.B. Folate, vitamin E, and acetyl-L-carnitine provide synergistic protection against oxidative stress resulting from exposure of human neuroblastoma cells to amyloid-beta. *Brain Res.* **2005**, *1061*, 114–117. [CrossRef] [PubMed]
32. Cazzaniga, E.; Bulbarelli, A.; Lonati, E.; Re, F.; Galimberti, G.; Gatti, E.; Pitto, M.; Ferrarese, C.; Masserini, M. Enhanced folate binding of cultured fibroblasts from Alzheimer's disease patients. *Neurosci. Lett.* **2008**, *436*, 317–320. [CrossRef] [PubMed]
33. Padilla, J.; Jenkins, N.T.; Thorne, P.K.; Martin, J.S.; Rector, R.S.; Davis, J.W.; Laughlin, M.H. Identification of genes whose expression is altered by obesity throughout the arterial tree. *Physiol. Genom.* **2014**, *46*, 821–832. [CrossRef] [PubMed]
34. Puig-Kröger, A.; Sierra-Filardi, E.; Domínguez-Soto, A.; Samaniego, R.; Corcuera, M.T.; Gómez-Aguado, F.; Ratnam, M.; Sánchez-Mateos, P.; Corbí, A.L. Folate Receptor β Is Expressed by Tumor-Associated Macrophages and Constitutes a Marker for M2 Anti-inflammatory/Regulatory Macrophages. *Cancer Res.* **2009**, *69*, 9395–9403. [CrossRef] [PubMed]
35. Nalio Ramos, R.; Missolo-Koussou, Y.; Gerber-Ferder, Y.; Bromley, C.P.; Bugatti, M.; Núñez, N.G.; Tosello Boari, J.; Richer, W.; Menger, L.; Denizeau, J.; et al. Tissue-resident FOLR2(+) macrophages associate with CD8(+) T cell infiltration in human breast cancer. *Cell* **2022**, *185*, 1189–1207.e1125. [CrossRef] [PubMed]
36. Chinju, A.; Moriyama, M.; Kakizoe-Ishiguro, N.; Chen, H.; Miyahara, Y.; Haque, A.; Furusho, K.; Sakamoto, M.; Kai, K.; Kibe, K.; et al. CD163+ M2 Macrophages Promote Fibrosis in IgG4-Related Disease Via Toll-like Receptor 7/Interleukin-1 Receptor-Associated Kinase 4/NF-κB Signaling. *Arthritis Rheumatol.* **2022**, *74*, 892–901. [CrossRef] [PubMed]
37. Escribese, M.M.; Sierra-Filardi, E.; Nieto, C.; Samaniego, R.; Sanchez-Torres, C.; Matsuyama, T.; Calderon-Gomez, E.; Vega, M.A.; Salas, A.; Sanchez-Mateos, P.; et al. The prolyl hydroxylase PHD3 identifies proinflammatory macrophages and its expression is regulated by activin A. *J. Immunol.* **2012**, *189*, 1946–1954. [CrossRef]
38. Yunna, C.; Mengru, H.; Lei, W.; Weidong, C. Macrophage M1/M2 polarization. *Eur. J. Pharmacol.* **2020**, *877*, 173090. [CrossRef]
39. Deza-Ponzio, R.; Herrera, M.L.; Bellini, M.J.; Virgolini, M.B.; Hereñú, C.B. Aldehyde dehydrogenase 2 in the spotlight: The link between mitochondria and neurodegeneration. *Neurotoxicology* **2018**, *68*, 19–24. [CrossRef]
40. Ueno, M.; Yoshino, Y.; Mori, H.; Funahashi, Y.; Kumon, H.; Ochi, S.; Ozaki, T.; Tachibana, A.; Yoshida, T.; Shimizu, H.; et al. Association Study and Meta-Analysis of Polymorphisms and Blood mRNA Expression of the ALDH2 Gene in Patients with Alzheimer's Disease. *J. Alzheimers Dis.* **2022**, *87*, 863–871. [CrossRef]
41. Marchitti, S.A.; Brocker, C.; Orlicky, D.J.; Vasiliou, V. Molecular characterization, expression analysis, and role of ALDH3B1 in the cellular protection against oxidative stress. *Free Radic. Biol. Med.* **2010**, *49*, 1432–1443. [CrossRef] [PubMed]
42. Cao, Y.; Su, N.; Zhang, D.; Zhou, L.; Yao, M.; Zhang, S.; Cui, L.; Zhu, Y.; Ni, J. Correlation between total homocysteine and cerebral small vessel disease: A Mendelian randomization study. *Eur. J. Neurol.* **2021**, *28*, 1931–1938. [CrossRef] [PubMed]
43. Kishi, N.; Tang, Z.; Maeda, Y.; Hirai, A.; Mo, R.; Ito, M.; Suzuki, S.; Nakao, K.; Kinoshita, T.; Kadesch, T.; et al. Murine homologs of deltex define a novel gene family involved in vertebrate Notch signaling and neurogenesis. *Int. J. Dev. Neurosci.* **2001**, *19*, 21–35. [CrossRef] [PubMed]
44. Takeyama, K.; Aguiar, R.C.; Gu, L.; He, C.; Freeman, G.J.; Kutok, J.L.; Aster, J.C.; Shipp, M.A. The BAL-binding protein BBAP and related Deltex family members exhibit ubiquitin-protein isopeptide ligase activity. *J. Biol. Chem.* **2003**, *278*, 21930–21937. [CrossRef] [PubMed]
45. Zhang, L.; Li, C.; Su, X. Emerging impact of the long noncoding RNA MIR22HG on proliferation and apoptosis in multiple human cancers. *J. Exp. Clin. Cancer Res.* **2020**, *39*, 271. [CrossRef] [PubMed]
46. Huang, C.; Yang, S.; Ge, R.; Sun, H.; Shen, F.; Wang, Y. ZNF23 induces apoptosis in human ovarian cancer cells. *Cancer Lett.* **2008**, *266*, 135–143. [CrossRef] [PubMed]
47. Weiner, M.W.; Veitch, D.P.; Aisen, P.S.; Beckett, L.A.; Cairns, N.J.; Cedarbaum, J.; Donohue, M.C.; Green, R.C.; Harvey, D.; Jack, C.R., Jr.; et al. Impact of the Alzheimer's Disease Neuroimaging Initiative, 2004 to 2014. *Alzheimer's Dement.* **2015**, *11*, 865–884. [CrossRef] [PubMed]
48. Kalaria, R.N.; Sepulveda-Falla, D. Cerebral Small Vessel Disease in Sporadic and Familial Alzheimer Disease. *Am. J. Pathol.* **2021**, *191*, 1888–1905. [CrossRef]

49. Sperber, C.; Hakim, A.; Gallucci, L.; Seiffge, D.; Rezny-Kasprzak, B.; Jäger, E.; Meinel, T.; Wiest, R.; Fischer, U.; Arnold, M.; et al. A typology of cerebral small vessel disease based on imaging markers. *J. Neurol.* **2023**, *270*, 4985–4994. [CrossRef]
50. Xia, Y.; Shen, Y.; Wang, Y.; Yang, L.; Wang, Y.; Li, Y.; Liang, X.; Zhao, Q.; Wu, J.; Chu, S.; et al. White matter hyperintensities associated with progression of cerebral small vessel disease: A 7-year Chinese urban community study. *Aging* **2020**, *12*, 8506–8522. [CrossRef]
51. Wang, J.; Wang, X.; Xia, M.; Liao, X.; Evans, A.; He, Y. GRETNA: A graph theoretical network analysis toolbox for imaging connectomics. *Front. Hum. Neurosci.* **2015**, *9*, 386. [CrossRef]
52. Jenkinson, M.; Beckmann, C.F.; Behrens, T.E.; Woolrich, M.W.; Smith, S.M. FSL. *Neuroimage* **2012**, *62*, 782–790. [CrossRef]
53. FMRIB, UK. FMRIB Software Library. Available online: https://fsl.fmrib.ox.ac.uk/fsl/fslwiki/ (accessed on 18 October 2023).
54. Ritchie, M.E.; Phipson, B.; Wu, D.; Hu, Y.; Law, C.W.; Shi, W.; Smyth, G.K. limma powers differential expression analyses for RNA-sequencing and microarray studies. *Nucleic Acids Res.* **2015**, *43*, e47. [CrossRef] [PubMed]
55. Wu, T.; Hu, E.; Xu, S.; Chen, M.; Guo, P.; Dai, Z.; Feng, T.; Zhou, L.; Tang, W.; Zhan, L.; et al. clusterProfiler 4.0: A universal enrichment tool for interpreting omics data. *Innovation* **2021**, *2*, 100141. [CrossRef]
56. Chin, C.H.; Chen, S.H.; Wu, H.H.; Ho, C.W.; Ko, M.T.; Lin, C.Y. cytoHubba: Identifying hub objects and sub-networks from complex interactome. *BMC Syst. Biol.* **2014**, *8* (Suppl. 4), S11. [CrossRef] [PubMed]
57. Kursa, M.B.; Rudnicki, W.R. Feature Selection with the Boruta Package. *J. Stat. Softw.* **2010**, *36*, 1–13. [CrossRef]
58. Percie du Sert, N.; Hurst, V.; Ahluwalia, A.; Alam, S.; Avey, M.T.; Baker, M.; Browne, W.J.; Clark, A.; Cuthill, I.C.; Dirnagl, U.; et al. The ARRIVE guidelines 2.0: Updated guidelines for reporting animal research. *BMJ Open Sci.* **2020**, *4*, e100115. [CrossRef] [PubMed]
59. Lee, S.; Lee, D.K. What is the proper way to apply the multiple comparison test? *Korean J. Anesthesiol.* **2018**, *71*, 353–360. [CrossRef] [PubMed]

Disclaimer/Publisher's Note: The statements, opinions and data contained in all publications are solely those of the individual author(s) and contributor(s) and not of MDPI and/or the editor(s). MDPI and/or the editor(s) disclaim responsibility for any injury to people or property resulting from any ideas, methods, instructions or products referred to in the content.

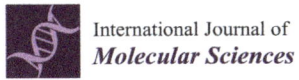

International Journal of Molecular Sciences

Article

Short- and Long-Term Regulation of HuD: A Molecular Switch Mediated by Folic Acid?

Nicoletta Marchesi [1,*,†], Pasquale Linciano [2,†], Lucrezia Irene Maria Campagnoli [1], Foroogh Fahmideh [1], Daniela Rossi [2], Giosuè Costa [3,4,5], Francesca Alessandra Ambrosio [3], Annalisa Barbieri [1], Simona Collina [2] and Alessia Pascale [1,*]

1. Department of Drug Sciences, Pharmacology Section, University of Pavia, 27100 Pavia, Italy; lucreziairenem.campagnoli01@universitadipavia.it (L.I.M.C.); foroogh.fahmidehtavako01@universitadipavia.it (F.F.); annalisa.barbieri@unipv.it (A.B.)
2. Department of Drug Sciences, Medicinal Chemistry Section, University of Pavia, 27100 Pavia, Italy; pasquale.linciano@unipv.it (P.L.); daniela.rossi@unipv.it (D.R.); simona.collina@unipv.it (S.C.)
3. Department of Experimental and Clinical Medicine, University "Magna Græcia" of Catanzaro, Campus "S. Venuta", 88100 Catanzaro, Italy; gcosta@unicz.it (G.C.); ambrosio@unicz.it (F.A.A.)
4. Net4Science Academic Spin-Off, University "Magna Græcia" of Catanzaro, 88100 Catanzaro, Italy
5. Associazione CRISEA-Centro di Ricerca e Servizi Avanzati per l'Innovazione Rurale, 88055 Catanzaro, Italy
* Correspondence: nicoletta.marchesi@unipv.it (N.M.); alessia.pascale@unipv.it (A.P.)
† These authors contributed equally to this work.

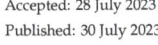

Citation: Marchesi, N.; Linciano, P.; Campagnoli, L.I.M.; Fahmideh, F.; Rossi, D.; Costa, G.; Ambrosio, F.A.; Barbieri, A.; Collina, S.; Pascale, A. Short- and Long-Term Regulation of HuD: A Molecular Switch Mediated by Folic Acid? *Int. J. Mol. Sci.* **2023**, 24, 12201. https://doi.org/10.3390/ijms241512201

Academic Editor: Ludmilla A. Morozova-Roche

Received: 28 June 2023
Revised: 25 July 2023
Accepted: 28 July 2023
Published: 30 July 2023

Copyright: © 2023 by the authors. Licensee MDPI, Basel, Switzerland. This article is an open access article distributed under the terms and conditions of the Creative Commons Attribution (CC BY) license (https://creativecommons.org/licenses/by/4.0/).

Abstract: The RNA-binding protein HuD has been shown to play a crucial role in gene regulation in the nervous system and is involved in various neurological and psychiatric diseases. In this study, through the creation of an interaction network on HuD and its potential targets, we identified a strong association between HuD and several diseases of the nervous system. Specifically, we focused on the relationship between HuD and the brain-derived neurotrophic factor (BDNF), whose protein is implicated in several neuronal diseases and is involved in the regulation of neuronal development, survival, and function. To better investigate this relationship and given that we previously demonstrated that folic acid (FA) is able to directly bind HuD itself, we performed in vitro experiments in neuron-like human SH-SY5Y cells in the presence of FA, also known to be a pivotal environmental factor influencing the nervous system development. Our findings show that FA exposure results in a significant increase in both HuD and BDNF transcripts and proteins after 2 and 4 h of treatment, respectively. Similar data were obtained after 2 h of FA incubation followed by 2 h of washout. This increase was no longer detected upon 24 h of FA exposure, probably due to a signaling shutdown mechanism. Indeed, we observed that following 24 h of FA exposure HuD is methylated. These findings indicate that FA regulates BDNF expression via HuD and suggest that FA can behave as an epigenetic modulator of HuD in the nervous system acting via short- and long-term mechanisms. Finally, the present results also highlight the potential of BDNF as a therapeutic target for specific neurological and psychiatric diseases.

Keywords: ELAV/HuD; BDNF; folic acid; neurodegenerative diseases; Alzheimer's disease

1. Introduction

Neurodegenerative diseases (NDs) are a heterogeneous group of diseases characterized by a progressive loss of function of the autonomic, peripheral, or central nervous system (CNS). These include Alzheimer's disease (AD), Parkinson's disease, multiple sclerosis, amyotrophic lateral sclerosis, and other neurological disorders. The WHO ranked NDs at 7th place in the leading causes of death worldwide. Moreover, the health, economic, and social burden caused by NDs is expected to dramatically rise in the next few decades as a result of the global population growth and aging. Therefore, the WHO recognized NDs as a global public health problem and included them in the top four challenging diseases that medicine and pharmacology should quickly address in the near future. The current, yet decade-old, pharmacological treatments for NDs are mainly symptomatic or focused on slowing down as much as possible the progression of the disease. For instance, concerning AD, in 2021, after 20 years of research failures in this field, FDA approved aducanumab, a monoclonal antibody able to target oligomeric and fibrillary beta-amyloid (Ab) protein aggregates in the brain, hence interrupting amyloid aggregation kinetics. However, reports of serious complications potentially related to the treatment have cast a shadow on that decision. Thus, research on new strategies, targets, and, consequently, new drugs to prevent neurodegeneration or to act as neurodegenerative disease-modifying therapies is still demanding [1]. Among the new putative therapeutic targets, RNA-binding proteins (RBPs), including the ELAV family, have gained attention. RBPs play a prominent role in modulating various aspects of RNA metabolism, including splicing, polyadenylation, nucleo-cytoplasmic shuttling, intracellular localization, stability, and translation of target mRNAs, thus contributing to a dynamic regulation of gene expression. This RBPs-mediated regulation has a strong impact on the levels of proteins that control key cellular functions such as proliferation, development, differentiation, and death. Indeed, a tight regulation of the expression of proteins involved in these biological processes is critical, and its dysregulation is linked to the pathogenesis of several diseases [2–6].

The ELAV family encompasses four members, namely HuR (ELAVL1), HuB (ELAVL2), HuC (ELAVL3), and HuD (ELAVL4) [7,8]. HuR is ubiquitously expressed, and it is mainly implicated in cell growth and cell cycle regulation [6]. Conversely, HuB, HuC, and HuD are the neuron-specific members of the family (nELAV), since they are mainly expressed in the nervous system, and they regulate the fate of target mRNAs coding for pivotal proteins taking part in key functions of neuronal cells. Among all the neuronal RBPs, HuD has been intensively investigated. A number of studies have leveraged the combination of mRNA-RBP complex purification methods and bioinformatic analyses, striving to identify the cellular targets regulated by HuD and thereby elucidating its biological function [9,10]. The gene ontology and the computational biological pathway analyses of identified HuD mRNA targets have unveiled the implication of this RBP in regulating neuronal differentiation and development, nerve regeneration, cellular response towards oxidative stress, repairing of the nervous tissue after nerve injury, as well as synaptic plasticity and memory processes [11–17]. Interestingly, recent research revealed that HuD may also indirectly regulate mRNA levels by controlling the expression of non-coding RNAs such as circular RNAs (circRNAs) and microRNAs (miRNAs). Indeed, deletion of HuD in the striatum has been observed to alter the levels of circRNAs and miRNAs and to affect their interactions with mRNAs. Bioinformatic analyses detected HuD-binding adenine/uracil-rich elements (ARE) in approximately 26% of brain-expressed circRNAs, indicating that HuD interactions with circRNAs might regulate their expression and transport. The subsequent alterations in HuD-regulated circRNA networks could thus influence neuronal differentiation and synaptic plasticity. Further bioinformatic examination of differentially expressed miRNAs revealed that the most likely mRNA targets of these miRNAs are associated with biological pathways and networks linked to transcriptional and epigenetic regulators (i.e., Jun, EGR3, MECP2, HDAC 1 and 9, and SMARC2), including BDNF and its associated proteins. Interestingly, the two foremost biological networks of these targets center on two proteins associated with neurodegeneration: the amyloid precursor protein (APP), which is linked to Alzheimer's disease, and Huntingtin (HTT), a genetic mutation associated with Huntington's disease [18].

As a result, alterations in the expression of HuD-targeted mRNAs are associated with neurodegeneration and mood disorders, epilepsy, schizophrenia, and intellectual disabilities [15,19,20]. Moreover, alterations in HuD activity through different post-translational modifications, including phosphorylation, ubiquitination, and sumoylation, can alter the binding affinity of HuD for its target mRNAs. As an example, phosphorylation of HuD in threonine residues by PKCα has been shown to modulate the stability of its down-stream target GAP-43 mRNA and to affect nELAV/HuD localization, also favoring HuD binding with polysomes [21,22]. Also, PKCα-mediated HuD phosphorylation is able to counteract an ADAM10 deficit following Aβ challenge [23]. Furthermore, methylation of HuD in arginine residues by CARM1 (coactivator-associated arginine methyltransferase 1) has been shown to reduce HuD function and the binding with its target mRNAs, leading to their decreased post-transcriptional regulation. Conversely, an increase in non-methylated, HuD favors binding with the neuronal mRNA targets, promoting differentiation and elongation of neurites, and contributing to the proper development of the nervous system [24].

Accordingly, these findings suggest HuD as a novel target for the development of brand-new pharmacological interventions aimed at counteracting NDs. In addition to the comprehensive biochemical and functional characterization of HuD, the availability of crystallographic structures for the first two RNA recognition motif (RRM) domains of the HuD protein in complex with C-FOS mRNA (PDB ID: 1FXL) and TNFα mRNA (PDB ID: 1G2E [25]), together with a combined NMR and in silico approaches, has contributed to the expansion of our understanding of the structural characteristics of the protein domains interacting with the target mRNAs and the postulation of a putative ligand-binding site [19,26–30]. These insights pave the way for Structure-based Drug Design.

Starting from these premises, we performed a drug repurposing study that allowed the identification of new ligands able to bind HuD, thus potentially influencing the formation of HuD-mRNA complexes. More in detail, by combining a virtual screening of natural compounds and FDA-approved drugs databases and STD-NMR studies, we selected folic acid (FA), rosmarinic acid, cefazolin, and enalapril maleate. Molecular dynamics studies performed to further investigate the ligand–protein interaction profile further support STD-NMR results, suggesting FA as the most attractive HuD binder (Figure 1; see also [31]).

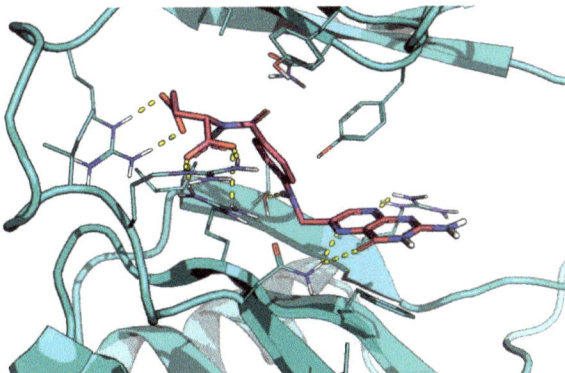

Figure 1. Predicted docking pose of folic acid (stick, violet carbon) at the HuD RNA-recognition motifs (RRMs)-1 and -2 binding site (teal cartoon). Important interacting residues are in the stick representation. Model atoms, except for carbons, are color-coded with oxygen (red) and nitrogen (blue). H-bonds are represented as yellow dotted lines.

FA, also known as vitamin B9, has fundamental roles in CNS function at all ages, and it has been recognized as a crucial environmental factor for the nervous system development. From the early fetal stages of the formation of the presumptive spinal cord and brain to the maturation and maintenance of the nervous system during infancy and childhood, as well as during the entire adult life, folate levels and their supplementation have been considered influential in the clinical outcomes of neurological diseases. Moreover, several studies proved the role of FA in the prevention of CNS developmental disorders, mood disorders, and dementias, including AD and vascular dementia. However, notwithstanding the vast epidemiological information recorded on folate function and neural tube defects, neural development, and neurodegenerative diseases, the mechanisms of folate action in the developing neural tissue is remaining still elusive.

Given the involvement of HuD in the maintenance and function of the CNS, our identification of FA as a potential ligand of HuD represented another brick in the wall to unravel the mechanism of action of FA at CNS level.

Accordingly, to gain a deeper insight into the effect of FA on HuD, in this study, we investigated at the cellular level the impact of FA on HuD expression, and we explored how this modulation influenced the regulation of specific HuD down-stream targets, crucial for maintaining a proper CNS function or for being involved in the development of NDs selected through the creation of a protein–protein interaction network.

2. Results

2.1. Protein–Protein Interaction Network of the Targets Controlled by HuD

The PPI network generated by STRING consisted of 33 nodes (Figure 2) and 76 edges. The number of edges is significantly larger than the one expected for a random network of the same size (degree $\leq$ 10–16); the nodes were more connected than randomly distributed. It suggested that the PPI network could be considered as a relatively small world in comparison with the random graph, and the proteins might be biologically relevant. The results of the topological analyses showed that BDNF was a hub extensively connected with their neighbors in the network (with the largest being k = 14) and the bottleneck had significant control over the network (BC = 0.151) in the PPI network. Moreover, BDNF is involved in 9 out of the 13 CNS-related pathological pathways examined (i.e., Huntington disease, amnestic disorder, toxic encephalopathy, cognitive disorder). BDNF is a neurotrophin that emerged as a key regulator of neuronal survival and differentiation, and it is strongly implicated in synaptic plasticity linked to learning and memory processes. Further, alterations in BDNF levels and signaling have been identified in various NDs and have been also associated with symptom onset and disease progression [32]. Among the 14 targets of HuD involved in neuronal and non–neuronal pathologies interconnected with BDNF, it is noteworthy to point out the interconnection with the Growth Associated Protein 43 (GAP43) [14,33,34], a primary contributor of neurite outgrowth, the Nerve Growth Factor (NGF) [35], which has an impact on neuronal differentiation, neurogenesis, dendritic maturation, neuronal plasticity, synaptic transmission, and neuronal signaling pathways, the Amyloid Precursor Protein (APP), whose abnormal processing leads to the production and accumulation of Aβ peptides, thus contributing to AD pathogenesis [36], and the Vascular Endothelial Growth Factor (VEGF), whose reduced levels or an impaired signaling may take part in NDs progression by compromising the neuroprotective mechanisms [37].

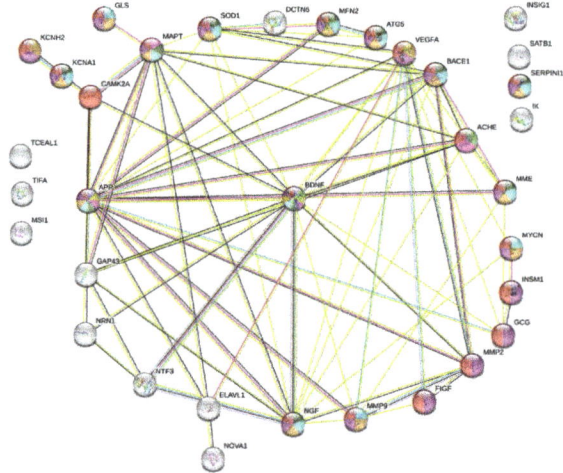

Figure 2. Protein–protein interaction network (PPIN) of the proteins whose mRNA is modulated by HuD and that are implicated in CNS diseases. PPIN was realized by the STRING tool. Nodes that

are strongly connected are positioned closely together and have a greater number of edges entering each node. The nodes of the same color represent the same disease-gene associations with HuD. ACHE: Acetylcholinesterase, APP: Amyloid Precursor Protein, ATG5: autophagy related 5, BACE1: Beta-Secretase 1, BDNF: Brain-derived neurotrophic factor, CAMK2A: Calcium/Calmodulin-Dependent Protein Kinase II Alpha, DCTN6: Dynactin Subunit 6, SOD1: superoxide dismutase 1, ELAVL1: ELAV-like protein 1, GAP43: Growth-Associated Protein 43, GCG: glucagon, GLS: Glutaminase, IK: Ikaros, INSIG1: Insulin-Induced Gene 1, INSM1: Insulinoma-associated protein 1, KCNA1: Potassium Voltage-Gated Channel Subfamily A Member 1, KCNH2: Potassium Voltage-Gated Channel Subfamily H Member 2, MAPT: Microtubule-associated protein tau, MFN2: mitofusin 2, MME: Membrane Metallo endopeptidase, MMP2: Matrix Metallopeptidase 2, MMP9: Matrix Metallopeptidase 9, MSI1: Musashi 1, MYCN: MYCN proto-oncogene, NGF: nerve growth factor, NOVA1: ventral neuron-specific protein 1, NTF3: Neurotrophin 3, NRN1: Neuritin 1, SATB1: special AT-rich sequence-binding protein-1, SERPINI1: Serpin Family I Member 1, TCEAL1: Transcription Elongation Factor A Like 1, TIFA: TRAF Interacting Protein With Forkhead-Associated Domain, VEGFA: Vascular endothelial growth factor A.

2.2. Effect of Folic Acid on Cell Viability and BDNF mRNA Content

The cytotoxicity of FA on human neuroblastoma SH-SY5Y cells was examined via MTT assay at different concentrations (100 nM, 1 µM, and 100 µM) and at both 24 and 48 h of exposure. The results, expressed as a percentage of cell viability, are reported in Figure S1. As expected, FA shows a good safety profile with no significant cell death vs. control at all the tested concentrations and times of exposure.

To identify the optimal concentration of FA to be used in the subsequent experiments, SH-SY5Y cells were treated with 100 nM, 1 µM, and 100 µM FA for 2 h. This timeframe was chosen based on previous experiments and on our own experience as being optimal for BDNF transcriptional activity, mRNA half-life ($t_{1/2}$ 132 ± 30 min) [38], and protein expression. As reported in Figure 3, FA induced a two-fold significative increase in BDNF mRNA levels at 100 nM, whereas no variation in BDNF transcript with respect to the control was detected at higher concentrations (1 and 100 mM). This profile likely indicates a concentration-dependent effect of FA on BDNF transcript content. Based on these results, 100 nM FA was chosen as the optimal concentration for the following experiments.

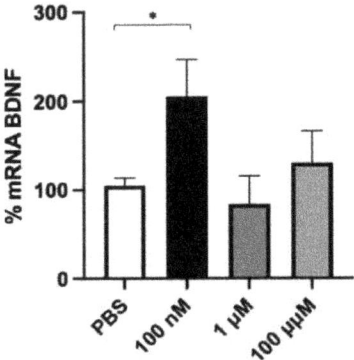

Figure 3. Effect of folic acid on BDNF transcript. SH-SY5Y cells were treated for 2 h with increasing concentrations of folic acid (0.1–1–100 µM) or phosphate-buffered saline (PBS) as vehicle control. mRNA levels were evaluated via RT-PCR. Each value represents the mean ± S.E.M. of independent experiments with respect to the control (100%). Statistical analysis was performed by two-way ANOVA followed by Dunnett's Multiple Comparisons test; * $p < 0.05$ vs. control, $n = 3$ independent samples.

2.3. Effect of Folic Acid on HuD and BDNF Expression

The effect of 100 nM FA on both HuD and BDNF mRNA content and the relative protein expression was evaluated at two timeframes, namely 2 and 4 h. As reported in Figure 4 (panels A and B), FA was able to significantly increase BDNF and HuD mRNA levels after 2 h of treatment, whereas a return to the baseline level for both transcripts was observed after 4 h of incubation.

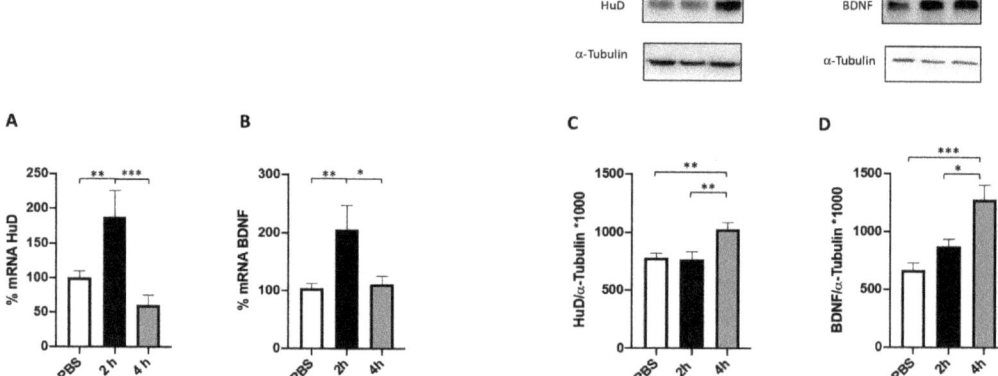

Figure 4. HuD and BDNF expression following 2 and 4 h of folic acid treatment. (**A,B**) Determination of HuD (**A**) and BDNF (**B**) mRNA levels via RT-PCR in SH-SY5Y cells exposed to solvent (phosphate-buffered saline; PBS) or to folic acid (FA) for 2 (2 h) and 4 h (4 h). The amounts of the total mRNA were normalized using the corresponding levels of GAPDH mRNA. The values are expressed as mean percentages ± S.E.M. with respect to the control (100%). * $p < 0.05$, ** $p < 0.01$, *** $p < 0.001$, Tukey's multiple comparisons test, $n = 3$ independent samples. (**C,D**) Representative cropped Western blotting (upper panel) and densitometric analysis (lower panel) of HuD (**C**) and BDNF (**D**) proteins and the respective a-tubulin in the total homogenates of SH-SY5Y cells following exposure to solvent (PBS) or FA for 2 h and 4 h. Results are expressed as mean grey levels ratios (mean ± S.E.M.) of HuD/a-tubulin (**C**) and BDNF/a-tubulin (**D**) ×1000. * $p < 0.05$, ** $p < 0.01$, *** $p < 0.001$, Tukey's multiple comparisons test, $n = 3$–7 independent samples.

To further investigate whether the observed increase in HuD and BDNF mRNA levels after FA treatment translates into an effective promotion of HuD and BDNF protein expression, their protein levels were measured after 2 and 4 h of FA exposure. The obtained results show a significant increase in the amount of both proteins after 4 h of FA exposure, while no changes were observed after 2 h compared to the control (Figure 4, panels C and D). This result is in line with the time lapse between gene transcription and protein expression.

Based on these findings, we then performed a washout period after 2 h of FA treatment to understand if this time of exposure is enough to activate the FA-dependent HuD/BDNF cascade.

The obtained data indicate that a 2-h FA treatment is sufficient to trigger the HuD/BDNF cascade (Figure 5). Indeed, as expected, at this time, we observed an increase in the amount of both HuD and BDNF transcripts with no changes in the corresponding protein content. However, following 2 h of washout, we could detect a significant rise in both HuD and BDNF protein levels, thus mirroring the profile previously observed following 4 h of FA incubation. Following 2 h of washout, we also found a further increase in the mRNA levels of both HuD and BDNF in comparison to the corresponding amounts detected after 2 h of FA only.

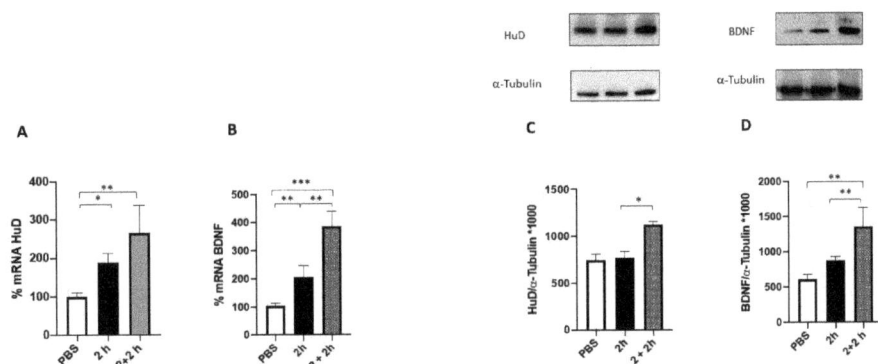

Figure 5. HuD and BDNF expression following 2 h + 2 h of washout of folic acid treatment. (**A,B**) Determination of HuD (**A**) and BDNF (**B**) mRNA levels via RT-PCR in SH-SY5Y cells exposed to solvent (phosphate-buffered saline; PBS) or to folic acid (FA) for 2 h (2 h) and 2 h + 2 h of washout (2 + 2 h). The amounts of the total mRNA were normalized with the corresponding levels of GAPDH mRNA. The values are expressed as mean percentages ± S.E.M. with respect to the control (100%). * $p < 0.05$, ** $p < 0.01$, *** $p < 0.001$, Tukey's multiple comparisons test, $n = 3$ independent samples. (**C,D**) Representative cropped Western blotting (upper panel) and densitometric analysis (lower panel) of HuD (**C**) and BDNF (**D**) proteins and the respective a-tubulin in the total homogenates of SH-SY5Y cells following exposure to solvent (PBS) or FA for 2 h and 2 + 2 h. Results are expressed as mean grey levels ratios (mean ± S.E.M.) of HuD/a-tubulin (**C**) and BDNF/a-tubulin (**D**) ×1000. * $p < 0.05$, ** $p < 0.01$, Tukey's multiple comparisons test, $n = 3$–7 independent samples.

To further investigate the effects of a prolonged FA treatment on BDNF and HuD expression, cells were exposed to FA for 24 h. As shown in Figure 6, no changes were observed in HuD and BDNF expression either at the transcript or protein level.

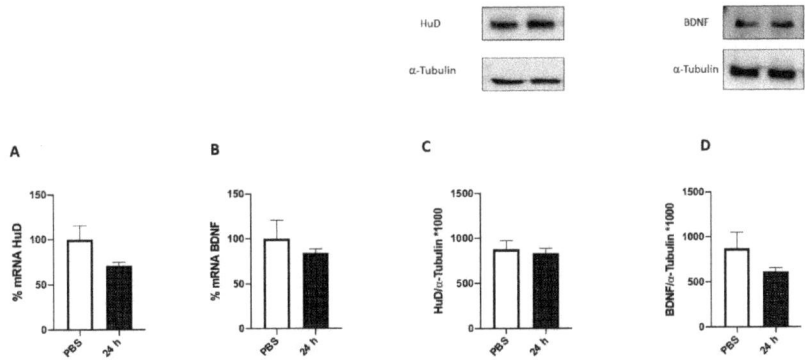

Figure 6. HuD and BDNF expression following 24 h of folic acid treatment. (**A,B**) Determination of HuD (**A**) and BDNF mRNA (**B**) levels via RT-PCR in SH-SY5Y cells exposed to solvent (phosphate-buffered saline; PBS) or folic acid (FA) for 24 h (24 h). The amounts of the total mRNA were normalized with the corresponding levels of GAPDH mRNA. The values are expressed as mean percentages ± S.E.M. with respect to the control (100%). (**C,D**) Representative cropped Western blotting (upper panel) and densitometric analysis (lower panel) of HuD (**C**) and BDNF (**D**) proteins and the respective a-tubulin in the total homogenates of SH-SY5Y cells following exposure to solvent (PBS) or FA for 24 h. Results are expressed as mean grey levels ratios (mean ± S.E.M.) of HuD/a-tubulin (**C**) and BDNF/a-tubulin (**D**) ×1000, $n = 3$–7 independent samples.

2.4. HuD Post-Translational Modification after Prolonged Folic Acid Treatment

Lastly, to obtain further insight into the mechanism by which a prolonged FA exposure might modulate HuD function, and given that FA is a methyl donor, we performed immunoprecipitation experiments to investigate FA-mediated potential post-translational modifications in the HuD protein. In particular, we focused on the implication of arginine methylation, as this modification affects the activity of proteins involved in various cellular pathways, including nuclear-cytoplasmic signaling, transcriptional activation, and posttranscriptional modulation [24,35,39]. As reported in Figure 7, a significant increase in mono-methyl arginine after 24 h of FA exposure, compared to the treatment with PBS alone, was observed. Conversely, no HuD methylation was observed at 2 h of treatment or after washout (2 + 2 h), suggesting that FA specifically induces arginine methylation only after a longer timeframe. In our experimental conditions, this methylation likely affects HuD activity.

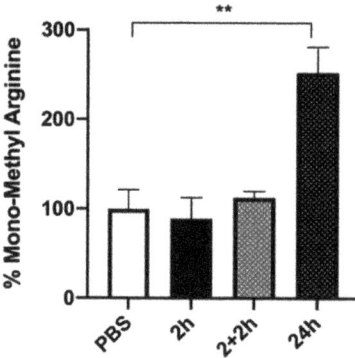

Figure 7. HuD methylation after folic acid treatment. Densitometric analysis of HuD methylation in arginine residues following folic acid exposure for 2 h (2 h), 2 h + 2 h of washout (2 + 2 h), or 24 h. The results are expressed as mean percentages $\pm$ S.E.M. with respect to the control (PBS, 100%). ** $p < 0.001$, Dunnett's multiple comparisons test, n = 3–6 independent samples. PBS: phosphate-buffered saline.

3. Discussion

RBPs are *trans*-acting factors involved in gene regulation at the post-transcriptional level. Through binding to target mRNA molecules, RBPs have a significant impact on their fate, primarily influencing their stability and/or translation [2,40,41]. One of the extensively studied RBPs is the ELAV family of proteins, also known as "Hu" proteins [42]. Among them, HuD activity has been extensively studied in neuronal development, plasticity, and regeneration. Further, in support of its key implication in the CNS, recent studies suggest that HuD misregulation might underlie neurological disorders, including neurodegenerative diseases such as Parkinson's disease, Alzheimer's disease, and amyotrophic lateral sclerosis. Thus, these discoveries emphasize the concept that HuD represents a promising focus for the creation of innovative pharmaceutical interventions intended to combat neurodegenerative disorders.

In this regard, in our previous study, we demonstrated that FA is a HuD binder [31]. Folic acid plays a crucial role in various aspects of CNS development, maintenance, and function. Substantial epidemiological evidence has been gathered on the role of folate in neural tube defects, neural development, and in counteracting neurodegenerative diseases. However, the specific mechanisms through which folate produces its effects have remained unclear, thus requiring further investigation. Based on our previous findings, in this study, we performed a deeper investigation into the effect of FA on HuD at the cellular level with possible future implications in the prevention of NDs. To this aim, the identification of the molecular targets whose expression and regulation is mediated by HuD, as well as a thorough understanding of their reciprocal interactions, was our first goal. Very recently, all the known transcripts controlled by HuD that play an important role in the CNS have been reviewed [43]. We processed the available data into a comprehensive PPI network (Figure 2). The analysis of this network revealed a remarkable degree of interconnections implicating the neuronal targets regulated by HuD. Among them, the BDNF stands out as the hub and bottleneck of the PPI network. Moreover, it is involved in 9 out of the 13 CNS-related pathological pathways examined (i.e., Huntington disease, amnestic disorder, toxic encephalopathy, cognitive disorder), and it is able to interact with an additional 14 targets, all under HuD control and also involved in CNS pathologies. In light of these considerations, we investigated the effects of FA on both the modulation of HuD and on the expression of the down-stream target BDNF.

Prior to conducting the experiments, we confirmed the non-toxic nature of FA through the assessment of mitochondrial activity, ensuring the safety of the concentrations used in the subsequent experiments performed in SHSY5Y neuronal cells. Notably, SH-SY5Y cells are commonly used as an in vitro model for studying neuronal function and disease. As depicted in Figure 4, the results demonstrated that FA exposure leads to a significant increase in both HuD and BDNF transcripts and proteins after 2 and 4 h of treatment, respectively. These data strongly indicate that HuD protein, once activated by FA, not only has a positive effect on its target transcript BDNF, but also acts on itself, thus boosting its own expression through a mechanism of auto-modulation.

Subsequently, we conducted additional experiments where the cells were exposed to folic acid for 2 h followed by a 2-h washout period (2 + 2 h; Figure 5) to assess whether this timeframe was sufficient to activate the HuD/BDNF cascade. Indeed, the results obtained in this experimental setting mirror, for both HuD and BDNF proteins, the profile previously observed following 4 h of FA incubation. Surprisingly, after 2 + 2 h treatment we found a further increase in the mRNA levels of both HuD and BDNF in comparison to the corresponding amounts detected after 2 h of FA only. This finding was unexpected when considering the results obtained following 4 h of FA treatment. In this regard, we may postulate that while a short exposure produces a long-lasting stimulation of the transcriptional phase, a prolonged incubation with FA (i.e., 4 h) can, instead, "freeze" the transcription process itself.

Moreover, the increase in HuD and BDNF expression was no longer detected after 24 h of folic acid exposure (Figure 6). This observation suggests the presence of a signaling shutdown mechanism occurring over time, probably acting on HuD functioning. To test this hypothesis, and given that FA is a methyl donor, which is a process requiring prolonged incubation times, we explored, via immunoprecipitation experiments, possible post-translational modifications in the HuD protein after 24 h of FA exposure. Intriguingly, we observed a methylation of HuD in arginine residues (Figure 7). As previously mentioned, the methylation of HuD in arginine residues has been shown to reduce HuD function and to negatively affect its activity on the down-stream targets [24]. Therefore, we can postulate that following 24 h of incubation, FA acts as an epigenetic modulator of HuD, switching off its activity.

Overall, the obtained results provide evidence for a time-dependent regulation of HuD mediated by folic acid. Namely, while a short-term exposure to FA leads to an increase in HuD activity, a long-term treatment induces a signaling shutdown, likely via methylation of HuD, with a consequent impact on the down-stream processes regulated by HuD, such as BDNF expression.

4. Material and Methods

4.1. Protein–Protein Interaction (PPI) Network

The Search Tool for Retrieval of Interacting Genes (STRING; https://string-db.org, accessed on 29 July 2022) database was exploited to build the PPI network among the CNS targets whose modulation is affected by HuD. Giving a list of proteins as an input, STRING can search for their neighbor interactors, namely the proteins that have direct interaction with the inputted proteins. Then, STRING can generate the PPI network consisting of all these proteins and all the interactions between them [43]. The interactions were analyzed by selecting "Homo sapiens" as organism and setting the confidence basis to 0.4 [44,45]. To evaluate the nodes in the PPI networks, it was imported in Cytoscape for the computing of several topological measures including degree (k) and between centrality (BC). The k and BC values are often used for detecting the hub or bottleneck in a network. The k of a node is defined as the number of edges linked to it. A node with a high k denotes a hub having many neighbors. The BC of a node is the proportion of the number of shortest paths passing through it to the number of all the shortest paths in the network, quantifying how often a node acts as a bridge along the shortest paths between two other nodes. A node with high BC has great influence on what flows in the network and has more control over the network. It can represent the bottleneck in the network. The protein nodes with high k or BC as the hubs or bottlenecks were considered.

4.2. Cell Culture

Human neuroblastoma SH-SY5Y cells were obtained from ATCC (Manassas, VA, USA) and cultured in a humidified incubator at 37 °C with 5% CO_2. The SH-SY5Y cells were grown in Eagle's minimum essential medium (EMEM) supplemented with 10% fetal bovine serum, 1% penicillin–streptomycin, L-glutamine (2 mM), nonessential amino acids (1 mM), and sodium pyruvate (1 mM).

4.3. MTT Assay

Mitochondrial enzymatic activity, as evaluation of the cell viability, was estimated via MTT [3-(4, 5-dimethylthiazol-2-yl)-2,5-diphenyltetrazolium bromide] assay (Sigma-Aldrich, Darmstadt, Germany). An amount of 200 mL of a suspension of 3.5×10^5 cells/well was seeded into 96-well plates. The cells were treated with 100 nM, 1 µM, and 100 µM FA (solubilized in phosphate-buffered saline, PBS) for 24 and 48 h and then subjected to MTT assay following the protocol published in our previous paper [46]. The absorbance values were measured at 595 nm using a Synergy HT microplate reader (BioTek Instruments, Santa Clara, CA, USA), and the results were expressed as % with respect to control.

4.4. Western Blotting

SH-SY5Y cells were treated with 100 nM FA for 2, 4, and 24 h, and then they were homogenized in a specific cell lysis buffer (Cell Signaling Technology, Denvers, CO, USA). Proteins were diluted in 2X sodium dodecyl sulphate (SDS) protein gel loading solution, boiled for 5 min, separated on 12% SDS-polyacrylamide gel electrophoresis (SDS-PAGE), and processed following standard procedures [47]. The mouse monoclonal antibodies were diluted as follows: the anti-ELAVL4/HuD antibody (Sigma-Aldrich, Darmstadt, Germany) at 1:1000; the anti-BDNF (anti-brain-derived neurotrophic factor; Sigma-Aldrich, Darmstadt, Germany) at 1:500; and the anti-α-tubulin (Sigma-Aldrich, Darmstadt, Germany) at 1:1000. The nitrocellulose membrane signals were detected via chemiluminescence (by using WesternBright® ECL HRP substrate, Advansta, San Jose, CA, USA) by means of an Imager Amersham 680 detection system. All the experiments were performed in duplicate. Alpha-tubulin was used for data normalization. Statistical analysis was performed on the densitometric values obtained with the ImageJ image processing program.

4.5. Real-Time Quantitative RT-PCR

RNA was extracted from total homogenates using RNeasy Micro Plus Kit (Qiagen, Hilden, Germany). The reverse transcription was performed following standard procedures. PCR amplifications were carried out using the Rotor-Gene Q (Qiagen, Hilden, Germany) in the presence of QuantiTect SYBR Green PCR mix (Qiagen, Hilden, Germany) with primers predesigned by SIGMA. Primer sequences used were as follows: forward: 5′-CATCGTCAACTATTTACCCC-3′ and reverse: 5′-GTCCTGTAATTTTGTCTCTCAC-3′ (for ELAVL4/HuD); forward: 5′-AACCATAAGGACGCGGACTT-3′ and reverse: 5′-TGCAGTCTTTTTATCTGCCG-3′ (for BDNF); forward: 5′-CAGCAAGAGCACAAGAGGA

AG-3′; and reverse: 5′-CAACTGTGAGGAGGGGAGATT-3′ (for GAPDH). The GAPDH mRNA was chosen as control since it is relatively stable during all the treatments, and it is unaffected by HuD because it does not possess ARE sequences (not shown). ELAVL4/HuD and BDNF mRNA expression was normalized over GAPDH mRNA.

4.6. Immunoprecipitation

Immunoprecipitation was performed according to a previously published protocol with minor modifications [48]. Immunoprecipitation was carried out at room temperature using 1 µg of an anti-HuD antibody (Sigma-Aldrich, Darmstadt, Germany) per 50 µg of total proteins diluted in the immunoprecipitation buffer (50 mM Tris pH7.4, 150 mM NaCl, 1 mM $MgCl_2$, 0.05% Igepal, 20 mM EDTA, 100 mM DTT, protease inhibitor cocktail, and RNAase inhibitor) in the presence of 50 µL A/G plus agarose (Santa Cruz Biotechnology Inc., Dallas, TX, USA). The sample, representing the immunoprecipitated HuD protein, was then subjected to Western blotting using an antibody recognizing methylated residues [Cell Signaling; Mono-Methyl Arginine (R*GG)]. An irrelevant antibody (Santa Cruz Biotechnology Inc., Dallas, TX, USA) with the same isotype as the specific immunoprecipitating antibody served as a negative control.

4.7. Statistical Analysis

The GraphPad Prism statistical package (version 9, San Diego, CA, USA) was used for the statistical analysis. The data were analyzed by analysis of variance (ANOVA) followed, when significant, by an appropriate post hoc comparison test, as detailed in the legends. Differences were considered statistically significant when p-value ≤ 0.05. The results are expressed as mean $\pm$ S.E.M.

5. Conclusions

In conclusion, our findings shed light on the potential neuroprotective effect of folic acid through the upregulation of HuD and BDNF expression. Of interest, considering that decreased levels of BDNF are associated with neurodegenerative diseases, including Alzheimer's and Parkinson's diseases, the observation that FA can increase BDNF expression holds promise for the prevention and treatment of these conditions. Furthermore, our findings also support HuD as a novel target of drugs focused on counteracting neurodegenerative diseases.

Supplementary Materials: The following supporting information can be downloaded at: https://www.mdpi.com/article/10.3390/ijms241512201/s1.

Author Contributions: Conceptualization, N.M. and A.P.; methodology, N.M., F.F. and G.C.; formal analysis, N.M., P.L. and A.B.; investigation, N.M., L.I.M.C., F.F., G.C. and F.A.A.; resources, S.C. and A.P.; data curation, N.M., P.L., S.C. and A.P.; writing—original draft preparation, N.M., P.L. and A.P.; writing—review and editing, N.M., P.L., G.C., D.R., S.C. and A.P. All authors have read and agreed to the published version of the manuscript.

Funding: N.M. has been granted a research fellowship from the University of Pavia (DFARMACO2020-A02).

Informed Consent Statement: Not applicable.

Data Availability Statement: The data presented in this study are available on request from the corresponding author.

Acknowledgments: We thank the Department of Drug Sciences of the University of Pavia for the research fellowship award to N.M.

Conflicts of Interest: The authors declare no conflict of interest.

References

1. Hussain, R.; Zubair, H.; Pursell, S.; Shahab, M. Neurodegenerative Diseases: Regenerative Mechanisms and Novel Therapeutic Approaches. *Brain Sci.* **2018**, *8*, E177. [CrossRef] [PubMed]
2. Varesi, A.; Campagnoli, L.I.M.; Barbieri, A.; Rossi, L.; Ricevuti, G.; Esposito, C.; Chirumbolo, S.; Marchesi, N.; Pascale, A. RNA Binding Proteins in Senescence: A Potential Common Linker for Age-Related Diseases? *Ageing Res. Rev.* **2023**, *88*. [CrossRef] [PubMed]
3. Lenzken, S.C.; Achsel, T.; Carrì, M.T.; Barabino, S.M.L. Neuronal RNA-Binding Proteins in Health, and Disease. *Wiley Interdiscip. Rev. RNA* **2014**, *5*, 565–576. [CrossRef]
4. Pascale, A.; Govoni, S. The Complex World of Post-Transcriptional Mechanisms: Is Their Deregulation a Common Link for Diseases? Focus on ELAV-like RNA-Binding Proteins. *Cell. Mol. Life Sci.* **2012**, *69*, 501–517. [CrossRef] [PubMed]
5. Prashad, S.; Gopal, P.P. RNA-Binding Proteins in Neurological Development and Disease. *RNA Biol.* **2021**, *18*, 972–987. [CrossRef]
6. Schieweck, R.; Ninkovic, J.; Kiebler, M.A. RNA-Binding Proteins Balance Brain Function in Health and Disease. *Physiol. Rev.* **2021**, *101*, 1309–1370. [CrossRef]
7. Colombrita, C.; Silani, V.; Ratti, A. ELAV Proteins along Evolution: Back to the Nucleus? *Mol. Cell. Neurosci.* **2013**, *56*, 447–455. [CrossRef]
8. Hinman, M.N.; Lou, H. Diverse Molecular Functions of Hu Proteins. *Cell Mol. Life Sci.* **2008**, *65*, 3168–3181. [CrossRef]
9. Bolognani, F.; Contente-Cuomo, T.; Perrone-Bizzozero, N.I. Novel Recognition Motifs and Biological Functions of the RNA-Binding Protein HuD Revealed by Genome-Wide Identification of Its Targets. *Nucleic Acids Res.* **2009**, *38*, 117–130. [CrossRef]
10. Wang, F.; Tidei, J.J.; Polich, E.D.; Gao, Y.; Zhao, H.; Perrone-Bizzozero, N.I.; Guo, W.; Zhao, X. Positive Feedback between RNA-Binding Protein HuD and Transcription Factor SATB1 Promotes Neurogenesis. *Proc. Natl. Acad. Sci. USA* **2015**, *112*, E4995–E5004. [CrossRef]
11. Abdelmohsen, K.; Hutchison, E.R.; Lee, E.K.; Kuwano, Y.; Kim, M.M.; Masuda, K.; Srikantan, S.; Subaran, S.S.; Marasa, B.S.; Mattson, M.P.; et al. MiR-375 Inhibits Differentiation of Neurites by Lowering HuD Levels. *Mol. Cell Biol.* **2010**, *30*, 4197–4210. [CrossRef] [PubMed]
12. Bronicki, L.M.; Jasmin, B.J. Emerging Complexity of the HuD/ELAVl4 Gene; Implications for Neuronal Development, Function, and Dysfunction. *RNA* **2013**, *19*, 1019–1037. [CrossRef] [PubMed]
13. Good, P.J. A Conserved Family of Elav-like Genes in Vertebrates. *Proc. Natl. Acad. Sci. USA* **1995**, *92*, 4557–4561. [CrossRef]
14. Pascale, A.; Gusev, P.A.; Amadio, M.; Dottorini, T.; Govoni, S.; Alkon, D.L.; Quattrone, A. Increase of the RNA-Binding Protein HuD and Posttranscriptional up-Regulation of the GAP-43 Gene during Spatial Memory. *Proc. Natl. Acad. Sci. USA* **2004**, *101*, 1217–1222. [CrossRef] [PubMed]
15. Perrone-Bizzozero, N.; Bird, C.W. Role of HuD in Nervous System Function and Pathology. *Front. Biosci.* **2013**, *5*, 554–563. [CrossRef] [PubMed]
16. Dell'Orco, M.; Sardone, V.; Gardiner, A.S.; Pansarasa, O.; Bordoni, M.; Perrone-Bizzozero, N.I.; Cereda, C. HuD Regulates SOD1 Expression during Oxidative Stress in Differentiated Neuroblastoma Cells and Sporadic ALS Motor Cortex. *Neurobiol. Dis.* **2021**, *148*, 105211. [CrossRef]
17. Tebaldi, T.; Zuccotti, P.; Peroni, D.; Köhn, M.; Gasperini, L.; Potrich, V.; Bonazza, V.; Dudnakova, T.; Rossi, A.; Sanguinetti, G.; et al. HuD Is a Neural Translation Enhancer Acting on MTORC1-Responsive Genes and Counteracted by the Y3 Small Non-Coding RNA. *Mol. Cell* **2018**, *71*, 256–270. [CrossRef]
18. Dell'Orco, M.; Oliver, R.J.; Perrone-Bizzozero, N. HuD Binds to and Regulates Circular RNAs Derived From Neuronal Development- and Synaptic Plasticity-Associated Genes. *Front. Genet.* **2020**, *11*, 790. [CrossRef]
19. Nasti, R.; Rossi, D.; Amadio, M.; Pascale, A.; Unver, M.Y.; Hirsch, A.K.H.; Collina, S. Compounds Interfering with Embryonic Lethal Abnormal Vision (ELAV) Protein-RNA Complexes: An Avenue for Discovering New Drugs. *J. Med. Chem.* **2017**, *60*, 8257–8267. [CrossRef]
20. Silvestri, B.; Mochi, M.; Garone, M.G.; Rosa, A. Emerging Roles for the RNA-Binding Protein HuD (ELAVL4) in Nervous System Diseases. *Int. J. Mol. Sci.* **2022**, *23*, 14606. [CrossRef]
21. Pascale, A.; Amadio, M.; Scapagnini, G.; Lanni, C.; Racchi, M.; Provenzani, A.; Govoni, S.; Alkon, D.L.; Quattrone, A. Neuronal ELAV Proteins Enhance MRNA Stability by a PKCalpha-Dependent Pathway. *Proc. Natl. Acad. Sci. USA* **2005**, *102*, 12065–12070. [CrossRef] [PubMed]
22. Talman, V.; Amadio, M.; Osera, C.; Sorvari, S.; Boije Af Gennäs, G.; Yli-Kauhaluoma, J.; Rossi, D.; Govoni, S.; Collina, S.; Ekokoski, E.; et al. The C1 Domain-Targeted Isophthalate Derivative HMI-1b11 Promotes Neurite Outgrowth and GAP-43 Expression through PKCα Activation in SH-SY5Y Cells. *Pharmacol. Res.* **2013**, *73*, 44–54. [CrossRef] [PubMed]
23. Marchesi, N.; Amadio, M.; Colombrita, C.; Govoni, S.; Ratti, A.; Pascale, A. PKC Activation Counteracts ADAM10 Deficit in HuD-Silenced Neuroblastoma Cells. *J. Alzheimer's Dis.* **2016**, *54*, 535–547. [CrossRef] [PubMed]
24. Fujiwara, T.; Mori, Y.; Chu, D.L.; Koyama, Y.; Miyata, S.; Tanaka, H.; Yachi, K.; Kubo, T.; Yoshikawa, H.; Tohyama, M. CARM1 Regulates Proliferation of PC12 Cells by Methylating HuD. *Mol. Cell Biol.* **2006**, *26*, 2273–2285. [CrossRef] [PubMed]
25. Wang, X.; Hall, T.M. Structural Basis for Recognition of AU-Rich Element RNA by the HuD Protein. *Nat. Struct. Biol.* **2001**, *8*, 141–145. [CrossRef]

26. Della Volpe, S.; Linciano, P.; Listro, R.; Tumminelli, E.; Amadio, M.; Bonomo, I.; Elgaher, W.A.M.; Adam, S.; Hirsch, A.K.H.; Boeckler, F.M.; et al. Identification of N,N-Arylalkyl-Picolinamide Derivatives Targeting the RNA-Binding Protein HuR, by Combining Biophysical Fragment-Screening and Molecular Hybridization. *Bioorg Chem.* **2021**, *116*, 105305. [CrossRef]
27. Della Volpe, S.; Nasti, R.; Queirolo, M.; Unver, M.Y.; Jumde, V.K.; Dömling, A.; Vasile, F.; Potenza, D.; Ambrosio, F.A.; Costa, G.; et al. Novel Compounds Targeting the RNA-Binding Protein HuR. Structure-Based Design, Synthesis, and Interaction Studies. *ACS Med. Chem. Lett.* **2019**, *10*, 615–620. [CrossRef] [PubMed]
28. Šponer, J.; Bussi, G.; Krepl, M.; Banáš, P.; Bottaro, S.; Cunha, R.A.; Gil-Ley, A.; Pinamonti, G.; Poblete, S.; Jurečka, P.; et al. RNA Structural Dynamics As Captured by Molecular Simulations: A Comprehensive Overview. *Chem. Rev.* **2018**, *118*, 4177–4338. [CrossRef] [PubMed]
29. Vasile, F.; Della Volpe, S.; Ambrosio, F.A.; Costa, G.; Unver, M.Y.; Zucal, C.; Rossi, D.; Martino, E.; Provenzani, A.; Hirsch, A.K.H.; et al. Exploration of Ligand Binding Modes towards the Identification of Compounds Targeting HuR: A Combined STD-NMR and Molecular Modelling Approach. *Sci. Rep.* **2018**, *8*, 13780. [CrossRef]
30. Uusitalo, J.J.; Ingólfsson, H.I.; Marrink, S.J.; Faustino, I. Martini Coarse-Grained Force Field: Extension to RNA. *Biophys. J.* **2017**, *113*, 246–256. [CrossRef]
31. Ambrosio, F.A.; Coricello, A.; Costa, G.; Lupia, A.; Micaelli, M.; Marchesi, N.; Sala, F.; Pascale, A.; Rossi, D.; Vasile, F.; et al. Identification of Compounds Targeting HuD. Another Brick in the Wall of Neurodegenerative Disease Treatment. *J. Med. Chem.* **2021**, *64*, 9989–10000. [CrossRef] [PubMed]
32. Gliwińska, A.; Czubilińska-Łada, J.; Więckiewicz, G.; Świętochowska, E.; Badeński, A.; Dworak, M.; Szczepańska, M. The Role of Brain-Derived Neurotrophic Factor (BDNF) in Diagnosis and Treatment of Epilepsy, Depression, Schizophrenia, Anorexia Nervosa and Alzheimer's Disease as Highly Drug-Resistant Diseases: A Narrative Review. *Brain Sci.* **2023**, *13*, 163. [CrossRef]
33. Beckel-Mitchener, A.C.; Miera, A.; Keller, R.; Perrone-Bizzozero, N.I. Poly(A) Tail Length-Dependent Stabilization of GAP-43 MRNA by the RNA-Binding Protein HuD. *J. Biol. Chem.* **2002**, *277*, 27996–28002. [CrossRef]
34. Bolognani, F.; Tanner, D.C.; Nixon, S.; Okano, H.J.; Okano, H.; Perrone-Bizzozero, N.I. Coordinated Expression of HuD and GAP-43 in Hippocampal Dentate Granule Cells during Developmental and Adult Plasticity. *Neurochem. Res.* **2007**, *32*, 2142–2151. [CrossRef]
35. Lim, C.S.; Alkon, D.L. Protein Kinase C Stimulates HuD-Mediated MRNA Stability and Protein Expression of Neurotrophic Factors and Enhances Dendritic Maturation of Hippocampal Neurons in Culture. *Hippocampus* **2012**, *22*, 2303–2319. [CrossRef]
36. Kang, M.-J.; Abdelmohsen, K.; Hutchison, E.R.; Mitchell, S.J.; Grammatikakis, I.; Guo, R.; Noh, J.H.; Martindale, J.L.; Yang, X.; Lee, E.K.; et al. HuD Regulates Coding and Noncoding RNA to Induce APP→Aβ Processing. *Cell Rep.* **2014**, *7*, 1401–1409. [CrossRef]
37. King, P.H. RNA-Binding Analyses of HuC and HuD with the VEGF and c-Myc 3′-Untranslated Regions Using a Novel ELISA-Based Assay. *Nucleic Acids Res.* **2000**, *28*, E20. [CrossRef] [PubMed]
38. Castrén, E.; Berninger, B.; Leingärtner, A.; Lindholm, D. Regulation of Brain-Derived Neurotrophic Factor MRNA Levels in Hippocampus by Neuronal Activity. *Prog. Brain Res.* **1998**, *117*, 57–64. [CrossRef]
39. Higashimoto, K.; Kuhn, P.; Desai, D.; Cheng, X.; Xu, W. Phosphorylation-Mediated Inactivation of Coactivator-Associated Arginine Methyltransferase 1. *Proc. Natl. Acad. Sci. USA* **2007**, *104*, 12318–12323. [CrossRef] [PubMed]
40. Doxakis, E. RNA Binding Proteins: A Common Denominator of Neuronal Function and Dysfunction. *Neurosci. Bull.* **2014**, *30*, 610–626. [CrossRef] [PubMed]
41. Bolognani, F.; Perrone-Bizzozero, N.I. RNA-Protein Interactions and Control of MRNA Stability in Neurons. *J. Neurosci. Res.* **2008**, *86*, 481–489. [CrossRef]
42. Hilgers, V. Regulation of Neuronal RNA Signatures by ELAV/Hu Proteins. *WIREs RNA* **2023**, *14*, e1733. [CrossRef]
43. Jung, M.; Lee, E.K. RNA–Binding Protein HuD as a Versatile Factor in Neuronal and Non–Neuronal Systems. *Biology* **2021**, *10*, 361. [CrossRef] [PubMed]
44. Liang, B.; Li, C.; Zhao, J. Identification of Key Pathways and Genes in Colorectal Cancer Using Bioinformatics Analysis. *Med. Oncol.* **2016**, *33*, 111. [CrossRef] [PubMed]
45. Zheng, D.; Wang, J.; Li, G.; Sun, Y.; Deng, Q.; Li, M.; Song, K.; Zhao, Z. Preliminary Therapeutic and Mechanistic Evaluation of S-Allylmercapto-N-Acetylcysteine in the Treatment of Pulmonary Emphysema. *Int. Immunopharmacol.* **2021**, *98*, 107913. [CrossRef] [PubMed]
46. Marchesi, N.; Barbieri, A.; Fahmideh, F.; Govoni, S.; Ghidoni, A.; Parati, G.; Vanoli, E.; Pascale, A.; Calvillo, L. Use of Dual-Flow Bioreactor to Develop a Simplified Model of Nervous-Cardiovascular Systems Crosstalk: A Preliminary Assessment. *PLoS ONE* **2020**, *15*, e0242627. [CrossRef] [PubMed]
47. Fahmideh, F.; Marchesi, N.; Campagnoli, L.I.M.; Landini, L.; Caramella, C.; Barbieri, A.; Govoni, S.; Pascale, A. Effect of Troxerutin in Counteracting Hyperglycemia-Induced VEGF Upregulation in Endothelial Cells: A New Option to Target Early Stages of Diabetic Retinopathy? *Front. Pharmacol.* **2022**, *13*, 951833. [CrossRef]
48. Mallucci, G.; Marchesi, N.; Campagnoli, L.I.M.; Boschi, F.; Fahmideh, F.; Fusco, S.; Tavazzi, E.; Govoni, S.; Bergamaschi, R.; Pascale, A. Evidence for Novel Cell Defense Mechanisms Sustained by Dimethyl Fumarate in Multiple Sclerosis Patients: The HuR/SOD2 Cascade. *Mult. Scler. Relat. Disord.* **2022**, *68*, 104197. [CrossRef]

Disclaimer/Publisher's Note: The statements, opinions and data contained in all publications are solely those of the individual author(s) and contributor(s) and not of MDPI and/or the editor(s). MDPI and/or the editor(s) disclaim responsibility for any injury to people or property resulting from any ideas, methods, instructions or products referred to in the content.

Case Report

Tako-Tsubo Syndrome in Amyotrophic Lateral Sclerosis: Single-Center Case Series and Brief Literature Review

Giovanni Napoli [1], Martina Rubin [1,2], Gianni Cutillo [1], Paride Schito [1,3], Tommaso Russo [1,3], Angelo Quattrini [3], Massimo Filippi [1,2,4] and Nilo Riva [1,3,*,†]

[1] Neurorehabilitation, Neurology Unit and Neurophysiology Unit, San Raffaele Scientific Institute, 20132 Milan, Italy; napoli.giovanni@hsr.it (G.N.); rubin.martina@hsr.it (M.R.); cutillo.gianni@hsr.it (G.C.); schito.paride@hsr.it (P.S.); russo.tommaso@hsr.it (T.R.); filippi.massimo@hsr.it (M.F.)
[2] Neuroimaging Research Unit, Institute of Experimental Neurology, Division of Neuroscience, San Raffaele Scientific Institute, 20132 Milan, Italy
[3] Experimental Neuropathology Unit, Institute of Experimental Neurology (INSPE), Division of Neuroscience, San Raffaele Scientific Institute, 20132 Milan, Italy; quattrini.angelo@hsr.it
[4] Vita-Salute San Raffaele University, 20132 Milan, Italy
* Correspondence: riva.nilo@hsr.it or nilo.riva@istituto-besta.it
† Current Address: 3rd Neurology Unit and Motor Neuron Disease Centre, Fondazione IRCCS Istituto Neurologico Carlo Besta, 20133 Milan, Italy.

Abstract: Amyotrophic lateral sclerosis (ALS) is a neurodegenerative disease with variable phenotypic expressions which has been associated with autonomic dysfunction. The cardiovascular system seems to be affected especially in the context of bulbar involvement. We describe four new cases of Tako-Tsubo syndrome (TTS) in ALS patients with an appraisal of the literature. We present a late-stage ALS patient with prominent bulbar involvement that presented TTS during hospitalization. We then retrospectively identify three additional ALS–TTS cases reporting relevant clinical findings. TTS cardiomyopathy has been observed in different acute neurological conditions, and the co-occurrence of ALS and TTS has already been reported. Cardiovascular autonomic dysfunctions have been described in ALS, especially in the context of an advanced diseases and with bulbar involvement. Noradrenergic hyperfunction linked to sympathetic denervation and ventilatory deficits coupled in different instances with a trigger event could play a synergistic role in the development of TTS in ALS. Sympathetic hyperfunctioning and ventilatory deficits in conjunction with cardiac autonomic nerves impairment may play a role in the development of TTS in a context of ALS.

Keywords: motor neuron disease; autonomic system; mortality; non-invasive ventilation; PEG; NIMV; vascular; cardio-vascular

1. Introduction

ALS is a fatal neurodegenerative disease that generally presents during the fifth to sixth decades, with concomitant upper motor neuron (UMN) and lower motor neuron (LMN) signs [1,2]. It causes progressive paralysis leading to respiratory failure within 3–5 years. In about 20% of cases, ALS presents with a bulbar onset, which is generally associated with an earlier development of nutritional and/or respiratory failure and, consequently, a poorer prognosis. However, up to 80% of ALS patients develop bulbar involvement regardless of the onset site [1,3]. While ALS has traditionally been considered a pure motor disease, recent advances in our understanding have revealed heterogeneous extra-motor involvement [2]. In addition to the well-recognized cognitive impairment, ALS is known to be associated with varying degrees of autonomic and cardiovascular dysfunction. These dysfunctions typically present during the advanced stages of the disease and are often associated with bulbar involvement [4–8]. However, they have also been described in early or even prodromal stages [5,9]. ALS has been linked to Tako-Tsubo syndrome (TTS) [7,10–13], an acute cardiomyopathy triggered by stress-related adrenergic dysregulation, mimicking acute coronary syndrome. TTS causes apical ballooning and transient left ventricular dysfunction. Although TTS is generally considered reversible, affected patients may experience persistent cardiac dysfunction even after the acute phase and the resolution of apical ballooning [14,15]. In this report, we present four new cases of ALS–TTS co-occurrence, focusing on autonomic dysfunction. We also provide an overview of the existing literature and speculate on the possible underlying pathophysiological mechanisms.

2. Case Presentation

A 59-year-old man with a 6-year history of ALS, diagnosed according to the revised El Escorial criteria [16] and the Awaji criteria [17], was admitted to the Neurorehabilitation Unit due to progressive development of dysphagia and respiratory failure in order to assess the need for non-invasive ventilation (NIV) or percutaneous endoscopic gastrostomy (PEG) placement.

At the time of diagnosis, the patient presented with a spinal onset, initially involving the lower limbs, and riluzole therapy was started. Two years later, he required a walker for ambulation, and three years later, he became wheelchair-bound. The upper limbs were gradually affected, with relatively preserved distal function.

In the two months leading up to admission, the patient reported progressive dysphagia, dyspnea with minimal effort or prolonged speech, orthopnea, and ineffective cough. One month prior, he underwent a cardiological assessment due to new-onset palpitations, and sporadic paroxysmal supraventricular tachycardia runs were observed on an electrocardiogram (ECG). Consequently, he was started on Flecainide. No other cardiac comorbidities were reported.

Upon admission, a routine ECG revealed a prolonged cQT interval (>530 ms), a right bundle branch block, and an anterior left hemiblock with T wave alterations suggestive of possible cardiac ischemia (Figure 1A). However, the patient was asymptomatic. Treatment with intravenous acetylsalicylate was initiated and later switched to a low-dose oral formulation, along with metoprolol and ramipril. Blood tests showed a mild elevation of troponin T and a severe elevation of pro-BNP. Echocardiography revealed concentric thickening of the left ventricle with a 45% ejection fraction (FE) and medial-apical dyskinesia, which was suggestive of Tako-Tsubo syndrome (TTS). To confirm the suspicion of TTS, a coronary CT scan was performed, which showed no stenosis in the coronary arteries. As a result, the previous therapy was discontinued, and Bisoprolol was initiated. In the following days, Troponin T and pro-BNP levels, as well as ECG findings (Figure 1B) and echocardiography results, progressively normalized.

2.1. Case Series

Reviewing a 10-year cohort of approximately 800 ALS patients, we retrospectively identified three additional cases of ALS–TTS (Table 1). The onset of TTS occurred at different disease durations, ranging from 38 to 73 months. Three out of the four patients had a spinal onset, with two presenting classical upper and lower motor neuron (UMN and LMN) signs, and one showing isolated LMN involvement. The fourth patient (pt.2) had a bulbar onset, characterized by dysarthria. All patients received treatment with riluzole and underwent testing for ALS-related genes, including a panel of 30 genes such as SOD1, TARDBP1, and FUS, as well as repeat-primed PCR for detecting the C9orf72 repeat expansion [18]. A C9orf72 mutation was detected only in the patient with bulbar onset, while no relevant mutations were found in the others. At the time of TTS diagnosis, two patients had a Revised Amyotrophic Lateral Sclerosis Functional Rating Scale score below 20, indicating functional impairment. Patient 2 (pt.2) had mild bulbar symptoms, including mild drooling, slight dysarthria, and dysphagia. All patients exhibited apical dyskinesia on echocardiography and elevated levels of Troponin T. ECG findings showed non-specific changes (Table 1). Three patients underwent coronary CT or angiography, which showed no evidence of coronary artery obstruction. Three patients had mild cardiovascular comorbidities, such as supraventricular tachycardia and hypertension, while patient 4 (pt.4) had coronary artery disease. Remarkably, pt.2, despite the bulbar onset, developed TTS without concomitant respiratory or nutritional failure. In contrast, pt.1 and pt.3 developed TTS concurrently with non-invasive ventilation (NIV) initiation, and pt.4 experienced TTS coinciding with tracheostomy and percutaneous endoscopic gastrostomy (PEG) placement. A potential trigger event for TTS was identified in pt.2 and pt.3, who were diagnosed with pulmonary embolism (PE) and a urinary tract infection, respectively. Pt.4 experienced TTS in association with tracheostomy and PEG placement, while in pt.1, TTS was an incidental finding.

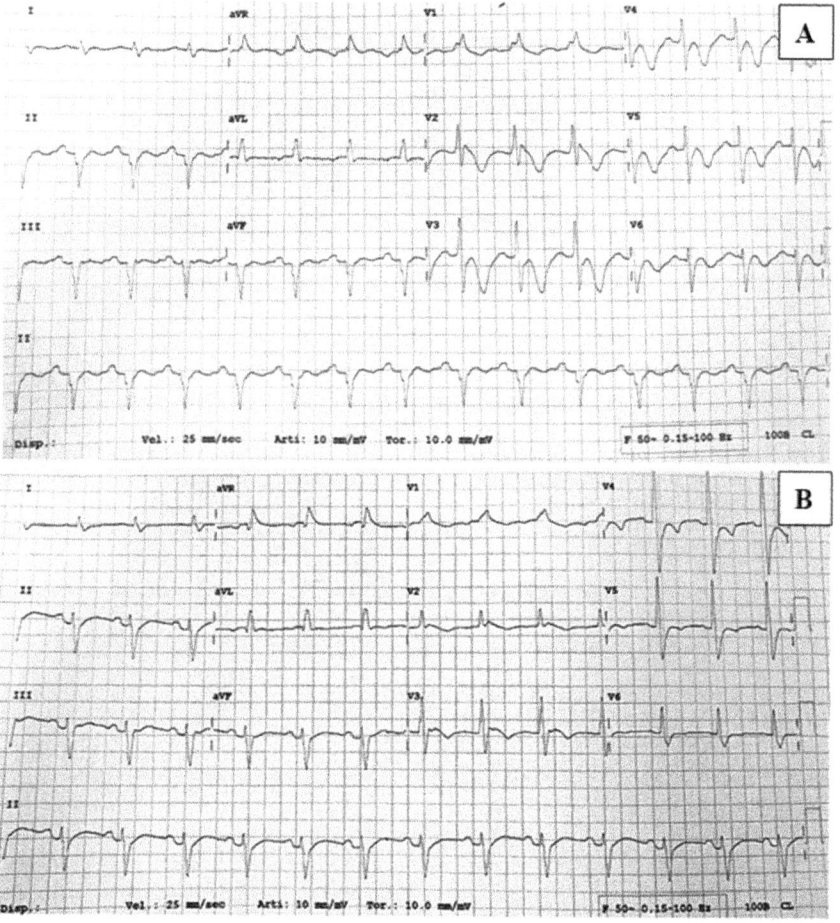

Figure 1. (**A**) ECG on admission revealed T-wave inversion on almost all leads, especially on precordial leads V2–V6, mimicking myocardial ischaemia. (**B**) ECG after 4 days revealed negative T-wave in anterior precordial leads, of smaller depth than previous one.

Table 1. Summary of the patient with ALS–TTS identified in our center. Abbreviations: ALS = amyotrophic lateral sclerosis; ALSFSR-R = Revised Amyotrophic Lateral Sclerosis Functional Rating Scale; CAD = coronary artery disease; CPK = creatine phosphokinase; HT = hypertension; LMN = lower motor neuron; M = male; MiToS = MiToS functional staging system; PE = pulmonary embolism; PEG = percutaneous endoscopic gastrostomy; PSVT = paroxysmal supraventricular tachycardia; T2DM = type 2 diabetes mellitus; TS = tracheostomy; TTS = Tako-Tsubo syndrome; UTI = urinary tract infection; † = exitus; * at TTS diagnosis.

Patient (Sex)	1 (Case Report, M)	2 (F)	3 (M)	4 (F)
ALS age of onset (years)	54	74	60	71
Site of onset	Upper limbs	Bulbar	Lower limbs	Lower limbs
ALS phenotype (according to Chiò, et al., 2011 [2])	Classic	Bulbar	LMN	Classic
ALS disease duration (from clinical onset)	73 months	19 months (†)	103 months (†)	38 months (†)
TTS (months after ALS onset)	73 months	11 months	86 months	38 months
Awaji at ALS diagnosis	Probable	Probable	Possible	Possible
ALSFRS-R *	15	45	19	18
KSS *	4	1	4	4
MiToS *	3	1	3	3
ALS genetics	/	C9orf72	/	/
Concomitant Medication	Riluzole, Acetyl-L-carnitine	Riluzole, Acetyl-L-carnitine, Baclofen	Riluzole	Riluzole
Time to Ventilation	73 months	N/A	86 months	32 months
Time to Tracheostomy	N/A	N/A	91 months	38 months
Time to PEG	75 months	N/A	N/A	38 months
Elevated ST/negative T at ECG	Prolonged QT, unspecific T wave alterations	Sinus tachycardia, VEBs	Negative antero-septal T	Aspecific conduction alterations
Troponin T (ng/dL)	231	421	459	316
pro-BNP (pg/mL)	939	34.309	3.074	/
CPK (U/L)	N/A	44	71	49
Ejection Fraction	45%	30%	35%	35%
Apical dyskinesia/ballooning at echocardiography	Yes	Yes	Yes	Yes
Coronary CT/coronarography	Heart angio-CT: negative	Coronarography: negative	N/A	Heart CT: negative
Pulmonary arterial Pressure	Normal	75 mmHg	Normal	Normal
Cardiovascular comorbidities	PSVT	HT	HT	T2DM, CAD
Intervening condition	Respiratory failure (adapted to NIV)	PE	PE + lower UTI	TS + PEG

2.2. Literature Review

The literature exploring the ALS–TTS association is heterogenous, and few reports could be retrieved. In our review, we found 10 relevant articles reporting on TTS in ALS, comprising a total of 32 patients (Table 2). In two cases [11,19], TTS was presented in association with overt bulbar signs, while Choi [20] reported nine patients with cervical or bulbar onset which developed TTS in late ALS stages. Data on respiratory failure were available for 13 patients. A TTS putative trigger was reported in all cases except for a single series [21].

Table 2. Summary of the ALS–TTS reported cases in the literature, focusing on bulbar impairment as TTS possible cause. Abbreviations: CR = case report; CS = case series; NIV = non-invasive ventilation; TIV = tracheostomy invasive ventilation; UTI = urinary tract infection.

Reference	Number of Cases	Type of Onset	Ventilatory Support	Bulbar Signs	Intervening Conditions
Takayama et al., 2004 [12]	1	Classic	N/A	N/A	Surgical gastrostomy; repair of incisional hernia (with tracheal intubation)
Mitani et al., 2005 [11]	1	Bulbar	NIV	Dysphagia, dysarthria.	Long-term NIV
Matsuyama et al., 2008 [10]	1	Classic	TIV	N/A	Tracheostomy
Massari et al., 2011 [19]	1	Classic	NIV	Dysphagia, dysarthria	Pneumonia
Peters, 2014 [22]	1	N/A	NIV	N/A	Respiratory distress syndrome, pneumonia
Santoro et al., 2016 [23]	1	N/A	N/A	N/A	Emotional distress (first episode); Femoral artery thrombosis (second episode)
Gdynia et al., 2006 [24]	1	Classic	N/A	N/A	Major surgery
Choi et al., 2017 [20]	9	Bulbar (pt.2,5,6) Cervical (pt.1,3,4,7,8) Respiratory (pt.9)	NIV (pt.2,5,7), TIV (pt.6,8)	N/A	N/A
Izumi et al., 2018 [13]	4	Bulbar (pt.1,4), Classic (pt.2,3)	TIV (pt.1,2)	N/A	UTI (pt.1); acute cholangitis (pt.2); pneumonia (pt.3)

3. Discussion

In our cohort, three ALS patients were diagnosed with TTS at relatively advanced stages, with increasingly evident bulbar impairment. Interestingly, the only patient with a bulbar onset developed TTS in an earlier disease stage, with only modest bulbar symptoms, but exhibited the most severe cardiac involvement. ALS has been associated with varying degrees of autonomic dysfunction. Parasympathetic hypofunctioning has been linked to altered salivary and gastrointestinal excretion, orthostatic or nocturnal hypotension, and decreased heart rate variability (HRV) [5,6]. On the other hand, sympathetic hyperfunctioning is associated with an increased risk of cardiac arrest [6,21,25]. While dysautonomia in ALS typically appears in late stages, it has rarely been reported early in cases with bulbar onset [4,8]. These manifestations may result from the involvement of cardiovascular and autonomic centers in the medulla oblongata. Pathological evidence has supported bulbar abnormalities in pTDP-43-related pathologies [26], possibly due to disease spread through contiguous anatomical structures rather than trans-synaptic propagation. This evidence might explain the co-occurrence of ALS–TTS, as previously described in several reports [10–12,19,20].

The relations between ALS and TTS and, more broadly, autonomic involvement in ALS have not been clearly understood and the currently available literature on this topic is heterogeneous and mostly based on case reports or small case series. In a Korean cohort study of 624 ALS patients, among 64 patients who underwent echocardiography after the presentation of cardiologic symptoms, TTS was detected in 9 cases, 8 of whom presented with bulbar or cervical onset and 1 with a respiratory onset, suggesting a potential role of bulbar involvement in TTS development [20]. Another retrospective analysis of a cohort of 250 ALS cases and 870 synucleinopathies found 4 TTS cases in the ALS group and none in the synucleinopathy group [13]. Interestingly, while Parkinson's disease, Lewy body dementia, and multiple system atrophy are known for their association with autonomic dysfunction [27], their co-occurrence with TTS seems rather uncommon, indicating a specific link between ALS-specific pathological mechanisms and cardiomyopathy development [24].

Several hypotheses on TTS pathophysiology have been proposed, involving neurochemical, hormonal, and genetic factors that point towards a stress-triggered catecholaminergic toxicity [14]. TTS has been observed not only in the context of pathologies compromising the medulla oblongata but also in several acute neurological conditions without clear evidence of bulbar involvement, such as traumatic brain or spinal injury, cerebral hemorrhages, stroke, seizures, cerebral surgery, neuromuscular diseases, and psychiatric comorbidities such as anxiety and depression [24,28,29]. This supports the etiopathogenetic hypothesis of an underlying stress-triggered mechanism causing an imbalance in plasma levels of epinephrine, norepinephrine, and cortisol and subsequent sympathetic dysfunction at the level of cardiac myocytes.

Autonomic disturbances related to bulbar involvement, necessitating tracheostomy, tracheal intubation, or long-term respiratory support, may exacerbate the physiological stress response, promoting the onset of TTS or even favoring TTS recurrence [23]. ALS-related autonomic dysfunctions have also been assessed in the context of cardiovascular involvement, with studies showing altered HRV related to impaired vagal response in resting conditions, particularly in patients with prominent bulbar signs [5]. Altered responses to orthostasis have also been demonstrated in ALS through spectral analysis of HRV and systolic arterial pressure [6], as well as through cardiological assessments with tilting-tests, transthoracic echocardiography, and Holter-ECG [21].

Sympathetic hyperfunctioning has been demonstrated even in early stages of ALS. A retrospective analysis showed a significant increase in QTc intervals and dispersion at terminal stages, inversely correlated with a decrease in neuronal density in the sympathetic intermediolateral nucleus of the upper thoracic cord, also correlating with an increased rate of sudden cardiac arrest [25]. A heart MRI study on 35 ALS patients without overt cardiac involvement showed a reduction of myocardial mass and volumes in 77% of patients and myocardial fibrosis in 23.5%, with these structural changes hypothesized to be caused by sympathetic hyperactivation secondary to denervation of autonomic cardiac nerves or respiratory weakness [30]. Moreover, a 123-I-MIBG-SPECT study on early-stage ALS demonstrated a significantly reduced MIBG uptake in the majority of subjects, associated with a reduction in HRV, supporting an early sympathetic denervation process as a possible cause of cardiac dysfunction [9]. Loss of adrenergic receptors due to myocardial denervation has been linked to an increased responsiveness of the remaining receptors, supporting the idea that compensatory noradrenergic hyperfunction due to sympathetic denervation and ventilatory deficits, frequently observed in the context of bulbar involvement, could play a synergistic role in the development of TTS cardiomyopathy [31]. As the bulbar phenotype is characterized by a more aggressive disease progression, the stressful conditions secondary to disability progression may also contribute to sympathetic surge and serve as triggering factors for TTS [5,9].

4. Conclusions

TTS is a rare stress-related cardiomyopathy that may arise in the context of ALS. Sympathetic hyperfunction may play a crucial role in its pathogenesis and may be related to bulbar structures involvement, independently of onset type. Bulbar onset seems to relate to an earlier TTS presentation and to a more severe cardiological prognosis. However, the relation between ALS and TTS, as well as its relationship with bulbar involvement, needs further investigations in order to reveal the potential underlying pathological mechanisms.

Author Contributions: Conceptualization, G.N., M.R., G.C. and N.R.; methodology G.N., M.R., G.C. and N.R.; investigation, G.N., M.R. and G.C.; resources, A.Q., M.F. and N.R.; data curation, G.N., M.R., G.C. and T.R.; writing—original draft preparation, G.N., M.R. and G.C.; writing—review and editing, T.R., P.S., M.F., N.R. and A.Q.; supervision, T.R., P.S., M.F., N.R. and A.Q.; funding acquisition, N.R. and A.Q. All authors have read and agreed to the published version of the manuscript.

Funding: This work was supported by the Giovanni Marazzina Foundation.

Institutional Review Board Statement: The study was conducted in accordance with the Declaration of Helsinki and approved by the Institutional Review Board of IRCCS Ospedale San Raffaele (protocol reference number DSAN 855-A-OS/3 2015-33, approved on 12 August 2018).

Informed Consent Statement: Informed consent was obtained from all subjects involved in the study.

Data Availability Statement: All data needed to evaluate the conclusions are present in the paper. Additional data related to this paper may be requested from the corresponding author upon reasonable request by qualified academic investigators.

Conflicts of Interest: The authors declare no conflict of interest related to this paper.

References

1. Swinnen, B.; Robberecht, W. The phenotypic variability of amyotrophic lateral sclerosis. *Nat. Rev. Neurol.* **2014**, *10*, 661–670. [CrossRef] [PubMed]
2. Chiò, A.; Calvo, A.; Moglia, C.; Mazzini, L.; Mora, G.; PARALS Study Group. Phenotypic heterogeneity of amyotrophic lateral sclerosis: A population based study. *J. Neurol. Neurosurg. Psychiatry* **2011**, *82*, 740–746. [CrossRef] [PubMed]
3. Hardiman, O.; Al-Chalabi, A.; Chio, A.; Corr, E.M.; Logroscino, G.; Robberecht, W.; Shaw, P.J.; Simmons, Z.; van den Berg, L.H. Amyotrophic lateral sclerosis. *Nat. Rev. Dis. Primers* **2017**, *3*, 17071. [CrossRef] [PubMed]
4. Piccione, E.A.; Sletten, D.M.; Staff, N.P.; Low, P.A. Autonomic system and amyotrophic lateral sclerosis. *Muscle Nerve* **2015**, *51*, 676–679. [CrossRef] [PubMed]
5. Merico, A.; Cavinato, M. Autonomic dysfunction in the early stage of ALS with bulbar involvement. *Amyotroph. Lateral Scler.* **2011**, *12*, 363–367. [CrossRef]
6. Vecchia, L.D.; De Maria, B.; Marinou, K.; Sideri, R.; Lucini, A.; Porta, A.; Mora, G. Cardiovascular neural regulation is impaired in amyotrophic lateral sclerosis patients. A study by spectral and complexity analysis of cardiovascular oscillations. *Physiol. Meas.* **2015**, *36*, 659–670. [CrossRef]
7. Chida, K.; Sakamaki, S.; Takasu, T. Alteration in autonomic function and cardiovascular regulation in amyotrophic lateral sclerosis. *J. Neurol.* **1989**, *236*, 127–130. [CrossRef] [PubMed]
8. Congiu, P.; Mariani, S.; Milioli, G.; Parrino, L.; Tamburrino, L.; Borghero, G.; Defazio, G.; Pereira, B.; Fantini, M.L.; Puligheddu, M. Sleep cardiac dysautonomia and EEG oscillations in amyotrophic lateral sclerosis. *Sleep* **2019**, *42*, zsz164. [CrossRef]
9. Drusehky, A.; Spitzer, A.; Platseh, G.; Claus, D.; Feistel, H.; Druschky, K.; Hilz, M.-J.; Neundörfer, B. Cardiac sympathetic denervation in early stages of amyotrophic lateral sclerosis demonstrated by ^{123}I-MIBG-SPECT. *Acta Neurol. Scand.* **1999**, *99*, 308–314. [CrossRef]
10. Matsuyama, Y.; Sasagasako, N.; Koike, A.; Matsuura, M.; Koga, T.; Kawajiri, M.; Ohyagi, Y.; Iwaki, T.; Kira, J.-I. An autopsy case of amyotrophic lateral sclerosis with ampulla cardiomyopathy. *Clin. Neurol.* **2008**, *48*, 249–254.
11. Mitani, M.; Funakawa, I.; Jinnai, K. Transient left ventricular apical ballooning, 'Takotsubo' cardiomyopathy, in an amyotrophic lateral sclerosis patient on long-term respiratory support. *Rinsho Shinkeigaku* **2005**, *45*, 740–743. [PubMed]
12. Takayama, N.; Iwase, Y.; Ohtsu, S.; Sakio, H. "Takotsubo" cardiomyopathy developed in the postoperative period in a patient with amyotrophic lateral sclerosis. *Masui. Jpn. J. Anesthesiol.* **2004**, *53*, 403–406.
13. Izumi, Y.; Miyamoto, R.; Fujita, K.; Yamamoto, Y.; Yamada, H.; Matsubara, T.; Unai, Y.; Tsukamoto, A.; Takamatsu, N.; Nodera, H.; et al. Distinct incidence of takotsubo syndrome between amyotrophic lateral sclerosis and synucleinopathies: A cohort study. *Front. Neurol.* **2018**, *9*, 1099. [CrossRef] [PubMed]
14. Templin, C.; Ghadri, J.R.; Diekmann, J.; Napp, L.C.; Bataiosu, D.R.; Jaguszewski, M.; Cammann, V.L.; Sarcon, A.; Geyer, V.; Neumann, C.A.; et al. Clinical Features and Outcomes of Takotsubo (Stress) Cardiomyopathy. *N. Engl. J. Med.* **2015**, *373*, 929–938. [CrossRef] [PubMed]
15. Scantlebury, D.C.; Prasad, A. Diagnosis of takotsubo cardiomyopathy—Mayo Clinic criteria. *Circ. J.* **2014**, *78*, 2129–2139. [CrossRef]
16. Brooks, B.R.; Miller, R.G.; Swash, M.; Munsat, T.L. El Escorial revisited: Revised criteria for the diagnosis of amyotrophic lateral sclerosis. *Amyotroph. Lateral Scler.* **2000**, *1*, 293–299. [CrossRef]
17. de Carvalho, M.; Dengler, R.; Eisen, A.; England, J.D.; Kaji, R.; Kimura, J.; Mills, K.; Mitsumoto, H.; Nodera, H.; Shefner, J.; et al. Electrodiagnostic criteria for diagnosis of ALS. *Clin. Neurophysiol.* **2008**, *119*, 497–503. [CrossRef]
18. Riva, N.; Pozzi, L.; Russo, T.; Pipitone, G.B.; Schito, P.; Domi, T.; Agosta, F.; Quattrini, A.; Carrera, P.; Filippi, M. NEK1 Variants in a Cohort of Italian Patients with Amyotrophic Lateral Sclerosis. *Front. Neurosci.* **2022**, *16*, 833051. [CrossRef]

19. Massari, F.M.; Tonella, T.; Tarsia, P.; Kirani, S.; Blasi, F.; Magrini, F. Sindrome tako-tsubo in giovane uomo affetto da sclerosi laterale amiotrofica. Descrizione di un caso clinico. *G. Ital. Cardiol.* **2011**, *12*, 388–391.
20. Choi, S.-J.; Hong, Y.-H.; Shin, J.-Y.; Yoon, B.-N.; Sohn, S.-Y.; Park, C.S.; Sung, J.-J. Takotsubo cardiomyopathy in amyotrophic lateral sclerosis. *J. Neurol. Sci.* **2017**, *375*, 289–293. [CrossRef]
21. Işcan, D.; Karaaslan, M.B.; Deveci, O.S.; Eker, R.A.; Koç, F. The importance of heart rate variability in predicting cardiac autonomic dysfunction in patients with amyotrophic lateral sclerosis. *Int. J. Clin. Pract.* **2021**, *75*, e14536. [CrossRef] [PubMed]
22. Peters, S. Tako tsubo cardiomyopathy in respiratory stress syndrome in amyotrophic lateral sclerosis. *Int. J. Cardiol.* **2014**, *177*, 187. [CrossRef] [PubMed]
23. Santoro, F.; Ieva, R.; Ferraretti, A.; Carapelle, E.; De Gennaro, L.; Specchio, L.M.; Di Biase, M.; Brunetti, N.D. Early recurrence of Tako-Tsubo cardiomyopathy in an elderly woman with amyotrophic lateral sclerosis: Different triggers inducing different apical ballooning patterns. *J. Cardiovasc. Med.* **2016**, *17*, e266–e268. [CrossRef]
24. Gdynia, H.J.; Kurt, A.; Endruhn, S.; Ludolph, A.C.; Sperfeld, A.D. Cardiomyopathy in motor neuron diseases. *J. Neurol. Neurosurg. Psychiatry* **2006**, *77*, 671–673. [CrossRef]
25. Asai, H.; Hirano, M.; Udaka, F.; Shimada, K.; Oda, M.; Kubori, T.; Nishinaka, K.; Tsujimura, T.; Izumi, Y.; Konishi, N.; et al. Sympathetic disturbances increase risk of sudden cardiac arrest in sporadic ALS. *J. Neurol. Sci.* **2007**, *254*, 78–83. [CrossRef] [PubMed]
26. Brettschneider, J.; Del Tredici, K.; Toledo, J.B.; Robinson, J.L.; Irwin, D.J.; Grossman, M.; Suh, E.R.; Van Deerlin, V.M.; Wood, E.M.; Baek, Y.; et al. Stages of pTDP-43 pathology in amyotrophic lateral sclerosis. *Ann. Neurol.* **2013**, *74*, 20–38. [CrossRef]
27. Mendoza-Velásquez, J.J.; Flores-Vázquez, J.F.; Barrón-Velázquez, E.; Sosa-Ortiz, A.L.; Illigens, B.M.W.; Siepmann, T. Autonomic Dysfunction in α-Synucleinopathies. *Front. Neurol.* **2019**, *10*, 363. [CrossRef] [PubMed]
28. Baker, C.; Muse, J.; Taussky, P. Takotsubo Syndrome in Neurologic Disease. *World Neurosurg.* **2021**, *149*, 26–31. [CrossRef]
29. Ziegelstein, R.C. Depression and tako-tsubo cardiomyopathy. *Am. J. Cardiol.* **2010**, *105*, 281–282. [CrossRef] [PubMed]
30. Rosenbohm, A.; Schmid, B.; Buckert, D.; Rottbauer, W.; Kassubek, J.; Ludolph, A.C.; Bernhardt, P. Cardiac Findings in Amyotrophic Lateral Sclerosis: A Magnetic Resonance Imaging Study. *Front. Neurol.* **2017**, *8*, 479. [CrossRef]
31. Hammond, H.K.; Roth, D.A.; Ford, C.E.; Stamnas, G.W.; Ziegler, M.G.; Ennis, C. Myocardial adrenergic denervation supersensitivity depends on a postreceptor mechanism not linked with increased cAMP production. *Circulation* **1992**, *85*, 666–679. [CrossRef] [PubMed]

Disclaimer/Publisher's Note: The statements, opinions and data contained in all publications are solely those of the individual author(s) and contributor(s) and not of MDPI and/or the editor(s). MDPI and/or the editor(s) disclaim responsibility for any injury to people or property resulting from any ideas, methods, instructions or products referred to in the content.

Review

Inhibition of Galectins and the P2X7 Purinergic Receptor as a Therapeutic Approach in the Neurovascular Inflammation of Diabetic Retinopathy

Caterina Claudia Lepre [1,†], Marina Russo [2,†], Maria Consiglia Trotta [2], Francesco Petrillo [3], Fabiana Anna D'Agostino [4], Gennaro Gaudino [5], Giovanbattista D'Amico [6], Maria Rosaria Campitiello [7], Erminia Crisci [4], Maddalena Nicoletti [4], Carlo Gesualdo [4,*], Francesca Simonelli [4], Michele D'Amico [2,‡], Anca Hermenean [1,‡] and Settimio Rossi [4,‡]

1 "Aurel Ardelean" Institute of Life Sciences, Vasile Goldis Western University of Arad, 310144 Arad, Romania
2 Department of Experimental Medicine, University of Campania "Luigi Vanvitelli", 80138 Naples, Italy
3 Ph.D. Course in Translational Medicine, Department of Experimental Medicine, University of Campania "Luigi Vanvitelli", 80138 Naples, Italy
4 Multidisciplinary Department of Medical, Surgical and Dental Sciences, University of Campania "Luigi Vanvitelli", 80138 Naples, Italy
5 School of Anesthesia and Intensive Care, University of Foggia, 71122 Foggia, Italy
6 School of Geriatrics, University of Studies of L'Aquila, 67010 L'Aquila, Italy
7 Department of Obstetrics and Gynecology and Physiopathology of Human Reproduction, ASL Salerno, 84124 Salerno, Italy
* Correspondence: carlo.gesualdo@unicampania.it
† These authors contributed equally to this work.
‡ These authors contributed equally to this work.

Abstract: Diabetic retinopathy (DR) is the most frequent microvascular retinal complication of diabetic patients, contributing to loss of vision. Recently, retinal neuroinflammation and neurodegeneration have emerged as key players in DR progression, and therefore, this review examines the neuroinflammatory molecular basis of DR. We focus on four important aspects of retinal neuroinflammation: (i) the exacerbation of endoplasmic reticulum (ER) stress; (ii) the activation of the NLRP3 inflammasome; (iii) the role of galectins; and (iv) the activation of purinergic 2X7 receptor (P2X7R). Moreover, this review proposes the selective inhibition of galectins and the P2X7R as a potential pharmacological approach to prevent the progression of DR.

Keywords: diabetic retinopathy; neuroinflammation; ROS; ER stress; NLRP3 inflammasome; galectins; P2X7R

1. Diabetic Retinopathy (DR): An Overview

Diabetes is known as a chronic disease with multiple complications [1]. One of the most harmful and common complications is diabetic retinopathy (DR) [2,3]. This is a leading cause of blindness worldwide [4], with 103.1 million adults affected by DR in 2020 and a predicted 160.5 million affected in 2045 [5]. Moreover, DR individuals often develop a visual impairment, leading to a poor quality of life for the patient and impacting on the health care system in terms of direct and indirect costs. Indeed, in 2020, there were 28.5 million patients affected by vision-threatening DR, and it is estimated this number will be 44.8 million by 2045 [5].

Historically, DR has been considered as a microangiopathy, and is characterized by increased retinal vascular permeability and endothelial damage [2,6,7]. In particular, the hallmarks of DR onset include the thickening of the basement membrane, the loss of pericytes, the alteration of tight junctions and the endothelial barrier, the formation of microaneurysms and the uncontrolled proliferation of endothelial cells [8–10]. These events later translate into capillary occlusion that anticipates retinal ischemia, which is, in turn, associated with vascular endothelial growth factor (VEGF) overexpression and neovascularization [9,11].

Accordingly, DR can be clinically classified as either non-proliferative diabetic retinopathy (NPDR) or proliferative diabetic retinopathy (PDR) [8], which are usually diagnosed by fluorescein angiography (FA) or mydriatic fundus camera examinations [12]. However, other imaging methods such as optical coherence tomography (OCT), Doppler OCT, OCT angiography and retinal imaging of the fundus can be used [12]. While NPDR is the early stage of the disease (which can be further classified as mild, moderate and severe), PDR represents the advanced stage of retinopathy. NPDR is characterized by progressive changes in retinal capillary microcirculation, resulting in microaneurysms, blood–retinal barrier (BRB) breakdown and intraretinal exudates [13]. Specifically, mild NPDR is diagnosed by the presence of few microaneurysms; moderate NPDR is characterized by microaneurysms, venous beading or intraretinal hemorrhages; severe NPDR is defined by the presence of hemorrhages or microaneurysms or both, venous beading or prominent intraretinal microvascular abnormalities (IRMAs) [14]. In contrast, PDR is characterized by the presence of numerous ischemic retinal areas, VEGF overproduction and neoangiogenesis [15,16], and is diagnosed by neovascularization of the disc retina and iris or by tractional retinal detachment or vitreous hemorrhage [14]. Indeed, PDR can evolve into more severe stages such as diabetic macular edema (DME), neovascular glaucoma and, in rare cases, retinal detachment [9,13,15,17].

While the glycemic, lipidic and blood pressure controls are needed for DR primary prevention, the current surgical and pharmacological options for DR management include pan-retinal laser photocoagulation in severe NPDR and PDR patients, focal retinal laser photocoagulation in patients with diabetic DME, anti-VEGF intravitreal injections in PDR and DME patients, and steroid intravitreal injections for non-responder DR patients or naïve patients when appropriate [18]. In particular, the early use of laser photocoagulation or intravitreal injections of glucocorticoids or anti-angiogenics drugs has proven effective in preventing the onset of blindness [19], while anti-VEGF intravitreal injections are considered the actual gold standard for DR therapy. However, DR management is still challenging, with the 40% of inadequately treated NPDR cases evolving to PDR within 12 months [13,20]. Therefore, several studies have been performed to identify new molecular pathways or circulating biomarkers as new potential pharmacological tools in DR prevention and/or treatment. Among these, an important role as predictive and therapeutic targets in DR progression has been proposed for melanocortin receptors, retinol binding protein 3 (RBP3), angiopoietin-like 3 (ANGPTL3), microRNAs, extracellular vesicles, metabolites as 12-hydroxyeicosatetraenoic acid and 2-piperidone, along with several mediators involved in the resolution of inflammation [21–27].

Currently, intraretinal inflammation and neurodegeneration have emerged as key processes in DR progression [16,28]. Indeed, along with microvascular damage, inflammatory and neurodegenerative processes contribute to alterations in the "retinal neurovascular unit", a functional unit composed of endothelial cells, glial cells and neurons [29]. In this regard, early retinal neurovascular alterations have been recently associated with specific serum microglial biomarkers such as ionized calcium-binding adapter molecule 1 (Iba-1), glucose transporter 5 (GLUT5), and translocator protein (TSPO) [27].

In this review, we focus on the importance of endoplasmic reticulum stress (ERS) and the consequent activation of the nucleotide-binding oligomerization domain-, leucine-rich repeat- and pyrin domain-containing 3 (NLRP3) inflammasome during retinal neuroinflammation. In particular, ERS modulation by specific proteins binding beta-galactoside residues on glycated proteins known as galectins is detailed. The galectin family consists of 15 identified members, all of which contain conserved carbohydrate-recognition domains (CRDs) of about 130 amino acids [30]. Based on the CRD organization of the polypeptide monomer, the galectins have been classified into three types: proto-type, chimera-type, and tandem-repeat-type [31]. The prototypical galectins have one CRD (galectin-1, -2, -5, -7, -10,

-11, -13, -14 and -15); the tandem-repeat-type galectins contain two homologous CRDs in a single polypeptide chain, separated by a linker of up to 70 amino acids (galectin-4, -6, -8, -9 and -12); galectin-3 contains a non-lectin N-terminal region (about 120 amino acids) connected to a CRD [32]. Outside the cell, galectins bind to cell-surface and extracellular matrix glycans; however, galectins are also detectable in the cytosol and nucleus. They may influence cellular signaling pathways, such as cell migration, autophagy, immune response, and inflammation [32].

Moreover, the importance of purinergic 2X7 receptor (P2X7R) in NLRP3 activation underlying neuroinflammation is analyzed, along with the options for their selective inhibition in several clinical settings. Specifically, the state of the art on galectins and P2X7R inhibitors in DR is described, along with their potential use as pharmacological tools to prevent DR progression.

2. The Role of Neuroinflammation in DR

The "retinal neurovascular unit" includes specific retinal glia elements, such as microglial cells and macroglia (Müller cells and astrocytes) [28,33,34]. These express marked ERS [35–37] and subsequent activation of NLRP3 inflammasome [38], as a consequence of advanced glycation end products (AGEs) and reactive oxygen species (ROS) formation, strongly induced by chronic hyperglycemia [39]. In this regard, increases in many pro-inflammatory cytokines and chemokines, such as interleukin 1 beta (IL-1β), interleukin 6 (IL-6), interleukin 8 (IL-8), tumor necrosis factor alpha (TNF-α) and monocyte chemoattractant protein-1 (MCP-1), have been found in serum and in ocular samples (vitreous and aqueous humor) of DR patients. The accumulation of these cytokines is mainly mediated by cells from the macroglia and microglia [40].

Microglial cells represent the first defense line in neural retina [41–43]. Specifically, the retinal inner layers are characterized by the presence of ramified microglial cells [44,45] controlling the regulation of retinal growth, blood vessel formation and the retinal endothelial cell–glia–neuron interactions [46–50]. When activated by hyperglycemia, retinal hypoxia, ischemia and ER stress [51–54], these cells are classified as M1 macrophages and release pro-inflammatory mediators such as IL-6 and IL-12, TNF-α and interferon gamma (IFN-γ), known inducers of inflammation, apoptosis and neurotoxicity [55–57]. Microglial cells can be alternatively classified as M2 macrophages and release anti-inflammatory mediators, thus exerting anti-inflammatory effects and neuroprotection [42,55,58].

Retinal microglia polarization directly influences Müller cells and macroglia cells, spanning the entire retinal width and connecting neurons and vascular components [59,60]. In healthy retina, Müller cells contribute to the BRB integrity, modulate retinal blood flow and regulate the production of ions, neurotransmitters and metabolites that favor retinal blood vessel dilatation or constriction [61]. As a consequence of hyperglycemia-induced ER stress [35,39], Müller cell activation leads to the release of pro-inflammatory cytokines and chemokines [62] which favor leucocytes recruitment [63], a phenomenon termed gliosis. Moreover, Müller cell inflammatory actions across the retinal laminal structure seems to favor microglia attraction and adhesion by modulating retinal injury response [60].

Lastly, astrocytes are the most abundant central nervous system (CNS) macroglial cell type, forming the inner retinal BRB [64]. These are prevalent in the retinal ganglion cell layer (GCL) and nerve fiber layer (NFL) and modulate the neuronal metabolism, neurotransmission, and the neurorepair process [65–67]. Astrocytes can exert either pro- or anti-inflammatory actions, depending on the microenvironment in which they are located and the received signal [68].

3. Mechanisms of DR Neuroinflammation

3.1. Endoplasmic Reticulum (ER) Stress

In the diabetic retina, hyperglycemia leads to elevated ROS production by various mechanisms, including the reduction of antioxidant enzymes [69] and the activation of hypoxia-inducible transcription factor 1 (HIF-1) [70,71].

During DR, the hyperglycemia-induced ER stress (ERS) affects all the components of the "neurovascular unit" and leads to the apoptosis of both vascular and neuronal cells [72,73]. In particular, the abnormal ERS causes the apoptosis of retinal pericytes [74] with BRB impairment and retinal neuroinflammation [75,76]. Among the ERS inducers, key roles are played by glycative stress and activation of the unfolded protein response (UPR) that are stimulated by AGEs and ROS formation, respectively [77]. Glycative stress is used to monitor the status of protein folding and ensure that only properly folded proteins are trafficked to the Golgi [78,79]. UPR is an adaptive signaling pathway which tends to enhance the ER capacity for protein folding and modification to restore an efficient protein-folding environment [77]. The main UPR actors are the inositol-requiring kinase 1 (IRE1), the protein kinase R (PKR)-like endoplasmic reticulum kinase (PERK) and the activating transcription factor 6 (ATF6) [77,80]. When the accumulation of protein aggregates exceeds the ER load capacity, the activation of UPR exacerbates ERS [81] (Figure 1).

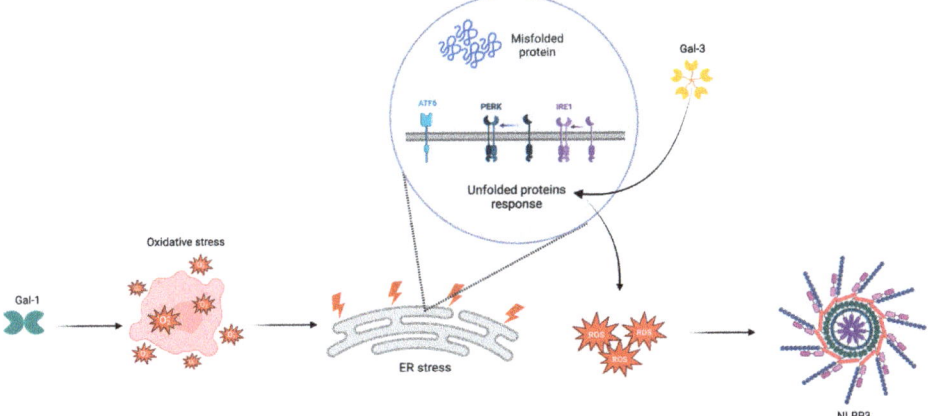

Figure 1. Involvement of galectins in ER stress. ATF6: activating transcription factor; ER: endoplasmic reticulum; Gal-1: galectin 1; Gal-3: galectin 3; IRE1: inositol-requiring kinase 1; NLRP3: nucleotide-binding domain, leucine-rich–containing family, pyrin domain–containing-3 inflammasome; PERK: protein kinase R-like endoplasmic reticulum kinase; ROS: reactive oxygen species. Arrow: increase. Created with BioRender.com, accessed on 2 May 2023.

ERS-induced microglial activation occurs during the different DR stages [27,47]. Indeed, activated microglial cells have been observed in the retinal plexiform layers (RPL) of NPDR patients and around the ischemic areas in PDR patients [82]. Notably, changes in M1/M2 microglia polarization can lead to visual loss by increasing the apoptosis of retinal neurons with consequent retinal NFL thinning [83].

Conversely, ERS-induced Müller cell activation seems to precede the DR vascular alterations [84], with NPDR patients showing Müller cell gliosis and swelling in the retinal inner nuclear layer (INL) and outer plexiform layer (OPL) [85], although PDR neuronal damage and DME cyst formation also characterize gliosis [86]. Lastly, retinal astrocytes are responsible for a sustained production of the pro-inflammatory IL-1β in response to hyperglycemia-induced ERS [87].

3.2. NLRP3 Inflammasome

ROS-induced ER stress leads to the activation of the NLRP3 inflammasome, a multi-proteic complex found as monomer when inactive [88–91] (Figure 1). In particular, ERS exacerbation leads to activation of the NLRP3 inflammasome [92] through the binding of thioredoxin-interacting protein (TXNIP) to NLRP3 [93,94].

The NLRP3 complex consists of a sensor component (NLRP3 protein), an effector component (caspase-1) and, in some cases, an adapter protein (known as apoptosis-associated speck-like protein—ASC) linking the sensor and the effector [93,95,96]. The NLRP3 sensor is characterized by three different domains known as cytosolic pattern recognition receptors (PRRs): an amino-terminal pyrin domain (PYD), a central nucleotide-binding and oligomerization domain (NOD domain), and a C-terminal leucine-rich repeat (LRR) domain. Through these, NLRP3 is known to sense an extremely broad range of both exogenous and endogenous stimuli, known as pathogen-associated molecular patterns (PAMPs) and danger-associated molecular patterns (DAMPs), including changes in the ion gradient across the cell, cellular stress mechanisms such as higher ROS production after lysosomal rupture, mitochondrial stress and ERS in response to the accumulation of misfolded proteins [97–100]. When activated, the pyrin domain of NLRP3 interacts with the ASC pyrin domain to initiate inflammasome assembly [100,101] (Figure 2).

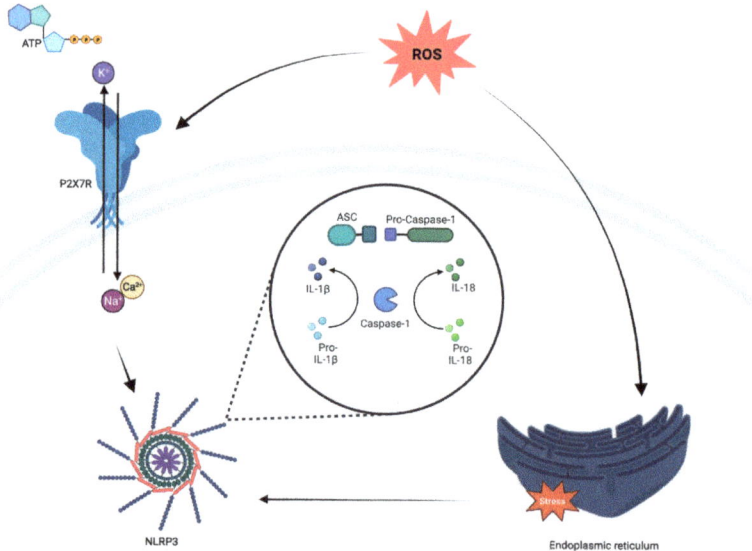

Figure 2. Involvement of P2X7R in NLRP3 activation. ASC: apoptosis-associated speck-like protein; ATP: adenosine triphosphate; Ca^{2+}: Calcium; IL-1β: interleukin 1 beta; IL-18: interleukin 18; P2X7R: purinergic 2X7 receptor; ROS: reactive oxygen species; Na^+: sodium; NLRP3: nucleotide-binding domain, leucine-rich-containing family, pyrin domain-containing-3 inflammasome; K^+: potassium. Arrow: increase. Created with BioRender.com, accessed on 2 May 2023.

The pyrene domain connects to the NLRP3 pyrene domain through an oligomerization process; in addition, the adaptor protein ASC brings pro-caspase 1 monomers near to each other through the CARD domain by inducing a proximity-mediated caspase-1 autoactivation [101]. Active caspase-1 can induce the release of pro-inflammatory cytokines, such as IL-1β and interleukin 18 (IL-18), favoring both apoptosis and pyroptosis, a cell death process during which some pro-inflammatory cytokines are released to attract and activate immune cells [93,95,102,103]. Moreover, active caspase-1 is also necessary for the proteolytic cleavage of Gasdermin D (GSDMD) and the consequent release of the GSDMD N-terminal fragment, which is necessary to mediate pyroptosis [104].

Similarly, NLRP3 is pivotal in DR progression [89,91,105–107]. Indeed, retinal NLRP3 levels were increased in serum and vitreous samples from patients affected by PDR compared with NPDR patients [40,106,107].

NLRP3 activation is shown by retinal epithelial [108–111] and endothelial cells [112–114]. However, it is evident also in retinal neuronal layers, such as retinal ganglion cells (RGC) in mouse models of retinal degeneration and in photoreceptors from a genetic mouse DR model [115–117]. Moreover, NLRP3 levels were increased in retinal microglial cells exposed to high glucose [118] and in retinal macroglia from a mouse model of ocular hypertension [119].

4. New Actors in Neuroinflammation
4.1. Galectins and ERS

Overall, galectin dysregulation has been linked to different pathological conditions, such as fibrosis, heart disease, cancer, and diabetes [32]. In this regard, Gal-1 has been associated with type 2 diabetes [120], while Gal-3 has been correlated to both type 1 and type 2 diabetes [121–123], with a suggested role for this galectin in mediating the chronic inflammation underlying the progression from prediabetes to the diabetic stage [124]. Moreover, in diabetic patients, diabetic nephropathy, diabetic foot, diabetic microvascular complications, and diabetic cardiomyopathy have been all related to changes in Gal-3 serum levels [125]. In particular, Galectin 1 (Gal-1) and Galectin 3 (Gal-3) seem to initiate the inflammatory response by acting as chemotactic agents towards the inflammatory site for the neutrophils, facilitating their binding to the endothelium and their trafficking through the extracellular matrix [126].

Galectins, induced by AGEs and considered as receptors for AGEs (RAGE), have emerged as ERS regulators. For example, the elevation of Galectin 9 (Gal-9) has been linked to inflammatory processes in both type 1 and type 2 diabetes [127,128]. However, an additional protective role against ERS has been described for Gal-9 [129], along with its importance in the facilitation of NLRP3 autophagic degradation [130].

In addition, Gal-1 and Gal-3 have also emerged as ERS regulators (Figure 1). Specifically, Gal-1 is upregulated in hypoxic microenvironments [131], resulting in increased ROS production and activation of the nuclear factor kappa B (NF-κB) signaling pathway [132]. This protein is considered a key regulator of endothelial cells functions and shows potent proangiogenic properties [133,134].

Gal-3 is localized at the ER-mitochondria interface and regulates the UPR [135]. It is involved in several processes underlying retinopathies, such as oxidative stress, proliferation, apoptosis, phagocytosis, oxidative stress, and angiogenesis [136]. Interestingly, Gal-3 may favor adaptive UPR following ERS by acting as both a pro- and anti-apoptotic regulator [135]. Tian and colleagues demonstrated that Gal-3 is also implicated in the process of activating the NLRP3 inflammasome, discovering a direct link of the N-terminal domain of Gal-3 to the NLRP3 inflammasome [137]. Several studies have shown alterations in the concentration of galectins in the brain and blood of patients with neurodegenerative diseases compared with healthy subjects. In particular, Gal-1 was found in neurofilamentous lesions of patients affected by amyotrophic lateral sclerosis (ALS) [138], while patients with multiple sclerosis showed a higher concentration of Galectin 4 (Gal-4) in chronic lesions of the brain [139]. However, Gal-3 can be considered as an indicator of prognosis, mortality or remission in neurodegenerative diseases [140] since its expression was found to be increased in patients with ALS, Alzheimer's and Parkinson's diseases (AD and PD, respectively) [141].

This could be firstly due to the high affinity showed by galectins for β-galactosides [142,143], which are involved in neuroprotection and neuroinflammation [144,145]. Moreover, galectins are expressed by glial cells. In particular, Gal-1 expression was reported in astrocytes and Müller cells, participating in the protection from axonal damage as it mediates T-cell activation and differentiation, whereas Gal-3 expression was mainly observed in M1 microglial cells and was associated with microglial activation in cell damage, ischemia, and encephalitis [30,140,146]. Particularly astrocyte-derived Gal-1 seems to play a key role in the modulation of inflammation, phagocytosis, axon growth and gliosis after spinal cord injury [147,148]. It was also found to be important in the modulation of microglia polarization and neuromodulation in a multiple sclerosis model [149], as well as modulation of axonal degeneration in a transgenic mouse model of ALS [150]. Regarding Gal-3, in primary rat microglia and macroglia, Gal-3 exposure increases the expression of TNF-α, IL-1β, IL-6 and INF-γ [151]. Accordingly, in a mouse model of Huntington's disease, Gal-3 increased the microglial expression of IL-1β [152]. Moreover, the suppression of Gal-3 in AD mice improved their cognitive performance, reducing amyloid plaques [153], as well as cognitive impairment, neuroinflammation and oxidative stress associated with diabetes in rats caused by modified citrus pectin (MCP) [154].

4.2. Purinergic 2X7 Receptor (P2X7R) and NLRP3 Inflammasome

P2X7R is a trimeric ion channel that belongs to the P2X family of ionotropic receptors preferably permeable to sodium, potassium and calcium, which are exclusively triggered by extracellular adenosine triphosphate (ATP) [96]. P2X receptors are widespread in different tissues and exert various functions: in some smooth muscle cells, activated P2X receptors mediate depolarization and contraction; in the CNS, activated P2X receptors allow calcium to enter neurons, leading to slower neuromodulatory responses; and in the cells of the immune system, activated P2X receptors trigger the release of pro-inflammatory cytokines [155].

P2X7R presents five domains: one extracellular domain; two transmembrane domains (classified as transmembrane 1 and 2); and two intracellular domains (N- and C-terminus), which form homotrimeric receptors after their activation [156,157]. Its signaling is important for regulating both the innate and adaptive immune response [156] and also inflammatory processes [96].

P2X7R is highly expressed in different cell types and tissues, such as retinal neural cells and the retinal vasculature [158], but also in immune cells [159]. In particular, in the human retina, P2X7R is localized in INL, OPL and GCL and is expressed by human retinal Müller cells, the native retinal pigment epithelium (RPE) and adult retinal pigment epithelial cell line-19 (ARPE-19) [160].

P2X7R has a key role in linking inflammation with purinergic signaling: this receptor and the NLRP3 inflammasome interact at distinct cytoplasmic sites, where changes in P2X7R-dependent ion concentrations (specifically a K+ efflux) occur [156,161,162], probably mediated by the cytoplasmic kinase never-in-mitosis A- related kinases (NEK) [156] (Figure 2). In particular, during NLRP3 inflammasome activation, the K+ efflux seems to be mediated by P2X7R following an increase in extracellular ATP [163]. This allows the release of pro-inflammatory cytokines associated with NLRP3 inflammasome activation [156]. In this regard, P2X7R is upregulated [162] in pathological conditions as a consequence of increased extracellular microglial ATP concentration [164]. This is indicative of the pro-inflammatory M1 phenotype microglia activation [164]. P2X7R is widely expressed in the CNS regions and is associated with neuroinflammation and neurodegeneration [164–166]. Therefore, P2X7R has been extensively investigated in order to develop small molecules that could act as potent blockers of the receptor [155].

Indeed, P2X7R activation in glial cells overall results in the release of the pro-inflammatory cytokines, thereby triggering or potentiating neuroinflammation [167]. This contributes to neurodegeneration by inducing microglia-mediated neuronal death [168], glutamate-mediated excitotoxicity and NLRP3 inflammasome activation, with the consequent release of IL-1β and IL-18 [96,164,169].

Several studies evidenced that P2X7R expression is upregulated in the activated microglia of AD patients and is concentrated in amyloid plaques [170,171]. Similarly, P2X7R was upregulated in the hippocampus of an AD animal model [172,173]. Furthermore, preclinical evidence suggests that P2X7R may have a role in the pathogenesis of Huntington's disease [174]. P2X7R also has a possible involvement in PD by mediating activation of the NLRP3 inflammasome [175]. This aspect is under investigation in an observational prospective study at the University of Pisa (Italy). This study is evaluating changes in P2X7R levels and their association with changes in NLRP3 inflammasome levels in patients with newly diagnosed PD or AD receiving routine treatment in comparison with an age- and gender-matched group [176]. P2X7R was also recently identified as a key contributor to cognitive impairment in a mouse model of migraine; activation of the NLRP3 inflammasome and P2X7R upregulation led to gliosis, neuronal loss and neuroinflammation [177]. Astrogliosis related to P2X7R has also been reported in a rat model of autoimmune encephalomyelitis [178].

5. Inhibition of Galectins and P2X7R and Its Potential Therapeutic Application for DR Neuroinflammation

It is well known that galectins and P2X7R are two key mediators in DR pathology and progression [84,157,179–189]. Therefore, these neuroinflammatory actors represent two potential pharmacological targets to prevent the onset of DR by their selective inhibition.

In this regard, different compounds inhibiting galectins have been evaluated in clinical trials. In particular, although Gal-1 inhibitor OTX0008 has been tested in patients with advanced solid tumors [190], Gal-3 inhibition has gained a wider application in several ongoing clinical trials. Indeed, both the Gal-3 inhibitors GR-MD-02 and GB1211 are in evaluation for liver fibrosis in non-alcoholic steatohepatitis (NASH) [143,191,192]. Administration of GB1211 alone has also been investigated for hepatic impairment [193], and its combination with atezolizumab (a monoclonal antibody targeting the Programmed Death Ligand-1) has been considered in non-small cell lung cancer patients [194]. Furthermore, the co-administration of GR-MD-02 with ipilimumab (a monoclonal antibody targeting the Cytotoxic T-Lymphocyte Antigen 4) or pembrolizumab (a monoclonal human antibody targeting the Programmed Cell Death protein 1) is undergoing evaluation in patients with metastatic melanoma [195] and in patients with advanced melanoma, non-small cell lung cancer and head and neck squamous cell cancer, respectively [196,197].

Gal-3 inhibition by GB0139 and TD139 compounds is under evaluation in idiopathic pulmonary fibrosis (IPF) [143,198,199], while MCP as a Gal-3 inhibitor has been considered for both hypertension and osteoarthritis [200,201].

Regarding P2X7R, different compounds have been tested on healthy volunteers to assess their safety and tolerability, bioavailability, pharmacokinetics, and pharmacodynamics as P2X7R antagonists. These include GSK1482160 [202], AZD9056 [203,204], and ce-224,535 [205,206]. In particular, ce-224,535 and AZD9056 have both been in evaluation for patients with rheumatoid arthritis (RA) [207,208], with ce-224,535 considered also for patients with knee osteoarthritis pain [209].

To date, none of these inhibitors has been considered for DR patients. However, several pre-clinical studies evidenced the potential role of galectin and P2X7R inhibition strategies in modulating diabetic retinal damage [179,181,183,184].

5.1. Galectin Inhibition in DR

Gal-1 and Gal-3 have been recently associated with the insurgence and progression of DR pathology (Table 1).

Table 1. Galectins in DR studies.

Study	Main Results	Treatments	Reference
Clinical Vitreous fluid samples from 36 patients with PDR (20 patients undergoing vitrectomy as controls)	VEGF and Gal-1 levels significantly higher in PDR patients compared with controls	-	[179]
Clinical Plasma samples from 20 PDR cases (20 non-diabetic, idiopathic macular diseases as controls)	Plasma levels of Gal-1, AGEs and IL-1β significantly increased in PDR patients	-	[185]

Table 1. *Cont.*

Study	Main Results	Treatments	Reference
Clinical 23 vitreous fluids aspirated from PDR (non-diabetic control eyes with idiopathic ERM and MH) Neovascular ocular tissues surgically excised from PDR patients (non-diabetic tissues as controls)	Gal-1 levels were significantly elevated in the vitreous fluids of PDR eyes compared with controls Gal-1 upregulated in PDR tissues and co-localized with VEGFR2	-	[186]
In vivo STZ-Sprague Dawley rats (non-diabetic rats as controls) STZ:55 mg/kg (single dose, i.v. injection) Vehicle: 10 mM sodium citrate buffer (single dose i.v. injection)	Retinal Gal-1 levels increased in diabetic rats compared with controls	-	[179]
In vivo Gal-3 knockout C57/BL6 mice (wild-type mice as controls)	Gal-3 knockout mice exhibited less activated inflammatory cells within the optic nerve after crush	-	[180]
In vivo Diabetic Gal-3 knockout C57/BL6 mice (wild-type diabetic mice as controls) STZ:160 mg/kg (single dose, i.p. injection) Vehicle: sodium citrate buffer (single dose i.p. injection)	Gal-3 knockout reduced RGC apoptosis, Iba-1 and GFAP in the distal optic nerve in diabetic mice; moreover, it prevented the loss of myelinated fibers	-	[188]
In vivo Diabetic Gal-3 knockout C57/BL6 mice (wild-type diabetic mice as controls) STZ:165 mg/kg (single dose, i.p. injection) Vehicle: sodium citrate buffer (single dose i.p. injection)	Gal-3 knockout reduced AGEs, VEGF and BRB breakdown in diabetic mice	-	[189]
In vitro Hypoxic ($CoCl_2$) human retinal Müller glial cells (non-hypoxic cells as controls) $CoCl_2$: 300 μM for 24 h	OTX008 attenuated the upregulation of Gal-1, VEGF and NF-κB in hypoxic retinal Müller cells	Gal-1 selective inhibitor OTX008 OTX008: 10 μM for 24 h	[179]
In vitro ARPE-19 cells exposed to HG (NG cells as controls) HG: 35 mM NG: 5 mM	OTX008 induced a significant increment in cell viability; while Gal-1 protein, ROS and TGF-β1 levels were reduced after OTX008	Gal-1 selective inhibitor OTX008 (2.5–5–10 μM)	[181]

Abbreviations. AGEs: advanced glycation end products; ARPE-19: adult retinal pigment epithelial cell line-19; BRB: blood-retinal barrier; $CoCl_2$: cobalt chloride; ERM: epiretinal membrane; Gal-1: galectin 1; Gal-3: galectin 3; GFAP: glial fibrillary acidic protein as activated macroglia marker; h: hours; HG: high glucose; Iba-1: ionized calcium-binding adapter molecule 1; IL-1β: interleukin 1 beta; i.p.: intraperitoneal; i.v.: intravenous; MH: macular hole; NF-kB: nuclear factor kappa-light-chain-enhancer of activated B cells; NG: normal glucose; OTX008: calixarene 0118; PDR: proliferative diabetic retinopathy; RGC: retinal ganglion cells; ROS: reactive oxygen species; STZ: streptozotocin; TGF-β1: transforming growth factor beta 1; VEGF: vascular-endothelial growth factor; VEGFR2: Vascular Endothelial Growth Factor Receptor 2.

In particular, Gal-1 levels were increased in the vitreous fluid and epiretinal fibrovascular membrane of PDR patients compared with non-diabetic controls [179]. This was probably due to the higher Gal-1 secretion induced in retinal Müller cells and astrocytes by hyperglycemic conditions [136]. The upregulation of Gal-1 protein levels in vitreous samples rose substantially with DR progression, being present from the pre-ischemic inflammatory stage [186]. Increased Gal-1 plasma levels were also detected in PDR patients compared with non-diabetic controls, along with a Gal-1 correlation with AGEs and IL-1β [185]. In line with this evidence, Gal-1 was also found to be upregulated in neovascular ocular tissues surgically excised from PDR patients, where it exhibited a colocalization with Vascular Endothelial Growth Factor Receptor 2 (VEGFR2) [186]. While in this study, Gal-1 exhibited no correlation with VEGFA, in a mouse model of oxygen induced-retinopathy (OIR), Gal-1 was shown to mediate vascular alterations concomitantly to VEGF up-regulation [187].

Gal-1 also seems to be involved in the regulation of the RPE that forms the BRB. Indeed, ARPE-19 cells exposed to high glucose exhibited high Gal-1 levels, which was associated with epithelial fibrosis and epithelial-mesenchymal transition [181]. Both processes were reduced by selective Gal-1 blocking with OTX008 [181].

Although Gal-1 has been associated with neuronal alterations in a mouse OIR model, and particularly with neuroglial injuries at post-natal day 26 [187], retinal neuroinflammatory actions have been specifically shown for Gal-3, whose pro-inflammatory role in diabetic optic neuropathy occurs through ROS-induced ERS [84]. Accordingly, within the neuronal retina, Gal-3 knockout resulted in reduced microglial activation and led to better preservation of RGC, nerve fibers, axons and cell bodies in diabetic mice [180]. This evidence was recently confirmed by Mendonça and colleagues [188], who showed that Gal-3 knockout in diabetic mice attenuated neuroinflammation in the retina and optic nerve. This effect was exerted by reducing the activation of retinal microglia and macroglia, and by increasing the number of myelinated fibers. Gal-3 knockout has also been associated with AGEs and VEGF reduction, along with the amelioration of BRB dysfunction, during short-term diabetes in mice [189].

5.2. P2X7R Inhibition in DR

Recent evidence suggests a role of the P2X7 receptor in controlling the BRB function and integrity [210,211]. Once P2X7R is activated, it mediates inflammatory vascular reactions induced by cytokines which degrade the BRB integrity and lead to retinal vascular occlusion and ischemia [182,210,212]. Moreover, P2X7R seems to mediate the accumulation of microglia and macrophages in the subretina [213].

A specific role for the P2X7R-NLRP3 inflammasome pathway in retinal endothelial inflammation and pericyte loss during the NPDR stage has been also described [182–184] (Table 2). Moreover, P2X7R stimulation or overexpression positively regulates VEGF secretion and accumulation, thus promoting DR neo-angiogenesis [157].

Therefore, a P2X7R inhibition strategy could represent a useful therapeutic tool to manage the early phase of DR. In this regard, the P2X7R selective inhibitor A74003 reduced the apoptosis of mice retinal endothelial cells (mRECs) stimulated with high glucose and lipopolysaccharide (LPS) [183]. Furthermore, Platania and colleagues analyzed the possible anti-inflammatory role of the selective P2X7R antagonist JNJ47965567 in diabetic human retinal pericytes [184]. While high glucose levels induced pericyte cell damage and a significant release of IL-1β, the treatment with JNJ47965567 decreased the IL-1β release by blocking P2X7R and consequently, NLRP3 inflammasome activation [184].

Table 2. P2X7R in DR studies.

Study	Treatment	Main Results	References
In vivo STZ-C57BL/6J mice (non-diabetic mice as controls) STZ: 50 mg/kg (daily, i.p. injection) for 5 days Vehicle: 0.1% mol/L citrate buffer (daily, i.p. injection) for 5 days	P2X7R selective inhibitor A74003 (100 μg/kg/d); NLRP3 inflammasome selective inhibitor MCC950 (100 μg/kg/d) A74003: 100 μg/kg/d, i.p. injection every alternate day from week 9 to week 12 MCC950: 100 μg/kg/d, i.p. injection daily for the first 3 days and then every alternate day from week 9 to week 12	P2X7R mRNA Significantly higher in the retinal tissues of STZ-mice; A74003 and MCC950 reduced retinal inflammation and apoptosis in STZ-mice	[183]
In vitro Pericyte-containing retinal microvessels from STZ-Long Evans rats (non-diabetic rats as controls) STZ: 75 mg/kg (single dose, i.p. injection) Vehicle: 0.8 mL (single dose, citrate buffer i.p. injection)	P2X7R agonist BzATP BzATP: 100 μM for 24 h	BzATP (100 μM) increased the apoptosis of pericyte-containing retinal microvessels from STZ-rats	[182]
In vitro mRECs exposed to HG, alone or in combination with LPS, (NG cells as controls) HG: 50 mM for 24 and 48 h LPS: 20 ng/mL for 48 h NG: 5.5 mM for 24 and 48 h	P2X7R selective inhibitor A74003; NLRP3 inflammasome selective inhibitor MCC950 A74003: 100 μmol/L 6 h before HG or HG + LPS, until 72 h MCC950: 100 μmol/L, 6 h before HG or HG + LPS, until 72 h	A74003 reduced apoptosis and pyroptosis in mRECS exposed to HG combined with LPS	[183]
In vitro Human retinal pericytes exposed to HG (NG cells as controls) HG: 25 mM for 48 h NG: 5 mM for 48 h	P2X7R agonist BzATP; P2X7R novel antagonist JNJ47965567 BzATP: 100 μM for 48 h JNJ47965567: 10–100 nM for 48 h	BzATP induced human retinal pericyte cell death and increased the pro-inflammatory cytokines levels; JNJ47965567 Protected pericytes viability and reduced pro-inflammatory cytokines	[184]

Abbreviations: BzATP: benzoylbenzoyl-adenosine triphosphate; h: hours; HG: high glucose; i.p.: intraperitoneal; LPS: lipopolysaccharide; mRECs: mice retinal endothelial cells; mRNA: messenger ribonucleic acid; NG: normal glucose; NLRP3: nucleotide-binding domain, leucine-rich–containing family, pyrin domain–containing-3 inflammasome; P2X7R: purinergic 2x7 receptors; STZ: streptozotocin.

6. Conclusions

Due to the role of galectins in ERS modulation and the role of P2X7R in NLRP3 inflammasome activation, both these mediators could represent two new potential targets, whose specific inhibition could help counteract the inflammatory process underlying DR progression, although evidence for a specific molecular relation and interlink between them is not available yet (Figure 3).

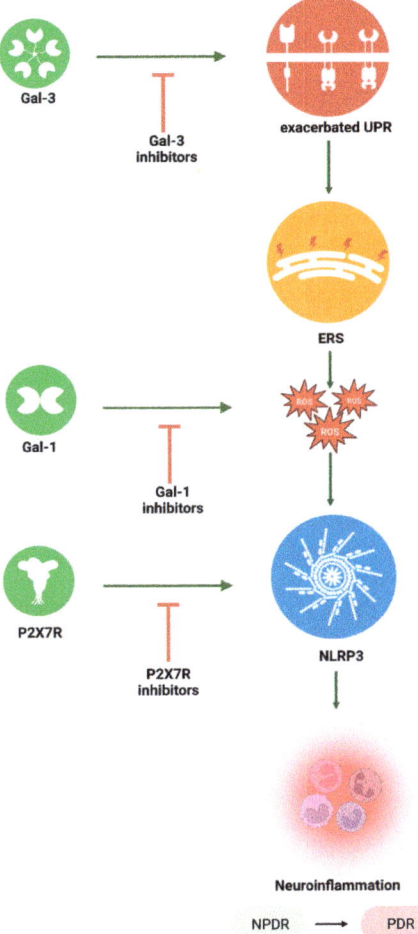

Figure 3. Diagram summarizing galectins, P2X7R and their inhibition of the ERS-NLRP3 inflammasome. ERS: endoplasmic reticulum stress; Gal-1: galectin 1; Gal-3: galectin 3; P2X7R: P2X7 receptor; NLRP3: nucleotide-binding domain, leucine-rich–containing family, pyrin domain–containing-3 inflammasome; NPDR: non-proliferative diabetic retinopathy; PDR: proliferative diabetic retinopathy; ROS: reactive oxygen species; UPR: unfolded protein response. Black arrow: progression; green arrow: increase; red arrow: decrease. Created with BioRender.com, accessed on 2 May 2023.

Author Contributions: Conceptualization, C.C.L., M.R. and M.C.T.; methodology, F.P. and F.A.D.; software, G.G. and G.D.; writing—original draft preparation, C.C.L., M.R., M.C.T. and C.G.; writing—review and editing, M.D., A.H. and S.R.; visualization, M.R.C., E.C. and M.N.; supervision, F.S. All authors have read and agreed to the published version of the manuscript.

Funding: This research was funded by the Italian Ministry of Education, University and Research, grant number PRIN 2020FR7TCL_002 and by the Roman Ministry of Research, Innovation and Digitalization, CNCS/CCCDI-UEFISCDI, project number PN-III-P4-ID-PCE-2020-1772, within PNCDI III.

Institutional Review Board Statement: Not applicable.

Informed Consent Statement: Not applicable.

Data Availability Statement: Not applicable.

Conflicts of Interest: The authors declare no conflict of interest.

References

1. Harding, J.L.; Pavkov, M.E.; Magliano, D.J.; Shaw, J.E.; Gregg, E.W. Global Trends in Diabetes Complications: A Review of Current Evidence. *Diabetologia* **2019**, *62*, 3–16. [CrossRef] [PubMed]
2. Ahmed, R.; Khalil, S.; Al-Qahtani, M. Diabetic Retinopathy and the Associated Risk Factors in Diabetes Type 2 Patients in Abha, Saudi Arabia. *J. Fam. Commun. Med.* **2016**, *23*, 18. [CrossRef] [PubMed]
3. Mahobia, A.; Sahoo, S.; Maiti, N.; Sathyanarayanan, R.; Aravinth, R.; Pandraveti, R.; Tiwari, H. Diabetic Retinopathy and Its Effect on Quality of Life: An Original Research. *J. Pharm. Bioall. Sci.* **2021**, *13*, 1365. [CrossRef] [PubMed]
4. Magliah, S.; Bardisi, W.; Al Attah, M.; Khorsheed, M. The Prevalence and Risk Factors of Diabetic Retinopathy in Selected Primary Care Centers during the 3-Year Screening Intervals. *J. Family Med. Prim. Care* **2018**, *7*, 975. [CrossRef]
5. Teo, Z.L.; Tham, Y.-C.; Yu, M.; Chee, M.L.; Rim, T.H.; Cheung, N.; Bikbov, M.M.; Wang, Y.X.; Tang, Y.; Lu, Y.; et al. Global Prevalence of Diabetic Retinopathy and Projection of Burden through 2045. *Ophthalmology* **2021**, *128*, 1580–1591. [CrossRef]
6. Zhang, X.; Saaddine, J.B.; Chou, C.-F.; Cotch, M.F.; Cheng, Y.J.; Geiss, L.S.; Gregg, E.W.; Albright, A.L.; Klein, B.E.K.; Klein, R. Prevalence of Diabetic Retinopathy in the United States, 2005–2008. *JAMA* **2010**, *304*, 649. [CrossRef]
7. Moreno, A.; Lozano, M.; Salinas, P. Retinopatia Diabetica. *Nutr. Hosp.* **2013**, *28* (Suppl. S2), 53–56. [CrossRef]
8. Kollias, A.N.; Ulbig, M.W. Diabetic Retinopathy. *Dtsch. Arztebl Int.* **2010**, *107*, 75–84. [CrossRef]
9. Beltramo, E.; Porta, M. Pericyte Loss in Diabetic Retinopathy: Mechanisms and Consequences. *CMC* **2013**, *20*, 3218–3225. [CrossRef]
10. Bernabeu, M.O.; Lu, Y.; Abu-Qamar, O.; Aiello, L.P.; Sun, J.K. Estimation of Diabetic Retinal Microaneurysm Perfusion Parameters Based on Computational Fluid Dynamics Modeling of Adaptive Optics Scanning Laser Ophthalmoscopy. *Front. Physiol.* **2018**, *9*, 989. [CrossRef]
11. Adornetto, A.; Gesualdo, C.; Laganà, M.L.; Trotta, M.C.; Rossi, S.; Russo, R. Autophagy: A Novel Pharmacological Target in Diabetic Retinopathy. *Front. Pharmacol.* **2021**, *12*, 695267. [CrossRef] [PubMed]
12. Das, D.; Biswas, S.K.; Bandyopadhyay, S. A Critical Review on Diagnosis of Diabetic Retinopathy Using Machine Learning and Deep Learning. *Multimed Tools Appl.* **2022**, *81*, 25613–25655. [CrossRef] [PubMed]
13. Wang, W.; Lo, A. Diabetic Retinopathy: Pathophysiology and Treatments. *Int. J. Mol. Sci.* **2018**, *19*, 1816. [CrossRef] [PubMed]
14. Wu, L. Classification of Diabetic Retinopathy and Diabetic Macular Edema. *World J. Diabetes* **2013**, *4*, 290. [CrossRef]
15. Nentwich, M.M. Diabetic Retinopathy—Ocular Complications of Diabetes Mellitus. *World J. Diabetes* **2015**, *6*, 489. [CrossRef]
16. Trotta, M.C.; Gesualdo, C.; Petrillo, F.; Lepre, C.C.; Della Corte, A.; Cavasso, G.; Maggiore, G.; Hermenean, A.; Simonelli, F.; D'Amico, M.; et al. Resolution of Inflammation in Retinal Disorders: Briefly the State. *Int. J. Mol. Sci.* **2022**, *23*, 4501. [CrossRef] [PubMed]
17. Cheung, N.; Mitchell, P.; Wong, T.Y. Diabetic Retinopathy. *Lancet* **2010**, *376*, 124–136. [CrossRef]
18. Gale, M.J.; Scruggs, B.A.; Flaxel, C.J. Diabetic Eye Disease: A Review of Screening and Management Recommendations. *Clin. Exp. Ophthalmol.* **2021**, *49*, 128–145. [CrossRef]
19. Romero-Aroca, P. Managing Diabetic Macular Edema: The Leading Cause of Diabetes Blindness. *World J. Diabetes* **2011**, *2*, 98. [CrossRef]
20. Hendrick, A.M.; Gibson, M.V.; Kulshreshtha, A. Diabetic Retinopathy. *Prim. Care Clin. Off. Pract.* **2015**, *42*, 451–464. [CrossRef]
21. Rossi, S.; Maisto, R.; Gesualdo, C.; Trotta, M.C.; Ferraraccio, F.; Kaneva, M.K.; Getting, S.J.; Surace, E.; Testa, F.; Simonelli, F.; et al. Corrigendum to "Activation of Melanocortin Receptors MC1 and MC5 Attenuates Retinal Damage in Experimental Diabetic Retinopathy". *Mediat. Inflamm.* **2021**, *2021*, 9861434. [CrossRef] [PubMed]
22. Kaushik, V.; Gessa, L.; Kumar, N.; Fernandes, H. Towards a New Biomarker for Diabetic Retinopathy: Exploring RBP3 Structure and Retinoids Binding for Functional Imaging of Eyes In Vivo. *Int. J. Mol. Sci.* **2023**, *24*, 4408. [CrossRef] [PubMed]
23. Yu, C.-G.; Yuan, S.-S.; Yang, L.-Y.; Ke, J.; Zhang, L.-J.; Lang, J.-N.; Zhang, D.-W.; Zhao, S.-Z.; Zhao, D.; Feng, Y.-M. Angiopoietin-like 3 Is a Potential Biomarker for Retinopathy in Type 2 Diabetic Patients. *Am. J. Ophthalmol.* **2018**, *191*, 34–41. [CrossRef] [PubMed]
24. Trotta, M.C.; Gesualdo, C.; Platania, C.B.M.; De Robertis, D.; Giordano, M.; Simonelli, F.; D'Amico, M.; Drago, F.; Bucolo, C.; Rossi, S. Circulating MiRNAs in Diabetic Retinopathy Patients: Prognostic Markers or Pharmacological Targets? *Biochem. Pharmacol.* **2021**, *186*, 114473. [CrossRef]
25. Xie, Z.; Xiao, X. Novel Biomarkers and Therapeutic Approaches for Diabetic Retinopathy and Nephropathy: Recent Progress and Future Perspectives. *Front. Endocrinol.* **2022**, *13*, 1065856. [CrossRef]
26. Xuan, Q.; Ouyang, Y.; Wang, Y.; Wu, L.; Li, H.; Luo, Y.; Zhao, X.; Feng, D.; Qin, W.; Hu, C.; et al. Multiplatform Metabolomics Reveals Novel Serum Metabolite Biomarkers in Diabetic Retinopathy Subjects. *Adv. Sci.* **2020**, *7*, 2001714. [CrossRef]
27. Trotta, M.C.; Gesualdo, C.; Petrillo, F.; Cavasso, G.; Corte, A.D.; D'Amico, G.; Hermenean, A.; Simonelli, F.; Rossi, S. Serum Iba-1, GLUT5, and TSPO in Patients With Diabetic Retinopathy: New Biomarkers for Early Retinal Neurovascular Alterations? A Pilot Study. *Trans. Vis. Sci. Tech.* **2022**, *11*, 16. [CrossRef]
28. Bianco, L.; Arrigo, A.; Aragona, E.; Antropoli, A.; Berni, A.; Saladino, A.; Battaglia Parodi, M.; Bandello, F. Neuroinflammation and Neurodegeneration in Diabetic Retinopathy. *Front. Aging Neurosci.* **2022**, *14*, 937999. [CrossRef]
29. Sorrentino, F.S.; Allkabes, M.; Salsini, G.; Bonifazzi, C.; Perri, P. The Importance of Glial Cells in the Homeostasis of the Retinal Microenvironment and Their Pivotal Role in the Course of Diabetic Retinopathy. *Life Sci.* **2016**, *162*, 54–59. [CrossRef]

30. Nio-Kobayashi, J.; Itabashi, T. Galectins and Their Ligand Glycoconjugates in the Central Nervous System Under Physiological and Pathological Conditions. *Front. Neuroanat.* **2021**, *15*, 767330. [CrossRef]
31. Vasta, G.R. Lectins as Innate Immune Recognition Factors: Structural, Functional, and Evolutionary Aspects. In *The Evolution of the Immune System*; Elsevier: Amsterdam, The Netherlands, 2016; pp. 205–224; ISBN 978-0-12-801975-7.
32. Johannes, L.; Jacob, R.; Leffler, H. Galectins at a Glance. *J. Cell Sci.* **2018**, *131*, jcs208884. [CrossRef]
33. Rathnasamy, G.; Foulds, W.S.; Ling, E.-A.; Kaur, C. Retinal Microglia—A Key Player in Healthy and Diseased Retina. *Prog. Neurobiol.* **2019**, *173*, 18–40. [CrossRef] [PubMed]
34. Vecino, E.; Rodriguez, F.D.; Ruzafa, N.; Pereiro, X.; Sharma, S.C. Glia–Neuron Interactions in the Mammalian Retina. *Prog. Retin. Eye Res.* **2016**, *51*, 1–40. [CrossRef] [PubMed]
35. Yang, J.; Chen, C.; McLaughlin, T.; Wang, Y.; Le, Y.-Z.; Wang, J.J.; Zhang, S.X. Loss of X-Box Binding Protein 1 in Müller Cells Augments Retinal Inflammation in a Mouse Model of Diabetes. *Diabetologia* **2019**, *62*, 531–543. [CrossRef] [PubMed]
36. Fernández, D.; Geisse, A.; Bernales, J.I.; Lira, A.; Osorio, F. The Unfolded Protein Response in Immune Cells as an Emerging Regulator of Neuroinflammation. *Front. Aging Neurosci.* **2021**, *13*, 682633. [CrossRef]
37. Sims, S.G.; Cisney, R.N.; Lipscomb, M.M.; Meares, G.P. The Role of Endoplasmic Reticulum Stress in Astrocytes. *Glia* **2022**, *70*, 5–19. [CrossRef]
38. Zheng, Q.; Ren, Y.; Reinach, P.S.; Xiao, B.; Lu, H.; Zhu, Y.; Qu, J.; Chen, W. Reactive Oxygen Species Activated NLRP3 Inflammasomes Initiate Inflammation in Hyperosmolarity Stressed Human Corneal Epithelial Cells and Environment-Induced Dry Eye Patients. *Exp. Eye Res.* **2015**, *134*, 133–140. [CrossRef]
39. Kang, Q.; Dai, H.; Jiang, S.; Yu, L. Advanced Glycation End Products in Diabetic Retinopathy and Phytochemical Therapy. *Front. Nutr.* **2022**, *9*, 1037186. [CrossRef]
40. Wu, H.; Hwang, D.-K.; Song, X.; Tao, Y. Association between Aqueous Cytokines and Diabetic Retinopathy Stage. *J. Ophthalmol.* **2017**, *2017*, 9402198. [CrossRef]
41. Sarlus, H.; Heneka, M.T. Microglia in Alzheimer's Disease. *J. Clin. Investig.* **2017**, *127*, 3240–3249. [CrossRef]
42. Guo, S.; Wang, H.; Yin, Y. Microglia Polarization From M1 to M2 in Neurodegenerative Diseases. *Front. Aging Neurosci.* **2022**, *14*, 815347. [CrossRef]
43. Wake, H.; Moorhouse, A.J.; Nabekura, J. Functions of Microglia in the Central Nervous System—Beyond the Immune Response. *Neuron. Glia Biol.* **2011**, *7*, 47–53. [CrossRef]
44. Santiago, A.R.; Baptista, F.I.; Santos, P.F.; Cristóvão, G.; Ambrósio, A.F.; Cunha, R.A.; Gomes, C.A. Role of Microglia Adenosine A$_{2A}$ Receptors in Retinal and Brain Neurodegenerative Diseases. *Mediators Inflamm.* **2014**, *2014*, 465694. [CrossRef] [PubMed]
45. Santos, A.M.; Martín-Oliva, D.; Ferrer-Martín, R.M.; Tassi, M.; Calvente, R.; Sierra, A.; Carrasco, M.-C.; Marín-Teva, J.L.; Navascués, J.; Cuadros, M.A. Microglial Response to Light-Induced Photoreceptor Degeneration in the Mouse Retina. *J. Comp. Neurol.* **2010**, *518*, 477–492. [CrossRef] [PubMed]
46. Huang, T.; Cui, J.; Li, L.; Hitchcock, P.F.; Li, Y. The Role of Microglia in the Neurogenesis of Zebrafish Retina. *Biochem. Biophy. Res. Commun.* **2012**, *421*, 214–220. [CrossRef] [PubMed]
47. Zeng, H. Microglial Activation in Human Diabetic Retinopathy. *Arch. Ophthalmol.* **2008**, *126*, 227. [CrossRef]
48. Jiao, H.; Natoli, R.; Valter, K.; Provis, J.; Rutar, M. Spatiotemporal Cadence of Macrophage Polarisation in a Model of Light-Induced Retinal Degeneration. *PLoS ONE* **2015**, *10*, e0143952. [CrossRef]
49. Arroba, A.I.; Álvarez-Lindo, N.; van Rooijen, N.; de la Rosa, E.J. Microglia-Mediated IGF-I Neuroprotection in the *Rd10* Mouse Model of Retinitis Pigmentosa. *Investig. Ophthalmol. Vis. Sci.* **2011**, *52*, 9124. [CrossRef]
50. Kettenmann, H.; Kirchhoff, F.; Verkhratsky, A. Microglia: New Roles for the Synaptic Stripper. *Neuron* **2013**, *77*, 10–18. [CrossRef]
51. Zhang, W.; Liu, H.; Al-Shabrawey, M.; Caldwell, R.W.; Caldwell, R.B. Inflammation and Diabetic Retinal Microvascular Complications. *J. Cardiovasc. Dis. Res.* **2011**, *2*, 96–103. [CrossRef]
52. Tang, J.; Kern, T.S. Inflammation in Diabetic Retinopathy. *Prog. Retin. Eye Res.* **2011**, *30*, 343–358. [CrossRef] [PubMed]
53. Fumagalli, S.; Perego, C.; Pischiutta, F.; Zanier, E.R.; De Simoni, M.-G. The Ischemic Environment Drives Microglia and Macrophage Function. *Front. Neurol.* **2015**, *6*, 81. [CrossRef]
54. Trotta, M.C.; Gesualdo, C.; Herman, H.; Gharbia, S.; Balta, C.; Lepre, C.C.; Russo, M.; Itro, A.; D'Amico, G.; Peluso, L.; et al. Systemic Beta-Hydroxybutyrate Affects BDNF and Autophagy into the Retina of Diabetic Mice. *Int. J. Mol. Sci.* **2022**, *23*, 10184. [CrossRef] [PubMed]
55. Yunna, C.; Mengru, H.; Lei, W.; Weidong, C. Macrophage M1/M2 Polarization. *Eur. J. Pharmacol.* **2020**, *877*, 173090. [CrossRef]
56. Wang, L.; Shang, X.; Qi, X.; Ba, D.; Lv, J.; Zhou, X.; Wang, H.; Shaxika, N.; Wang, J.; Ma, X. Clinical Significance of M1/M2 Macrophages and Related Cytokines in Patients with Spinal Tuberculosis. *Dis. Markers* **2020**, *2020*, 2509454. [CrossRef] [PubMed]
57. Colonna, M.; Butovsky, O. Microglia Function in the Central Nervous System During Health and Neurodegeneration. *Annu. Rev. Immunol.* **2017**, *35*, 441–468. [CrossRef]
58. Grigsby, J.G.; Cardona, S.M.; Pouw, C.E.; Muniz, A.; Mendiola, A.S.; Tsin, A.T.C.; Allen, D.M.; Cardona, A.E. The Role of Microglia in Diabetic Retinopathy. *J. Ophthalmol.* **2014**, *2014*, 705783. [CrossRef]
59. Coughlin, B.A.; Feenstra, D.J.; Mohr, S. Müller Cells and Diabetic Retinopathy. *Vision Res.* **2017**, *139*, 93–100. [CrossRef]
60. Wang, M.; Ma, W.; Zhao, L.; Fariss, R.N.; Wong, W.T. Adaptive Müller Cell Responses to Microglial Activation Mediate Neuroprotection and Coordinate Inflammation in the Retina. *J. Neuroinflamm.* **2011**, *8*, 173. [CrossRef]

61. Carpi-Santos, R.; De Melo Reis, R.A.; Gomes, F.C.A.; Calaza, K.C. Contribution of Müller Cells in the Diabetic Retinopathy Development: Focus on Oxidative Stress and Inflammation. *Antioxidants* **2022**, *11*, 617. [CrossRef]
62. Liu, X.; Ye, F.; Xiong, H.; Hu, D.; Limb, G.A.; Xie, T.; Peng, L.; Yang, W.; Sun, Y.; Zhou, M.; et al. IL-1β Upregulates IL-8 Production in Human Müller Cells Through Activation of the P38 MAPK and ERK1/2 Signaling Pathways. *Inflammation* **2014**, *37*, 1486–1495. [CrossRef] [PubMed]
63. Bringmann, A.; Wiedemann, P. Müller Glial Cells in Retinal Disease. *Ophthalmologica* **2012**, *227*, 1–19. [CrossRef] [PubMed]
64. Tang, Y.; Chen, Y.; Chen, D. The Heterogeneity of Astrocytes in Glaucoma. *Front. Neuroanat.* **2022**, *16*, 995369. [CrossRef] [PubMed]
65. Yu, Y.; Chen, H.; Su, S.B. Neuroinflammatory Responses in Diabetic Retinopathy. *J. Neuroinflamm.* **2015**, *12*, 141. [CrossRef]
66. Chiareli, R.A.; Carvalho, G.A.; Marques, B.L.; Mota, L.S.; Oliveira-Lima, O.C.; Gomes, R.M.; Birbrair, A.; Gomez, R.S.; Simão, F.; Klempin, F.; et al. The Role of Astrocytes in the Neurorepair Process. *Front. Cell Dev. Biol.* **2021**, *9*, 665795. [CrossRef]
67. García-Cáceres, C.; Balland, E.; Prevot, V.; Luquet, S.; Woods, S.C.; Koch, M.; Horvath, T.L.; Yi, C.-X.; Chowen, J.A.; Verkhratsky, A.; et al. Role of Astrocytes, Microglia, and Tanycytes in Brain Control of Systemic Metabolism. *Nat. Neurosci.* **2019**, *22*, 7–14. [CrossRef]
68. Giovannoni, F.; Quintana, F.J. The Role of Astrocytes in CNS Inflammation. *Trends Immunol.* **2020**, *41*, 805–819. [CrossRef]
69. Maisto, R.; Gesualdo, C.; Trotta, M.C.; Grieco, P.; Testa, F.; Simonelli, F.; Barcia, J.M.; D'Amico, M.; Di Filippo, C.; Rossi, S. Melanocortin Receptor Agonists MCR$_{1-5}$ Protect Photoreceptors from High-Glucose Damage and Restore Antioxidant Enzymes in Primary Retinal Cell Culture. *J. Cell Mol. Med.* **2017**, *21*, 968–974. [CrossRef]
70. Costagliola, C.; Romano, V.; De Tollis, M.; Aceto, F.; dell'Omo, R.; Romano, M.R.; Pedicino, C.; Semeraro, F. TNF-Alpha Levels in Tears: A Novel Biomarker to Assess the Degree of Diabetic Retinopathy. *Mediators Inflamm.* **2013**, *2013*, 629529. [CrossRef]
71. Lazzara, F.; Trotta, M.C.; Platania, C.B.M.; D'Amico, M.; Petrillo, F.; Galdiero, M.; Gesualdo, C.; Rossi, S.; Drago, F.; Bucolo, C. Stabilization of HIF-1α in Human Retinal Endothelial Cells Modulates Expression of MiRNAs and Proangiogenic Growth Factors. *Front. Pharmacol* **2020**, *11*, 1063. [CrossRef]
72. Kong, D.-Q.; Li, L.; Liu, Y.; Zheng, G.-Y. Association between Endoplasmic Reticulum Stress and Risk Factors of Diabetic Retinopathy. *Int. J. Ophthalmol.* **2018**, *11*, 1704–1710. [CrossRef]
73. Rinaldi, C.; Donato, L.; Alibrandi, S.; Scimone, C.; D'Angelo, R.; Sidoti, A. Oxidative Stress and the Neurovascular Unit. *Life* **2021**, *11*, 767. [CrossRef]
74. Zhong, Y.; Wang, J.J.; Zhang, S.X. Intermittent but Not Constant High Glucose Induces ER Stress and Inflammation in Human Retinal Pericytes. *Adv. Exp. Med. Biol.* **2012**, *723*, 285–292. [CrossRef]
75. Shi, X.; Li, P.; Liu, H.; Prokosch, V. Oxidative Stress, Vascular Endothelium, and the Pathology of Neurodegeneration in Retina. *Antioxidants* **2022**, *11*, 543. [CrossRef] [PubMed]
76. Yang, X.; Yu, X.-W.; Zhang, D.-D.; Fan, Z.-G. Blood-Retinal Barrier as a Converging Pivot in Understanding the Initiation and Development of Retinal Diseases. *Chin. Med. J.* **2020**, *133*, 2586–2594. [CrossRef]
77. Cao, S.S.; Kaufman, R.J. Endoplasmic Reticulum Stress and Oxidative Stress in Cell Fate Decision and Human Disease. *Antioxid. Redox Signal.* **2014**, *21*, 396–413. [CrossRef] [PubMed]
78. Araki, K.; Nagata, K. Protein Folding and Quality Control in the ER. *Cold Spring Harb. Perspec. Biol.* **2011**, *3*, a007526. [CrossRef] [PubMed]
79. *The Plant Endoplasmic Reticulum: Methods and Protocols*; Hawes, C.; Kriechbaumer, V. (Eds.) Methods in Molecular Biology; Springer: New York, NY, USA, 2018; Volume 1691, ISBN 978-1-4939-7388-0.
80. Martino, E.; Balestrieri, A.; Mele, L.; Sardu, C.; Marfella, R.; D'Onofrio, N.; Campanile, G.; Balestrieri, M.L. Milk Exosomal MiR-27b Worsen Endoplasmic Reticulum Stress Mediated Colorectal Cancer Cell Death. *Nutrients* **2022**, *14*, 5081. [CrossRef]
81. Li, W.; Cao, T.; Luo, C.; Cai, J.; Zhou, X.; Xiao, X.; Liu, S. Crosstalk between ER Stress, NLRP3 Inflammasome, and Inflammation. *Appl. Microbiol. Biotechnol.* **2020**, *104*, 6129–6140. [CrossRef]
82. Karlstetter, M.; Scholz, R.; Rutar, M.; Wong, W.T.; Provis, J.M.; Langmann, T. Retinal Microglia: Just Bystander or Target for Therapy? *Prog. Retin. Eye Res.* **2015**, *45*, 30–57. [CrossRef]
83. Altmann, C.; Schmidt, M.H.H. The Role of Microglia in Diabetic Retinopathy: Inflammation, Microvasculature Defects and Neurodegeneration. *Int. J. Mol. Sci.* **2018**, *19*, 110. [CrossRef] [PubMed]
84. Mendonca, H.; Carpi-Santos, R.; da Costa Calaza, K.; Blanco Martinez, A. Neuroinflammation and Oxidative Stress Act in Concert to Promote Neurodegeneration in the Diabetic Retina and Optic Nerve: Galectin-3 Participation. *Neural Regen. Res.* **2020**, *15*, 625. [CrossRef] [PubMed]
85. Rübsam, A.; Parikh, S.; Fort, P. Role of Inflammation in Diabetic Retinopathy. *Int. J. Mol. Sci.* **2018**, *19*, 942. [CrossRef]
86. Udaondo, P.; Adan, A.; Arias-Barquet, L.; Ascaso, F.J.; Cabrera-López, F.; Castro-Navarro, V.; Donate-López, J.; García-Layana, A.; Lavid, F.J.; Rodríguez-Maqueda, M.; et al. Challenges in Diabetic Macular Edema Management: An Expert Consensus Report. *OPTH* **2021**, *15*, 3183–3195. [CrossRef] [PubMed]
87. Liu, Y.; Biarnés Costa, M.; Gerhardinger, C. IL-1β Is Upregulated in the Diabetic Retina and Retinal Vessels: Cell-Specific Effect of High Glucose and IL-1β Autostimulation. *PLoS ONE* **2012**, *7*, e36949. [CrossRef] [PubMed]
88. Kim, Y.K.; Shin, J.-S.; Nahm, M.H. NOD-Like Receptors in Infection, Immunity, and Diseases. *Yonsei Med. J.* **2016**, *57*, 5. [CrossRef]

89. Trotta, M.C.; Maisto, R.; Guida, F.; Boccella, S.; Luongo, L.; Balta, C.; D'Amico, G.; Herman, H.; Hermenean, A.; Bucolo, C.; et al. The Activation of Retinal HCA2 Receptors by Systemic Beta-Hydroxybutyrate Inhibits Diabetic Retinal Damage through Reduction of Endoplasmic Reticulum Stress and the NLRP3 Inflammasome. *PLoS ONE* **2019**, *14*, e0211005. [CrossRef] [PubMed]
90. Abrishami, M.; Tohidinezhad, F.; Daneshvar, R.; Omidtabrizi, A.; Amini, M.; Sedaghat, A.; Amini, S.; Reihani, H.; Allahyari, A.; Seddigh-Shamsi, M.; et al. Ocular Manifestations of Hospitalized Patients with COVID-19 in Northeast of Iran. *Ocul. Immunol. Inflamm.* **2020**, *28*, 739–744. [CrossRef]
91. Kuo, C.Y.-J.; Maran, J.J.; Jamieson, E.G.; Rupenthal, I.D.; Murphy, R.; Mugisho, O.O. Characterization of NLRP3 Inflammasome Activation in the Onset of Diabetic Retinopathy. *Int. J. Mol. Sci.* **2022**, *23*, 14471. [CrossRef]
92. Chen, X.; Guo, X.; Ge, Q.; Zhao, Y.; Mu, H.; Zhang, J. ER Stress Activates the NLRP3 Inflammasome: A Novel Mechanism of Atherosclerosis. *Oxidative Med. Cell. Longev.* **2019**, *2019*, 3462530. [CrossRef]
93. Zheng, D.; Liwinski, T.; Elinav, E. Inflammasome Activation and Regulation: Toward a Better Understanding of Complex Mechanisms. *Cell Discov.* **2020**, *6*, 36. [CrossRef] [PubMed]
94. Zhou, R.; Tardivel, A.; Thorens, B.; Choi, I.; Tschopp, J. Thioredoxin-Interacting Protein Links Oxidative Stress to Inflammasome Activation. *Nat. Immunol.* **2010**, *11*, 136–140. [CrossRef] [PubMed]
95. Lu, A.; Wu, H. Structural Mechanisms of Inflammasome Assembly. *FEBS J.* **2015**, *282*, 435–444. [CrossRef] [PubMed]
96. Pelegrin, P. P2X7 Receptor and the NLRP3 Inflammasome: Partners in Crime. *Biochem. Pharmacol.* **2021**, *187*, 114385. [CrossRef] [PubMed]
97. Abais, J.M.; Xia, M.; Zhang, Y.; Boini, K.M.; Li, P.-L. Redox Regulation of NLRP3 Inflammasomes: ROS as Trigger or Effector? *Antioxid. Redox Signal.* **2015**, *22*, 1111–1129. [CrossRef]
98. Snezhkina, A.V.; Kudryavtseva, A.V.; Kardymon, O.L.; Savvateeva, M.V.; Melnikova, N.V.; Krasnov, G.S.; Dmitriev, A.A. ROS Generation and Antioxidant Defense Systems in Normal and Malignant Cells. *Oxidative Med. Cell. Longev.* **2019**, *2019*, 6175804. [CrossRef]
99. Swanson, K.V.; Deng, M.; Ting, J.P.-Y. The NLRP3 Inflammasome: Molecular Activation and Regulation to Therapeutics. *Nat. Rev. Immunol.* **2019**, *19*, 477–489. [CrossRef]
100. Kelley, N.; Jeltema, D.; Duan, Y.; He, Y. The NLRP3 Inflammasome: An Overview of Mechanisms of Activation and Regulation. *Int. J. Mol. Sci.* **2019**, *20*, 3328. [CrossRef]
101. Prather, E.R.; Gavrilin, M.A.; Wewers, M.D. The Central Inflammasome Adaptor Protein ASC Activates the Inflammasome after Transition from a Soluble to an Insoluble State. *J. Biol. Chem.* **2022**, *298*, 102024. [CrossRef]
102. Yu, P.; Zhang, X.; Liu, N.; Tang, L.; Peng, C.; Chen, X. Pyroptosis: Mechanisms and Diseases. *Sig. Transduct. Target. Ther.* **2021**, *6*, 128. [CrossRef]
103. de Zoete, M.R.; Palm, N.W.; Zhu, S.; Flavell, R.A. Inflammasomes. *Cold Spring Harb. Perspect. Biol.* **2014**, *6*, a016287. [CrossRef]
104. He, W.; Wan, H.; Hu, L.; Chen, P.; Wang, X.; Huang, Z.; Yang, Z.-H.; Zhong, C.-Q.; Han, J. Gasdermin D Is an Executor of Pyroptosis and Required for Interleukin-1β Secretion. *Cell Res.* **2015**, *25*, 1285–1298. [CrossRef]
105. Raman, K.S.; Matsubara, J.A. Dysregulation of the NLRP3 Inflammasome in Diabetic Retinopathy and Potential Therapeutic Targets. *Ocul. Immunol. Inflamm.* **2022**, *30*, 470–478. [CrossRef] [PubMed]
106. Loukovaara, S.; Piippo, N.; Kinnunen, K.; Hytti, M.; Kaarniranta, K.; Kauppinen, A. NLRP3 Inflammasome Activation Is Associated with Proliferative Diabetic Retinopathy. *Acta Ophthalmol.* **2017**, *95*, 803–808. [CrossRef] [PubMed]
107. Kuo, C.Y.J.; Murphy, R.; Rupenthal, I.D.; Mugisho, O.O. Correlation between the Progression of Diabetic Retinopathy and Inflammasome Biomarkers in Vitreous and Serum—A Systematic Review. *BMC Ophthalmol.* **2022**, *22*, 238. [CrossRef] [PubMed]
108. Tseng, W.A.; Thein, T.; Kinnunen, K.; Lashkari, K.; Gregory, M.S.; D'Amore, P.A.; Ksander, B.R. NLRP3 Inflammasome Activation in Retinal Pigment Epithelial Cells by Lysosomal Destabilization: Implications for Age-Related Macular Degeneration. *Investig. Ophthalmol. Vis. Sci.* **2013**, *54*, 110. [CrossRef] [PubMed]
109. Mohr, L.K.M.; Hoffmann, A.V.; Brandstetter, C.; Holz, F.G.; Krohne, T.U. Effects of Inflammasome Activation on Secretion of Inflammatory Cytokines and Vascular Endothelial Growth Factor by Retinal Pigment Epithelial Cells. *Invest. Ophthalmol. Vis. Sci.* **2015**, *56*, 6404. [CrossRef] [PubMed]
110. Doktor, F.; Prager, P.; Wiedemann, P.; Kohen, L.; Bringmann, A.; Hollborn, M. Hypoxic Expression of NLRP3 and VEGF in Cultured Retinal Pigment Epithelial Cells: Contribution of P2Y2 Receptor Signaling. *Purinergic Signal.* **2018**, *14*, 471–484. [CrossRef]
111. Ebeling, M.C.; Fisher, C.R.; Kapphahn, R.J.; Stahl, M.R.; Shen, S.; Qu, J.; Montezuma, S.R.; Ferrington, D.A. Inflammasome Activation in Retinal Pigment Epithelium from Human Donors with Age-Related Macular Degeneration. *Cells* **2022**, *11*, 2075. [CrossRef]
112. Jiang, Y.; Liu, L.; Curtiss, E.; Steinle, J.J. Epac1 Blocks NLRP3 Inflammasome to Reduce IL-1β in Retinal Endothelial Cells and Mouse Retinal Vasculature. *Mediat. Inflamm.* **2017**, *2017*, 2860956. [CrossRef]
113. Zou, W.; Luo, S.; Zhang, Z.; Cheng, L.; Huang, X.; Ding, N.; Pan, Y.; Wu, Z. ASK1/P38-mediated NLRP3 Inflammasome Signaling Pathway Contributes to Aberrant Retinal Angiogenesis in Diabetic Retinopathy. *Int. J. Mol. Med.* **2020**, *47*, 732–740. [CrossRef] [PubMed]
114. Ding, X.; Xie, H.; Shan, W.; Li, L. Agonism of GPR120 Prevented High Glucose-Induced Apoptosis of Retinal Endothelial Cells through Inhibiting NLRP3 Inflammasome. *Klin. Monbl. Augenheilkd* **2022**. [CrossRef] [PubMed]

115. Viringipurampeer, I.A.; Metcalfe, A.L.; Bashar, A.E.; Sivak, O.; Yanai, A.; Mohammadi, Z.; Moritz, O.L.; Gregory-Evans, C.Y.; Gregory-Evans, K. NLRP3 Inflammasome Activation Drives Bystander Cone Photoreceptor Cell Death in a P23H Rhodopsin Model of Retinal Degeneration. *Hum. Mol. Genet.* **2016**, *25*, 1501–1516. [CrossRef]
116. Wooff, Y.; Fernando, N.; Wong, J.H.C.; Dietrich, C.; Aggio-Bruce, R.; Chu-Tan, J.A.; Robertson, A.A.B.; Doyle, S.L.; Man, S.M.; Natoli, R. Caspase-1-Dependent Inflammasomes Mediate Photoreceptor Cell Death in Photo-Oxidative Damage-Induced Retinal Degeneration. *Sci. Rep.* **2020**, *10*, 2263. [CrossRef] [PubMed]
117. Chaurasia, S.S.; Lim, R.R.; Parikh, B.H.; Wey, Y.S.; Tun, B.B.; Wong, T.Y.; Luu, C.D.; Agrawal, R.; Ghosh, A.; Mortellaro, A.; et al. The NLRP3 Inflammasome May Contribute to Pathologic Neovascularization in the Advanced Stages of Diabetic Retinopathy. *Sci. Rep.* **2018**, *8*, 2847. [CrossRef]
118. Huang, L.; You, J.; Yao, Y.; Xie, M. High Glucose Induces Pyroptosis of Retinal Microglia through NLPR3 Inflammasome Signaling. *Arq. Bras. Oftalmol.* **2021**, *84*, 67–73.
119. Pronin, A.; Pham, D.; An, W.; Dvoriantchikova, G.; Reshetnikova, G.; Qiao, J.; Kozhekbaeva, Z.; Reiser, A.E.; Slepak, V.Z.; Shestopalov, V.I. Inflammasome Activation Induces Pyroptosis in the Retina Exposed to Ocular Hypertension Injury. *Front. Mol. Neurosci.* **2019**, *12*, 36. [CrossRef]
120. Fryk, E.; Strindberg, L.; Lundqvist, A.; Sandstedt, M.; Bergfeldt, L.; Mattsson Hultén, L.; Bergström, G.; Jansson, P.-A. Galectin-1 Is Inversely Associated with Type 2 Diabetes Independently of Obesity—A SCAPIS Pilot Study. *Metabolism Open* **2019**, *4*, 100017. [CrossRef]
121. Bobronnikova, L. Galectin-3 as a Potential Biomarker of Metabolic Disorders and Cardiovascular Remodeling in Patients with Hypertension and Type 2 Diabetes. *Vessel Plus.* **2017**, *1*, 61–67. [CrossRef]
122. Vora, A.; de Lemos, J.A.; Ayers, C.; Grodin, J.L.; Lingvay, I. Association of Galectin-3 With Diabetes Mellitus in the Dallas Heart Study. *J. Clin. Endocrinol. Metab.* **2019**, *104*, 4449–4458. [CrossRef]
123. Souza, I.D.P.; Rodrigues, K.F.; Pietrani, N.T.; Bosco, A.A.; Gomes, K.B.; Alves, M.T. Evaluation of Galectin-3 Levels in Patients with Type 2 Diabetes Mellitus and Chronic Kidney Disease. *J. Bras. De Patol. E Med. Lab.* **2021**, *57*, 1–9. [CrossRef]
124. Atalar, M.N.; Abuşoğlu, S.; Ünlü, A.; Tok, O.; İpekçi, S.H.; Baldane, S.; Kebapcılar, L. Assessment of Serum Galectin-3, Methylated Arginine and Hs-CRP Levels in Type 2 Diabetes and Prediabetes. *Life Sci.* **2019**, *231*, 116577. [CrossRef] [PubMed]
125. Li, Y.; Li, T.; Zhou, Z.; Xiao, Y. Emerging Roles of Galectin-3 in Diabetes and Diabetes Complications: A Snapshot. *Rev. Endocr. Metab. Disord.* **2022**, *23*, 569–577. [CrossRef] [PubMed]
126. Jeethy Ram, T.; Lekshmi, A.; Somanathan, T.; Sujathan, K. Galectin-3: A Factotum in Carcinogenesis Bestowing an Archery for Prevention. *Tumor Biol.* **2021**, *43*, 77–96. [CrossRef]
127. Kanzaki, M.; Wada, J.; Sugiyama, K.; Nakatsuka, A.; Teshigawara, S.; Murakami, K.; Inoue, K.; Terami, T.; Katayama, A.; Eguchi, J.; et al. Galectin-9 and T Cell Immunoglobulin Mucin-3 Pathway Is a Therapeutic Target for Type 1 Diabetes. *Endocrinology* **2012**, *153*, 612–620. [CrossRef]
128. Kurose, Y.; Wada, J.; Kanzaki, M.; Teshigawara, S.; Nakatsuka, A.; Murakami, K.; Inoue, K.; Terami, T.; Katayama, A.; Watanabe, M.; et al. Serum Galectin-9 Levels Are Elevated in the Patients with Type 2 Diabetes and Chronic Kidney Disease. *BMC Nephrol.* **2013**, *14*, 23. [CrossRef]
129. Sudhakar, J.N.; Lu, H.-H.; Chiang, H.-Y.; Suen, C.-S.; Hwang, M.-J.; Wu, S.-Y.; Shen, C.-N.; Chang, Y.-M.; Li, F.-A.; Liu, F.-T.; et al. Lumenal Galectin-9-Lamp2 Interaction Regulates Lysosome and Autophagy to Prevent Pathogenesis in the Intestine and Pancreas. *Nat. Commun.* **2020**, *11*, 4286. [CrossRef] [PubMed]
130. Wang, W.; Qin, Y.; Song, H.; Wang, L.; Jia, M.; Zhao, C.; Gong, M.; Zhao, W. Galectin-9 Targets NLRP3 for Autophagic Degradation to Limit Inflammation. *J. Immunol.* **2021**, *206*, 2692–2699. [CrossRef] [PubMed]
131. Kuo, P.; Le, Q.-T. Galectin-1 Links Tumor Hypoxia and Radiotherapy. *Glycobiology* **2014**, *24*, 921–925. [CrossRef] [PubMed]
132. Morgan, M.J.; Liu, Z. Crosstalk of Reactive Oxygen Species and NF-KB Signaling. *Cell Res.* **2011**, *21*, 103–115. [CrossRef]
133. Astorgues-Xerri, L.; Riveiro, M.E.; Tijeras-Raballand, A.; Serova, M.; Rabinovich, G.A.; Bieche, I.; Vidaud, M.; de Gramont, A.; Martinet, M.; Cvitkovic, E.; et al. OTX008, a Selective Small-Molecule Inhibitor of Galectin-1, Downregulates Cancer Cell Proliferation, Invasion and Tumour Angiogenesis. *Eur. J. Cancer* **2014**, *50*, 2463–2477. [CrossRef]
134. Griffioen, A.W.; Thijssen, V.L. Galectins in Tumor Angiogenesis. *Ann. Transl. Med.* **2014**, *2*, 90. [PubMed]
135. Coppin, L.; Jannin, A.; Ait Yahya, E.; Thuillier, C.; Villenet, C.; Tardivel, M.; Bongiovanni, A.; Gaston, C.; de Beco, S.; Barois, N.; et al. Galectin-3 Modulates Epithelial Cell Adaptation to Stress at the ER-Mitochondria Interface. *Cell Death Dis.* **2020**, *11*, 360. [CrossRef]
136. Caridi, B.; Doncheva, D.; Sivaprasad, S.; Turowski, P. Galectins in the Pathogenesis of Common Retinal Disease. *Front. Pharmacol.* **2021**, *12*, 687495. [CrossRef] [PubMed]
137. Tian, J.; Yang, G.; Chen, H.; Hsu, D.K.; Tomilov, A.; Olson, K.K.A.; Dehnad, A.; Fish, S.R.; Cortopassi, G.; Zhao, K.B.; et al. Galectin-3 Regulates Inflammasome Activation in Cholestatic Liver Injury. *FASEB J.* **2016**, *30*, 4202–4213. [CrossRef] [PubMed]
138. Kato, T.; Kurita, K.; Seino, T.; Kadoya, T.; Horie, H.; Wada, M.; Kawanami, T.; Daimon, M.; Hirano, A. Galectin-1 Is a Component of Neurofilamentous Lesions in Sporadic and Familial Amyotrophic Lateral Sclerosis. *Biochem. Biophys. Res. Commun.* **2001**, *282*, 166–172. [CrossRef]
139. de Jong, C.G.H.M.; Stancic, M.; Pinxterhuis, T.H.; van Horssen, J.; van Dam, A.-M.; Gabius, H.-J.; Baron, W. Galectin-4, a Negative Regulator of Oligodendrocyte Differentiation, Is Persistently Present in Axons and Microglia/Macrophages in Multiple Sclerosis Lesions. *J. Neuropathol. Exp. Neurol.* **2018**, *77*, 1024–1038. [CrossRef]

140. Hara, A.; Niwa, M.; Noguchi, K.; Kanayama, T.; Niwa, A.; Matsuo, M.; Hatano, Y.; Tomita, H. Galectin-3 as a Next-Generation Biomarker for Detecting Early Stage of Various Diseases. *Biomolecules* **2020**, *10*, 389. [CrossRef]
141. Ramos-Martínez, E.; Ramos-Martínez, I.; Sánchez-Betancourt, I.; Ramos-Martínez, J.C.; Peña-Corona, S.I.; Valencia, J.; Saucedo, R.; Almeida-Aguirre, E.K.P.; Cerbón, M. Association between Galectin Levels and Neurodegenerative Diseases: Systematic Review and Meta-Analysis. *Biomolecules* **2022**, *12*, 1062. [CrossRef]
142. Hermenean, A.; Oatis, D.; Herman, H.; Ciceu, A.; D'Amico, G.; Trotta, M.C. Galectin 1—A Key Player between Tissue Repair and Fibrosis. *Int. J. Mol. Sci.* **2022**, *23*, 5548. [CrossRef]
143. Oatis, D.; Simon-Repolski, E.; Balta, C.; Mihu, A.; Pieretti, G.; Alfano, R.; Peluso, L.; Trotta, M.C.; D'Amico, M.; Hermenean, A. Cellular and Molecular Mechanism of Pulmonary Fibrosis Post-COVID-19: Focus on Galectin-1, -3, -8, -9. *Int. J. Mol. Sci.* **2022**, *23*, 8210. [CrossRef] [PubMed]
144. Chen, H.-L.; Liao, F.; Lin, T.-N.; Liu, F.-T. Galectins and Neuroinflammation. In *Glycobiology of the Nervous System*; Yu, R.K., Schengrund, C.-L., Eds.; Advances in Neurobiology; Springer: New York, NY, USA, 2014; Volume 9, pp. 517–542; ISBN 978-1-4939-1153-0.
145. Ramírez Hernández, E.; Alanis Olvera, B.; Carmona González, D.; Guerrero Marín, O.; Pantoja Mercado, D.; Valencia Gil, L.; Hernández-Zimbrón, L.F.; Sánchez Salgado, J.L.; Limón, I.D.; Zenteno, E. Neuroinflammation and Galectins: A Key Relationship in Neurodegenerative Diseases. *Glycoconj J.* **2022**, *39*, 685–699. [CrossRef]
146. Bonsack, F.; Sukumari-Ramesh, S. Differential Cellular Expression of Galectin-1 and Galectin-3 After Intracerebral Hemorrhage. *Front. Cell. Neurosci.* **2019**, *13*, 157. [CrossRef]
147. Gaudet, A.D.; Sweet, D.R.; Polinski, N.K.; Guan, Z.; Popovich, P.G. Galectin-1 in Injured Rat Spinal Cord: Implications for Macrophage Phagocytosis and Neural Repair. *Mol. Cell. Neurosci.* **2015**, *64*, 84–94. [CrossRef] [PubMed]
148. Quintá, H.R.; Pasquini, J.M.; Rabinovich, G.A.; Pasquini, L.A. Glycan-Dependent Binding of Galectin-1 to Neuropilin-1 Promotes Axonal Regeneration after Spinal Cord Injury. *Cell Death Differ.* **2014**, *21*, 941–955. [CrossRef] [PubMed]
149. Rubinstein, N.; Alvarez, M.; Zwirner, N.W.; Toscano, M.A.; Ilarregui, J.M.; Bravo, A.; Mordoh, J.; Fainboim, L.; Podhajcer, O.L.; Rabinovich, G.A. Targeted Inhibition of Galectin-1 Gene Expression in Tumor Cells Results in Heightened T Cell-Mediated Rejection. *Cancer Cell* **2004**, *5*, 241–251. [CrossRef]
150. Kobayakawa, Y.; Sakumi, K.; Kajitani, K.; Kadoya, T.; Horie, H.; Kira, J.; Nakabeppu, Y. Galectin-1 Deficiency Improves Axonal Swelling of Motor Neurones in SOD1 [G93A] Transgenic Mice: Galectin-1 Is Associated with Axonal Degeneration in SOD1 [G93A] Mice. *Neuropathol. Appl. Neurobiol.* **2015**, *41*, 227–244. [CrossRef]
151. Jeon, S.-B.; Yoon, H.J.; Chang, C.Y.; Koh, H.S.; Jeon, S.-H.; Park, E.J. Galectin-3 Exerts Cytokine-Like Regulatory Actions through the JAK–STAT Pathway. *J. Immunol.* **2010**, *185*, 7037–7046. [CrossRef]
152. Siew, J.J.; Chen, H.-M.; Chen, H.-Y.; Chen, H.-L.; Chen, C.-M.; Soong, B.-W.; Wu, Y.-R.; Chang, C.-P.; Chan, Y.-C.; Lin, C.-H.; et al. Galectin-3 Is Required for the Microglia-Mediated Brain Inflammation in a Model of Huntington's Disease. *Nat. Commun.* **2019**, *10*, 3473. [CrossRef]
153. Boza-Serrano, A.; Ruiz, R.; Sanchez-Varo, R.; García-Revilla, J.; Yang, Y.; Jimenez-Ferrer, I.; Paulus, A.; Wennström, M.; Vilalta, A.; Allendorf, D.; et al. Galectin-3, a Novel Endogenous TREM2 Ligand, Detrimentally Regulates Inflammatory Response in Alzheimer's Disease. *Acta Neuropathol.* **2019**, *138*, 251–273. [CrossRef]
154. Yin, Q.; Chen, J.; Ma, S.; Dong, C.; Zhang, Y.; Hou, X.; Li, S.; Liu, B. Pharmacological Inhibition of Galectin-3 Ameliorates Diabetes-Associated Cognitive Impairment, Oxidative Stress and Neuroinflammation in Vivo and in Vitro. *JIR* **2020**, *13*, 533–542. [CrossRef] [PubMed]
155. North, R.A. P2X Receptors. *Philos. Trans. R. Soc. B* **2016**, *371*, 20150427. [CrossRef]
156. Martínez-Cuesta, M.Á.; Blanch-Ruiz, M.A.; Ortega-Luna, R.; Sánchez-López, A.; Álvarez, Á. Structural and Functional Basis for Understanding the Biological Significance of P2X7 Receptor. *Int. J. Mol. Sci.* **2020**, *21*, 8454. [CrossRef]
157. Tassetto, M.; Scialdone, A.; Solini, A.; Di Virgilio, F. The P2X7 Receptor: A Promising Pharmacological Target in Diabetic Retinopathy. *Int. J. Mol. Sci.* **2021**, *22*, 7110. [CrossRef] [PubMed]
158. Platania, C.B.M.; Lazzara, F.; Fidilio, A.; Fresta, C.G.; Conti, F.; Giurdanella, G.; Leggio, G.M.; Salomone, S.; Drago, F.; Bucolo, C. Blood-Retinal Barrier Protection against High Glucose Damage: The Role of P2X7 Receptor. *Biochem. Pharmacol.* **2019**, *168*, 249–258. [CrossRef] [PubMed]
159. Di Virgilio, F.; Sarti, A.C.; Grassi, F. Modulation of Innate and Adaptive Immunity by P2X Ion Channels. *Curr. Opin. Immunol.* **2018**, *52*, 51–59. [CrossRef] [PubMed]
160. Yang, D. Targeting the P2X7 Receptor in Age-Related Macular Degeneration. *Vision* **2017**, *1*, 11. [CrossRef]
161. Franceschini, A.; Capece, M.; Chiozzi, P.; Falzoni, S.; Sanz, J.M.; Sarti, A.C.; Bonora, M.; Pinton, P.; Di Virgilio, F. The P2X7 Receptor Directly Interacts with the NLRP3 Inflammasome Scaffold Protein. *FASEB J.* **2015**, *29*, 2450–2461. [CrossRef]
162. Andrejew, R.; Oliveira-Giacomelli, Á.; Ribeiro, D.E.; Glaser, T.; Arnaud-Sampaio, V.F.; Lameu, C.; Ulrich, H. The P2X7 Receptor: Central Hub of Brain Diseases. *Front. Mol. Neurosci.* **2020**, *13*, 124. [CrossRef]
163. Xu, Z.; Chen, Z.; Wu, X.; Zhang, L.; Cao, Y.; Zhou, P. Distinct Molecular Mechanisms Underlying Potassium Efflux for NLRP3 Inflammasome Activation. *Front. Immunol.* **2020**, *11*, 609441. [CrossRef]
164. Territo, P.R.; Zarrinmayeh, H. P2X7 Receptors in Neurodegeneration: Potential Therapeutic Applications From Basic to Clinical Approaches. *Front. Cell. Neurosci.* **2021**, *15*, 617036. [CrossRef] [PubMed]

165. Monif, M.; Burnstock, G.; Williams, D.A. Microglia: Proliferation and Activation Driven by the P2X7 Receptor. *Int. J. Biochem. Cell Biol.* **2010**, *42*, 1753–1756. [CrossRef]
166. Illes, P.; Khan, T.M.; Rubini, P. Neuronal P2X7 Receptors Revisited: Do They Really Exist? *J. Neurosci.* **2017**, *37*, 7049–7062. [CrossRef]
167. Sidoryk-Węgrzynowicz, M.; Strużyńska, L. Astroglial and Microglial Purinergic P2X7 Receptor as a Major Contributor to Neuroinflammation during the Course of Multiple Sclerosis. *Int. J. Mol. Sci.* **2021**, *22*, 8404. [CrossRef]
168. Leeson, H.; Chan-Ling, T.; Lovelace, M.; Brownlie, J.; Gu, B.; Weible, M. P2X7 Receptor Signaling during Adult Hippocampal Neurogenesis. *Neural. Regen. Res.* **2019**, *14*, 1684. [CrossRef] [PubMed]
169. Beamer, E.; Gölöncsér, F.; Horváth, G.; Bekő, K.; Otrokocsi, L.; Koványi, B.; Sperlágh, B. Purinergic Mechanisms in Neuroinflammation: An Update from Molecules to Behavior. *Neuropharmacology* **2016**, *104*, 94–104. [CrossRef] [PubMed]
170. Lee, H.G.; Won, S.M.; Gwag, B.J.; Lee, Y.B. Microglial P2X$_7$ Receptor Expression Is Accompanied by Neuronal Damage in the Cerebral Cortex of the APP$_{swe}$/PS1dE9 Mouse Model of Alzheimer's Disease. *Exp. Mol. Med.* **2011**, *43*, 7. [CrossRef]
171. Francistiová, L.; Bianchi, C.; Di Lauro, C.; Sebastián-Serrano, Á.; de Diego-García, L.; Kobolák, J.; Dinnyés, A.; Díaz-Hernández, M. The Role of P2X7 Receptor in Alzheimer's Disease. *Front. Mol. Neurosci.* **2020**, *13*, 94. [CrossRef]
172. Parvathenani, L.K.; Tertyshnikova, S.; Greco, C.R.; Roberts, S.B.; Robertson, B.; Posmantur, R. P2X7 Mediates Superoxide Production in Primary Microglia and Is Up-Regulated in a Transgenic Mouse Model of Alzheimer's Disease. *J. Biol. Chem.* **2003**, *278*, 13309–13317. [CrossRef]
173. McLarnon, J.G.; Ryu, J.K.; Walker, D.G.; Choi, H.B. Upregulated Expression of Purinergic P2X$_7$ Receptor in Alzheimer Disease and Amyloid-β Peptide-Treated Microglia and in Peptide-Injected Rat Hippocampus. *J. Neuropathol. Exp. Neurol.* **2006**, *65*, 1090–1097. [CrossRef]
174. Ollà, I.; Santos-Galindo, M.; Elorza, A.; Lucas, J.J. P2X7 Receptor Upregulation in Huntington's Disease Brains. *Front. Mol. Neurosci.* **2020**, *13*, 567430. [CrossRef] [PubMed]
175. Solini, A.; Rossi, C.; Santini, E.; Giuntini, M.; Raggi, F.; Parolini, F.; Biancalana, E.; Del Prete, E.; Bonuccelli, U.; Ceravolo, R. P2X7 Receptor/NLRP3 Inflammasome Complex and A-synuclein in Peripheral Blood Mononuclear Cells: A Prospective Study in Neo-diagnosed, Treatment-naïve Parkinson's Disease. *Eur. J. Neurol.* **2021**, *28*, 2648–2656. [CrossRef] [PubMed]
176. University of Pisa. P2X7 Receptor, Inflammation and Neurodegenerative Diseases (NeuroInfiam). Available online: https://clinicaltrials.gov/ct2/show/NCT03918616 (accessed on 2 May 2023).
177. Wang, Y.; Shan, Z.; Zhang, L.; Fan, S.; Zhou, Y.; Hu, L.; Wang, Y.; Li, W.; Xiao, Z. P2X7R/NLRP3 Signaling Pathway-Mediated Pyroptosis and Neuroinflammation Contributed to Cognitive Impairment in a Mouse Model of Migraine. *J. Headache Pain* **2022**, *23*, 75. [CrossRef] [PubMed]
178. Grygorowicz, T.; Wełniak-Kamińska, M.; Strużyńska, L. Early P2X7R-Related Astrogliosis in Autoimmune Encephalomyelitis. *Mol. Cell. Neurosci.* **2016**, *74*, 1–9. [CrossRef] [PubMed]
179. Abu El-Asrar, A.M.; Ahmad, A.; Allegaert, E.; Siddiquei, M.M.; Alam, K.; Gikandi, P.W.; De Hertogh, G.; Opdenakker, G. Galectin-1 Studies in Proliferative Diabetic Retinopathy. *Acta Ophthalmol.* **2020**, *98*, e1–e12. [CrossRef] [PubMed]
180. Abreu, C.A.; De Lima, S.V.; Mendonça, H.R.; Oliveira Goulart, C.d.; Blanco Martinez, A.M. Absence of Galectin-3 Promotes Neuroprotection in Retinal Ganglion Cells after Optic Nerve Injury. *Histol. Histopathol.* **2017**, *32*, 253–262. [CrossRef]
181. Trotta, M.C.; Petrillo, F.; Gesualdo, C.; Rossi, S.; Corte, A.D.; Váradi, J.; Fenyvesi, F.; D'Amico, M.; Hermenean, A. Effects of the Calix[4]Arene Derivative Compound OTX008 on High Glucose-Stimulated ARPE-19 Cells: Focus on Galectin-1/TGF-β/EMT Pathway. *Molecules* **2022**, *27*, 4785. [CrossRef]
182. Sugiyama, T.; Kobayashi, M.; Kawamura, H.; Li, Q.; Puro, D.G. Enhancement of P2X$_7$-Induced Pore Formation and Apoptosis: An Early Effect of Diabetes on the Retinal Microvasculature. *Investig. Ophthalmol. Vis. Sci.* **2004**, *45*, 1026. [CrossRef]
183. Kong, H.; Zhao, H.; Chen, T.; Song, Y.; Cui, Y. Targeted P2X7/NLRP3 Signaling Pathway against Inflammation, Apoptosis, and Pyroptosis of Retinal Endothelial Cells in Diabetic Retinopathy. *Cell Death Dis.* **2022**, *13*, 336. [CrossRef]
184. Platania, C.B.M.; Giurdanella, G.; Di Paola, L.; Leggio, G.M.; Drago, F.; Salomone, S.; Bucolo, C. P2X7 Receptor Antagonism: Implications in Diabetic Retinopathy. *Biochem. Pharmacol.* **2017**, *138*, 130–139. [CrossRef]
185. Hase, K.; Kanda, A.; Noda, K.; Ishida, S. Increased Plasma Galectin-1 Correlates with Advanced Glycation End Products and Interleukin-1β in Patients with Proliferative Diabetic Retinopathy. *Int. J. Ophthalmol.* **2019**, *12*, 692. [CrossRef]
186. Kanda, A.; Noda, K.; Saito, W.; Ishida, S. Aflibercept Traps Galectin-1, an Angiogenic Factor Associated with Diabetic Retinopathy. *Sci. Rep.* **2015**, *5*, 17946. [CrossRef] [PubMed]
187. Ridano, M.E.; Subirada, P.V.; Paz, M.C.; Lorenc, V.E.; Stupirski, J.C.; Gramajo, A.L.; Luna, J.D.; Croci, D.O.; Rabinovich, G.A.; Sánchez, M.C. Galectin-1 Expression Imprints a Neurovascular Phenotype in Proliferative Retinopathies and Delineates Responses to Anti-VEGF. *Oncotarget* **2017**, *8*, 32505–32522. [CrossRef] [PubMed]
188. Mendonça, H.R.; Carvalho, J.N.A.; Abreu, C.A.; Mariano de Souza Aguiar dos Santos, D.; Carvalho, J.R.; Marques, S.A.; da Costa Calaza, K.; Martinez, A.M.B. Lack of Galectin-3 Attenuates Neuroinflammation and Protects the Retina and Optic Nerve of Diabetic Mice. *Brain Res.* **2018**, *1700*, 126–137. [CrossRef]
189. Canning, P.; Glenn, J.V.; Hsu, D.K.; Liu, F.-T.; Gardiner, T.A.; Stitt, A.W. Inhibition of Advanced Glycation and Absence of Galectin-3 Prevent Blood-Retinal Barrier Dysfunction during Short-Term Diabetes. *Exp. Diabetes Res.* **2007**, *2007*, 51837. [CrossRef] [PubMed]

190. Oncoethix GmbH. A Phase I, First-in-Man Study of OTX008 Given Subcutaneously as a Single Agent to Patients With Advanced Solid Tumors. Available online: https://clinicaltrials.gov/ct2/show/NCT01724320 (accessed on 2 May 2023).
191. Galectin Therapeutics Inc. Phase 2 Study to Evaluate Non-Invasive Imaging Methods in Efficacy Assessment of GR-MD-02 for the Treatment of Liver Fibrosis in Patients With NASH With Advanced Fibrosis. 2020. Available online: https://clinicaltrials.gov/ct2/show/NCT02421094 (accessed on 2 May 2023).
192. Galecto Biotech AB. A Study to Evaluate the Safety, Tolerability, Pharmacokinetics and Pharmacodynamics of Orally Administered GB1211 in Participants With Suspected or Confirmed Non-Alcoholic Steatohepatitis (NASH) and Liver Fibrosis. 2020. Available online: https://clinicaltrials.gov/ct2/show/NCT04607655 (accessed on 2 May 2023).
193. Galecto Biotech. A Single and Repeat Dose Trial in Participants with Hepatic Impairment. 2021. Available online: https://clinicaltrials.gov/ct2/show/NCT05009680 (accessed on 2 May 2023).
194. A Study to Investigate the Safety and Efficacy of GB1211 (a Galectin-3 Inhibitor) in Combination with Atezolizumab in Patients With Non-Small Cell Lung Cancer (NSCLC). Available online: https://clinicaltrials.gov/ct2/show/NCT05240131 (accessed on 2 May 2023).
195. Galectin Inhibitor (GR-MD-02) and Ipilimumab in Patients With Metastatic Melanoma. Available online: https://clinicaltrials.gov/ct2/show/NCT02117362 (accessed on 2 May 2023).
196. GR-MD-02 + Pembrolizumab Versus Pembrolizumab Monotherapy in Melanoma and Squamous Cell Head and Neck Cancer Patients. Available online: https://clinicaltrials.gov/ct2/show/NCT04987996 (accessed on 2 May 2023).
197. GR-MD-02 Plus Pembrolizumab in Melanoma, Non-Small Cell Lung Cancer, and Squamous Cell Head and Neck Cancer Patients. Available online: https://clinicaltrials.gov/ct2/show/NCT02575404 (accessed on 2 May 2023).
198. Galecto Biotech AB. A Study to Test the Efficacy and Safety of Inhaled GB0139 in Subjects With Idiopathic Pulmonary Fibrosis (IPF). 2019. Available online: https://clinicaltrials.gov/ct2/show/NCT03832946 (accessed on 2 May 2023).
199. Galecto Biotech AB. A Placebo-Controlled RCT in HV's Investigating the Safety, Tolerability and PK (Pharmacokinetic) of TD139, a Galectin-3 Inhibitor, Followed by an Expansion Cohort Treating Subjects With Idiopathic Pulmonary Fibrosis (IPF). 2021. Available online: https://clinicaltrials.gov/ct2/show/NCT02257177 (accessed on 2 May 2023).
200. Galectin-3 Blockade in Patients With High Blood Pressure. Available online: https://clinicaltrials.gov/ct2/show/NCT01960946 (accessed on 2 May 2023).
201. Massachusetts General Hospital. Blocking Extracellular Galectin-3 in Patients With Osteoarthritis. 2016. Available online: https://clinicaltrials.gov/ct2/show/NCT02800629 (accessed on 2 May 2023).
202. GlaxoSmithKline. First Time in Human Study Evaluating the Safety, Tolerability, Pharmacokinetics, Pharmacodynamics and the Effect of Food of Single Assending Doses of GSK1482160. 2009. Available online: https://clinicaltrials.gov/ct2/show/results/NCT00849134 (accessed on 2 May 2023).
203. AstraZeneca. A Study to Assess Co-Administered AZD9056 (Steady State) and Simvastatin (Single Dose) in Healthy Volunteers. 2008. Available online: https://www.clinicaltrials.gov/ct2/show/NCT00736606 (accessed on 2 May 2023).
204. AstraZeneca. Cross-over Study to Investigate Retinal Function Following Administration of a Single Dose of AZD9056. 2008. Available online: https://www.clinicaltrials.gov/ct2/show/NCT00700986 (accessed on 2 May 2023).
205. Pfizer. Study of Controlled Release Formulations of CE-224,535 Against the Immediate Release Formulation in Normal Volunteers. 2008. Available online: https://clinicaltrials.gov/ct2/show/NCT00782600 (accessed on 2 May 2023).
206. Pfizer. A Study in Normal Healthy People, Testing Different Versions of a Pill That Will Be Used to Treat Rheumatoid Arthritis. 2009. Available online: https://clinicaltrials.gov/ct2/show/NCT00838058 (accessed on 2 May 2023).
207. Pfizer. Study of CE-224,535 A Twice Daily Pill to Control Rheumatoid Arthritis in Patients Who Have not Totally Improved with Methotrexate. 2008. Available online: https://clinicaltrials.gov/ct2/show/NCT00628095 (accessed on 2 May 2023).
208. AstraZeneca. A 6-Month Randomised, Double-Blind, Open Arm Comparator, Phase IIb, with AZD9056, in Patients with Rheumatoid Arthritis (RA). 2007. Available online: https://clinicaltrials.gov/ct2/show/NCT00520572 (accessed on 2 May 2023).
209. Pfizer. A Study of the Effect of CE-224535 on Knee OA (Osteoarthritis) Pain. Available online: https://clinicaltrials.gov/ct2/show/NCT00418782 (accessed on 2 May 2023).
210. Liou, G.I. Diabetic Retinopathy: Role of Inflammation and Potential Therapies for Anti-Inflammation. *World J. Diabetes* **2010**, *1*, 12–18. [CrossRef]
211. Campbell, M.; Humphries, P. The Blood-Retina Barrier: Tight Junctions and Barrier Modulation. *Adv. Exp. Med. Biol.* **2012**, *763*, 70–84.
212. Sugiyama, T. Role of P2X$_7$ Receptors in the Development of Diabetic Retinopathy. *World J. Diabetes* **2014**, *5*, 141–145. [CrossRef]
213. Carver, K.A.; Lin, C.M.; Bowes Rickman, C.; Yang, D. Lack of the P2X7 Receptor Protects against AMD-like Defects and Microparticle Accumulation in a Chronic Oxidative Stress-Induced Mouse Model of AMD. *Biochem. Biophys. Res. Commun.* **2017**, *482*, 81–86. [CrossRef]

Disclaimer/Publisher's Note: The statements, opinions and data contained in all publications are solely those of the individual author(s) and contributor(s) and not of MDPI and/or the editor(s). MDPI and/or the editor(s) disclaim responsibility for any injury to people or property resulting from any ideas, methods, instructions or products referred to in the content.

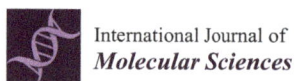

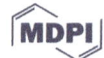

Article

After Ischemic Stroke, Minocycline Promotes a Protective Response in Neurons via the RNA-Binding Protein HuR, with a Positive Impact on Motor Performance

Katarzyna Pawletko [1,2,*], Halina Jędrzejowska-Szypułka [1,*], Katarzyna Bogus [3], Alessia Pascale [4], Foroogh Fahmideh [4], Nicoletta Marchesi [4], Aniela Grajoszek [1,2], Daria Gendosz de Carrillo [1,5] and Jarosław Jerzy Barski [1,2]

1. Department of Physiology, Faculty of Medical Sciences in Katowice, Medical University of Silesia, Medyków 18, 40-752 Katowice, Poland; agrajoszek@sum.edu.pl (A.G.); dariagendosz@gmail.com (D.G.d.C.); jbarski@sum.edu.pl (J.J.B.)
2. Department for Experimental Medicine, Medical University of Silesia, Medyków 4, 40-752 Katowice, Poland
3. Department of Histology, Faculty of Medical Sciences in Katowice, Medical University of Silesia, Medyków 18, 40-752 Katowice, Poland; kasiabogus@outlook.com
4. Department of Drug Sciences, Pharmacology Section, University of Pavia, Viale Taramelli 14, 27100 Pavia, Italy; alessia.pascale@unipv.it (A.P.); foroogh.ft@gmail.com (F.F.); nicoletta.marchesi@unipv.it (N.M.)
5. Department of Histology and Cell Pathology, Faculty of Medical Sciences in Zabrze, Medical University of Silesia, Poniatowskiego 15, 40-055 Katowice, Poland
* Correspondence: kpawletko@sum.edu.pl (K.P.); hszypulka@sum.edu.pl (H.J.-S.)

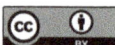

Abstract: Ischemic stroke is the most common cause of adult disability and one of the leading causes of death worldwide, with a serious socio-economic impact. In the present work, we used a new thromboembolic model, recently developed in our lab, to induce focal cerebral ischemic (FCI) stroke in rats without reperfusion. We analyzed selected proteins implicated in the inflammatory response (such as the RNA-binding protein HuR, TNFα, and HSP70) via immunohistochemistry and western blotting techniques. The main goal of the study was to evaluate the beneficial effects of a single administration of minocycline at a low dose (1 mg/kg intravenously administered 10 min after FCI) on the neurons localized in the penumbra area after an ischemic stroke. Furthermore, given the importance of understanding the crosstalk between molecular parameters and motor functions following FCI, motor tests were also performed, such as the Horizontal Runway Elevated test, CatWalk™ XT, and Grip Strength test. Our results indicate that a single administration of a low dose of minocycline increased the viability of neurons and reduced the neurodegeneration caused by ischemia, resulting in a significant reduction in the infarct volume. At the molecular level, minocycline resulted in a reduction in TNFα content coupled with an increase in the levels of both HSP70 and HuR proteins in the penumbra area. Considering that both HSP70 and TNF-α transcripts are targeted by HuR, the obtained results suggest that, following FCI, this RNA-binding protein promotes a protective response by shifting its binding towards HSP70 instead of TNF-α. Most importantly, motor tests showed that reduced inflammation in the brain damaged area after minocycline treatment directly translated into a better motor performance, which is a fundamental outcome when searching for new therapeutic options for clinical practice.

Keywords: ischemic stroke; penumbra; minocycline; HuR; RNA-binding protein; inflammation; motor test

1. Introduction

Stroke is the most common cause of adult disability and one of the leading causes of death worldwide. Approximately 87% are ischemic [1–5], with a serious socio-economic impact [6]. The therapeutic actions aimed at saving the hypoxic area (the penumbra)

must be balanced with the risks of negative consequences associated with the undertaken treatment. Moreover, a very important factor within the therapeutic approach, primarily based on thrombolysis or thrombectomy, is the narrow "time window" available. This drawback renders the use of the most effective therapies (i.e., alteplase) ineffective in protecting against secondary damage [7,8]. Therefore, due to these limitations, only a small percentage of patients (<10%) affected by ischemic stroke qualify for this type of intervention [9,10]. Hence, the search for new therapeutic approaches for patients affected by ischemic stroke is a compelling medical need [11,12]. Within this context, the use of animal models is one of the most valid strategies to develop effective therapies [11,13]. Notably, the animal model of focal cerebral ischemia (FCI) allows for more reproducible results compared to other models [14–16] and closely mimics what happens in humans (i.e., the ischemic area takes a relatively small area of the entire cerebral cortex) [17,18]. Furthermore, this model is characterized by a low burden on the animals and enables the verification of the tested substance's effect through motor tests [17,19]. A poor prognosis in ischemic stroke results from the irreversible loss of neurons [20], which is due to an abrupt blood flow shortage and excitotoxicity. Inflammation persists over an extended period, beginning at the time of stroke. Consequently, an increased level of pro-inflammatory cytokines and chemokines is observed, together with the infiltration of leukocytes into the areas affected by ischemia. Several studies have reported that pro-inflammatory cytokines (i.e., interleukin-1, interleukin-6 and TNFα (tumor necrosis factor alpha)) play a major role in the development of inflammation after stroke [21–24]. This suggests that anti-inflammatory treatments could expand the "therapeutic window" and facilitate the implementation of current clinical interventions [25]. Moreover, post-stroke inflammation plays an important role in the survival and regeneration of nerve cells, exerting a beneficial effect on brain tissue [26,27]. Therefore, in the search for new pharmacological strategies, the modulation of inflammation has been identified as a promising therapeutic option [28]. Antibiotics, especially tetracyclines, have gained a growing interest in this regard. Minocycline is a broad-spectrum antibiotic belonging to the tetracycline group with anti-inflammatory, antioxidant, and anti-apoptotic effects [29–32]. Previous studies on stroke have shown that the administration of minocycline attenuates neurological deficits and reduces ischemic infarct volume [8]. The anti-inflammatory properties of minocycline have been identified as an important feature of the action of this drug in various models of ischemic stroke [14,33–35]. Therefore, in the present study, we investigated the effect of minocycline on selected proteins implicated in the inflammatory response after ischemic stroke, including TNFα, HSP70, and the RNA-binding protein HuR.

TNFα is produced by various cell types, including neurons, microglia, astrocytes, and endothelial cells [28,36]. Previous studies have indicated that the prompt induction of TNFα mRNA in the photothrombotic model likely originates from ischemic neurons and not from activated glial cells [37]. In addition, TNFα is one of the earliest cytokines to appear in the context of the inflammatory reaction after ischemic brain injury, contributing to the stimulation of the inflammatory process in the cerebrospinal fluid and blood serum [38,39]. In contrast to TNFα protein, HSP70 (Heat Shock Protein 70) plays a protective role during the inflammatory process by inhibiting the response of pro-inflammatory cytokines such as TNFα and interleukin-1 [40]. Moreover, published research has shown that HSP70 regulates inflammation both intracellularly, where it exhibits anti-inflammatory properties, and extracellularly, where it may enhance immune responses [41–44]. Within this context, RNA-binding proteins (RBP) of the ELAV (embryonic lethal abnormal visual) family, which include the ubiquitously expressed HuR protein (also known as ELAV1) and three neuron-specific members (HuB, HuC, and HuD), may also play an important role. These RBPs act post-transcriptionally and influence the post-synthesis fate of the target transcripts, thereby regulating gene expression by binding to distinct signatures (known as ARE, adenine-uracil-rich elements) [45]. HuR, the most extensively studied member, is primarily localized in the nucleus and is known to affect the stability, translation, pre-mRNA splicing, and nuclear export of target mRNAs [42,45–47]. Within the general context of inflammation, HuR can play a dual role by participating in both non-inflammatory and inflammatory pathways. For example, HuR can bind to HSP70 mRNA in both in the nuclear and cytoplasmic compartments [48,49]. Under conditions of oxidative stress [50], it can promote a defense response in vulnerable neurons, thus directly blocking or delaying neuronal death [46,51]. On the other hand, HuR protein may also promote inflammation by interacting with mRNAs that encode pro-inflammatory cytokines such as TNFα [45,52–55]. Considering that both HSP70 and TNF-α transcripts are targeted by HuR, it was of interest to examine the role of this RBP following FCI and explore the effect of minocycline on its protein expression.

Finally, given the importance of understanding the crosstalk between molecular parameters and motor functions following FCI, motor tests were also carried out in this work (Figure 1). Specifically, our goal was to assess whether minocycline can modulate inflammation and whether possible improvement at the molecular level translates into a better motor performance after non-reperfusion ischemic stroke. This outcome holds considerable importance and relevance in the pursuit of novel and more effective therapies for clinical intervention.

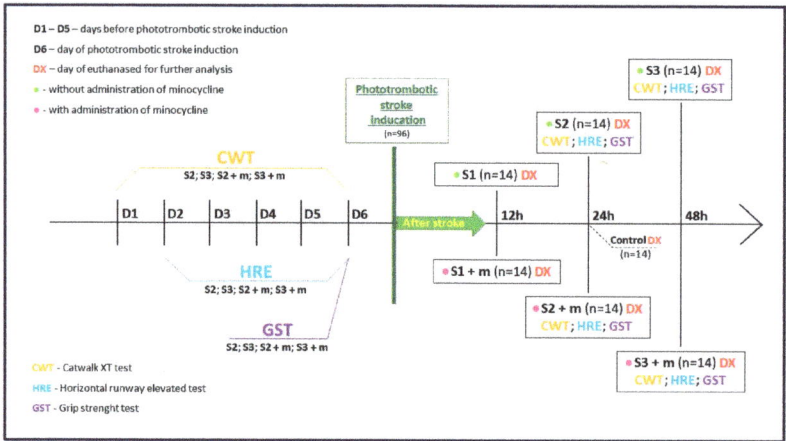

Figure 1. Graphical flowchart providing an overview of the study. Groups S1, S2, and S3 consisted of animals without minocycline administration; the time elapsed between ischemic stroke induction and euthanasia was equal to 12 h, 24 h, and 48 h, respectively. Groups S1 + m, S2 + m, S3 + m included animals with minocycline administration; the time elapsed between ischemic stroke induction and euthanasia (DX) was equal to 12 h, 24 h, and 48 h, respectively. In order to verify the effect of minocycline administration on the level of motility after stroke induction, the following motor tests were also performed on the animals: CatWalk™ XT (CWT), Grip Strength test (GST), and the Horizontal Runway Elevated (HRE) test.

2. Results

In total, six rats died immediately after anesthesia administration, resulting in a mortality rate of 6.25% for the entire study. No complications were observed at the sites of inflammation and necrosis within the skin incision or at dye injection sites.

2.1. Characterization of the Peri-Infarct Area following Ischemic Stroke

Nissl staining was performed to localize the necrotic and the penumbra areas after ischemic stroke in rats in the ipsilateral hemisphere. This staining allowed an easy localization of the ischemic area, which appeared much brighter compared to the healthy tissues. In order to compare the dynamics of the necrosis and the peri-infarct tissue changes among all groups (n = 5), the following parameters were measured: brain area (the entire area of the slice), necrosis area in relation to the brain area, necrosis width, and necrosis depth. For each rat, three measurements were made for each variable, and the mean was calculated.

Then, variable statistic was performed for the "brain area" variable (ANOVA, $p = 0.838$). This result confirmed the lack of statistical significance of the "brain area" variable, regardless of the administration of minocycline and the time interval. For the control group (n = 6) statistical calculations were also made for the "brain area" variable (ANOVA, $p = 0.091$).

Infarct formation was already well advanced at 12 h (S1 and S1 + m groups) after the induction of the photothrombotic stroke, as evidenced by the increase in the volume of the "necrosis area to brain area" (Figure 2b). The infarct volume reached its maximum after 24 h (S2 and S2 + m groups); then, the infarction volume decreased significantly on the second day (S3 and S3 + m groups). Statistical analysis revealed significant differences (the Mann Whitney U test, $p = 0.008$) in all tested variables, including "necrosis area to brain area", "necrosis width", and "necrosis depth" at each time interval between the groups without administration of minocycline (S1, S2 and S3) and with administration of minocycline (S1 + m, S2 + m and S3 + m). The greatest decrease in infarct volume was observed between the S2 and S2 + m groups, where the administration of minocycline resulted in an average decrease of 0.8% in the volume of the infarcted area compared to the group without the administration of minocycline (Figure 2b).

2.2. Effect of Minocycline on Inflammation in the Peri-Infarct Area following Ischemic Stroke

Immunohistochemical staining was used to characterize the morphological and biochemical responses in the peri-infarct area immediately adjacent to the necrosis. By labeling the neurons with the NeuN neuronal marker, we were able to determine the extent of the necrosis after stroke induction. Only living neurons were labeled with NeuN, while dead neurons were not. The images showed that the necrotic area had already formed 12 h after the stroke, reaching its maximum extension at 24 h (S2 group).e NeuN labeling was retained at the edge of the infarct focus and in the healthy tissue (see Figure S1 in the Supplementary Materials). Next, we studied the expression of HuR, TNFα, and HSP70 proteins in living neurons by performing double immunolabelling in brain sections (HuR+NeuN, TNFα+NeuN, HSP70+NeuN) and analyzing five regions of interest (ROIs), as shown in Figure 2a. Concerning HuR protein, the variables "nNeuN", "nHuR" and "relative HuR" were examined for the Ipsi1, Ipsi2, Ipsi3, Cont4, and Cont5 regions in all the experimental groups. The Control group showed the same level of "relative HuR", approximately 71%, in five ROIs (Figure 3a). The "relative HuR" variable was similar in the S1 and S1 + m groups, decreased slightly in the S2 + m group, and decreased drastically in the S2 group (reaching a level similar to the Control group at 24 h). At 48 h post-stroke induction, the expression of "relative Hurt" in the S3 + m group did not fall below 82% (Figure 3a). A comparison between the groups without the administration of minocycline and the groups with minocycline at each time point showed a statistically significant difference for all the three variables in favor of the groups with minocycline (the Mann-Whitney U test, $p = 0.002$; Figure 3a). With respect to the TNFα protein, the variables "nNeuN", "nTNFα", and "relative TNFα" were examined for the Ipsi1, Ipsi2, Ipsi3, Cont4, and Cont5 regions in all experimental groups. The Cont4 and Cont5 regions did not show any signal in any of the experimental group. The Control group exhibited a very low level of "relative TNFα", approximately 0.02%, in all ROIs (Figure 3b). A comparison between the groups without minocycline versus those with minocycline at each time point (the Mann-Whitney U test, $p = 0.002$) showed a more significant increase in TNFα expression in the groups without minocycline (Figure 3b). Concerning the HSP70 protein, the variables "nNeuN", "nHSP70" and "relative HSP70" were examined for the Ipsi1, Ipsi2, Ipsi3, Cont4, and Cont5 regions. There were no HSP70-positive cells in the Cont4 and Cont5 regions in any experimental group (Figure 3c). The results revealed statistically significant differences between the groups without the administration of minocycline and those with minocycline at all time points examined for all the "nNeuN", "nHSP70", and "relative HSP70" variables (Mann-Whitney U test, $p = 0.002$). HSP70 expression in the minocycline groups was statistically significantly higher than in the groups without the administration of minocycline. The "relative HSP70" variable peaked 24 h after stroke induction in both groups (Figure 3c).

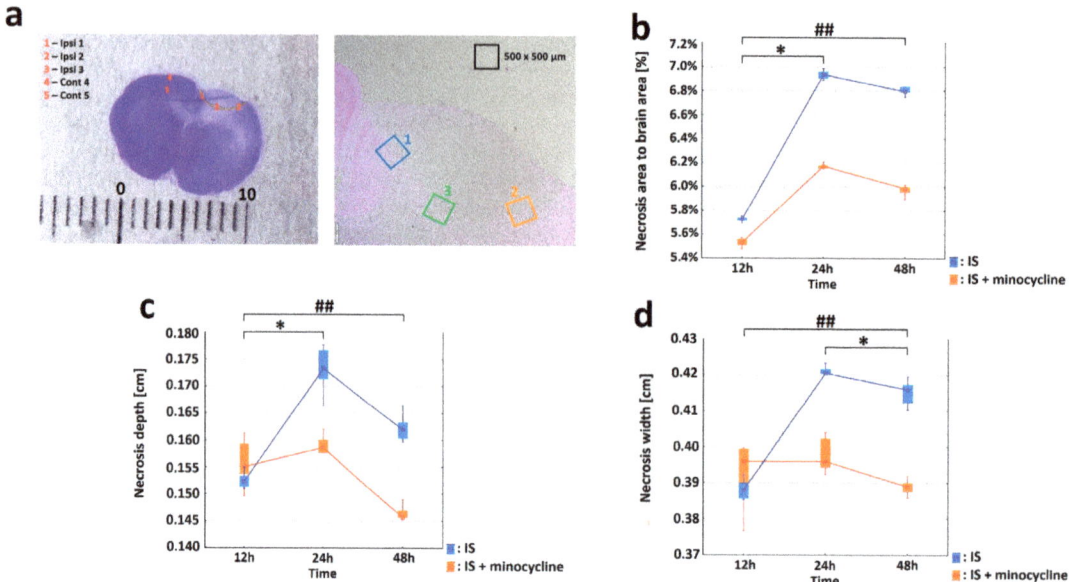

Figure 2. Effect of minocycline on infarct volume. Comparison of dynamics of volume, width, and depth of the necrotic area after ischemic stroke induction in rats: Nissl staining. Administration of minocycline caused less intense histopathological changes compared to the groups without minocycline (IS: ischemic stroke groups, IS + minocycline: ischemic stroke + minocycline groups). (**a**) A Nissl-stained coronal section of a rat brain 24 h after the induction of a photothrombotic stroke showing a clearly defined infarct area (left panel) and the ROIs (right panel). The scale is in millimeters (Ipsi: ipsilaterally hemisphere, Cont: contralateral hemisphere). (**b**) Changes in the average necrosis area (%) over time and the relative effect of minocycline. The results for the variable "necrosis area to brain area" for groups without minocycline (Kruskall-Wallis test, $p = 0.005$) and groups with minocycline (Kruskall-Wallis test, $p = 0.002$). For the pairs S1 + m vs. S2 + m and S1 vs. S2, a statistically significant difference was demonstrated (Dunn's *post hoc* test, $p < 0.05$), where * $p < 0.05$ for intragroup comparisons. For each time interval, the differences between the studied groups were significant (Mann-Whitney U test, $p = 0.008$), where ## $p < 0.01$ for the comparison of groups without versus groups with the administration of minocycline. (**c**) The necrosis width spread after stroke induction. Within the groups: with minocycline (Kruskall-Wallis test; $p = 0.0652$), groups without minocycline (the Kruskall-Wallis test, $p = 0.004$). For S1 vs. S2, a statistically significant difference was demonstrated (Dunn's *post hoc* test, $p < 0.05$), where * $p < 0.05$ for intragroup comparisons. For each time interval, the differences between the studied groups were significant (Mann-Whitney U test, $p = 0.008$), where ## $p < 0.01$ for the comparison of groups without versus groups with the administration of minocycline. The analyses for groups S1 and S1 + m did not show any statistically significant differences. (**d**) The necrosis depth deepened after stroke induction. Within the groups: with minocycline (Kruskall-Wallis test, $p = 0.008$), without minocycline (Kruskall-Wallis test, $p = 0.003$). For the pairs S2 + m vs. S3 + m and S1 vs. S2, a statistically significant difference was demonstrated (Dunn's *post hoc* test, $p < 0.05$), where * $p < 0.05$ for intragroup comparisons. For each time interval, the differences between the studied groups were significant (Mann-Whitney U test, $p = 0.008$), where ## $p < 0.01$ for the comparison of groups without versus groups with the administration of minocycline. The analysis between groups S1 and S1 + m did not show any statistically significant differences.

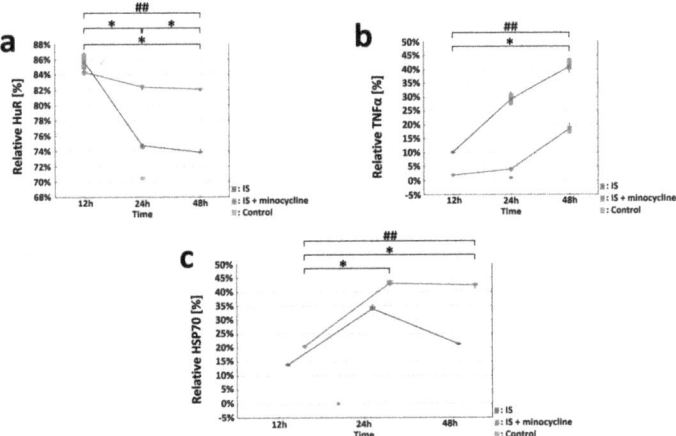

Figure 3. Effect of minocycline on selected parameters of inflammation after the induction of ischemic stroke in rats. HuR, TNFα, and HSP70 were investigated in the peri-infarct area after ischemic stroke induction: immunohistochemistry (IS: ischemic stroke groups; IS + minocycline: ischemic stroke + minocycline groups; Control: control group). (**a**) HuR and NeuN double - immunolabeled neurons. The variables "nNeuN", "nHuR", and "relative HuR" show statistically significant difference (KruskalWallis test, $p = 0.0002$). S1 vs. Control, S2 vs. Control, S3 vs. Control, S1 vs. S3, and S1 + m vs. S3 + m showed a statistically significant difference (Dunn's *post hoc* test, $p < 0.05$). S1 + m vs. Control, S2 + m vs. Control, S3 + m vs. Control, S1 vs. S3, and S1 + m vs. S3 + m showed a statistically significant difference for the relative "HuR" variable (Dunn's *post hoc* test, $p < 0.05$), where * $p < 0.05$ for intragroup comparisons and comparisons with the control group. Comparing the groups without the administration of minocycline and with the administration of minocycline at each time point revealed the presence of statistically significant differences for all the three examined variables, "nNeuN", "nHuR", and "relative HuR", in favor of the minocycline groups (Mann-Whitney U test, $p = 0.002$), where ## $p < 0.01$ for the comparison of groups without versus groups with the administration of minocycline. (**b**) TNFα and NeuN double-immunolabeled neurons. The obtained results for the "nNeuN", "nTNFα", and "relative TNFα" variables showed statistically significant differences for all variables only between the S2 vs. Control groups (Kruskall-Wallis, $p = 0.0005$; Dunn's *post hoc* test, $p < 0.05$). For each studied variable, the pairs S1 vs. S3 and S1 + m *vs*. S3 + m were statistically significant (Dunn's *post hoc* test, $p < 0.05$), where * $p < 0.05$ for intragroup comparisons and comparisons with the control group. The occurrence of differences between the groups without minocycline and with minocycline at each time point were compared for the "nNeuN", "nTNFα", and "relative TNFα" variables. All three variables were statistically significantly different at each time point between the groups without minocycline and with minocycline (Mann-Whitney U test, $p = 0.002$), where ## $p < 0.01$ for the comparison of groups without versus groups with the administration of minocycline. (**c**) HSP70 and NeuN double-immunolabeled neurons. The values of the "nNeuN", "nHSP70", and "relative HSP70" variables showed a statistically significant difference between all groups without minocycline and those with minocycline (Kruskall-Wallis test, $p = 0.0001$). The pairs S1 vs. S3 and S1 + m vs. S3 + m showed a statistically significant difference (Dunn's *post hoc* test, $p < 0.05$) for the "nNeuN" and "nHSP70" variables. The pairs S1 vs. S3, S1 + m vs. S2 + m, and S1 + m vs. S3 + m showed a statistically significant difference in the "relative HSP70" variable (Dunn's *post hoc* test, $p < 0.05$), where * $p < 0.05$ for intragroup comparisons and comparisons with the control group. The "nNeuN", "nHSP70", and "relative HSP70" variables results showed statistically significant differences (Mann-Whitney U test, $p = 0.002$) between the groups without minocycline and those with minocycline at all time points examined, where ## $p < 0.01$ for the comparison of groups without versus groups with the administration of minocycline.

The effect minocycline on the amount of HuR, TNFα, and HSP70 proteins in peri-infarct and infarct tissues was evaluated using the Western blotting technique. Concerning HuR protein, there was a significantly higher HuR protein expression in rats from the S3 + m group compared to the S3 group after FCI induction. There were no statistically significant differences for the other groups (Mann-Whitney U test, $p = 0.041$; Figure 4a). With respect to the HSP70 protein, there was a statistically significant difference in the level of HSP70 protein expression between the S3 and S3 + m groups. There were no statistically significant differences in the other groups (Mann-Whitney U test, $p = 0.025$; Figure 4b). With respect to the TNFα protein, a non-parametric analysis was performed. After inducing FCI in the rats, the level of TNFα protein was statistically significantly higher in the S3 group than in the S3 + m group (Kruskall-Wallis test, $p = 0.004$; Dunn's post hoc test, $p = 0.0362$). There were no statistically significant differences in the other groups (Figure 4c).

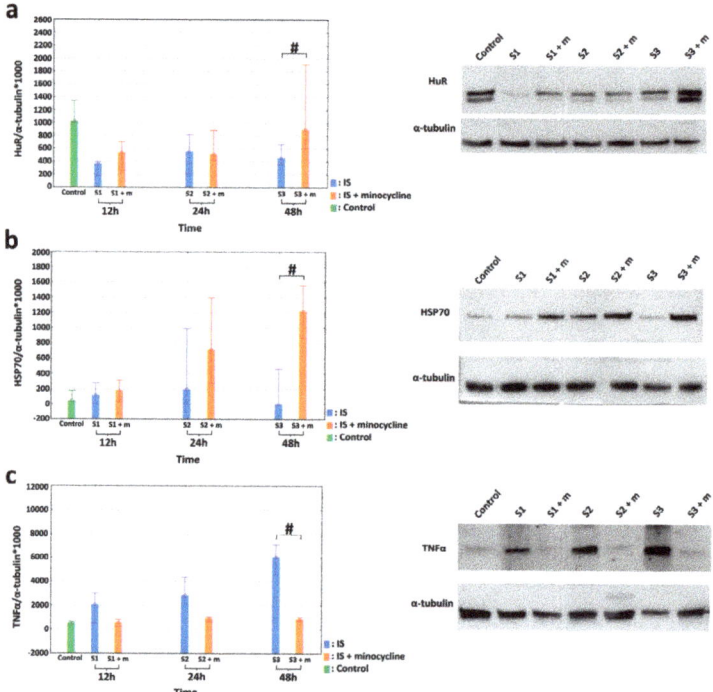

Figure 4. Effects of minocycline administration on selected markers of inflammation after photothrombotic stroke in rats. HuR, TNFα, and HSP70 levels in the peri-infarct area after ischemic stroke induction; Western blotting (IS: ischemic stroke groups; IS + minocycline: ischemic stroke + minocycline groups; Control: control group). (**a**) HuR protein levels: the results confirmed a significantly higher HuR protein expression in the S3 + m rats compared to the S3 group after FCI induction (the Mann Whitney U, $p = 0.041$), where # $p < 0.05$ for the comparison of groups without versus groups with the administration of minocycline. (**b**) HSP70 protein levels: the results confirmed a statistically significant difference in HSP70 protein expression between the S3 and S3 + m groups (Mann Whitney U, $p = 0.025$), where # $p < 0.05$ for the comparison of groups without versus groups with the administration of minocycline. (**c**) TNFα protein levels: there was a statistically significant difference between the S3 and S3 + m groups (Kruskall-Wallis test, $p = 0.004$; Dunn's *post hoc* test, $p = 0.0362$), where # $p < 0.05$ for the comparison of groups without versus groups with the administration of minocycline.

2.3. Effect of Minocycline on the Level of Motor Performance in Rats after FCI

In our study, we also aimed to assess whether the administration of minocycline can improve motor performance in rats after the induction of ischemic stroke. For this purpose, all the stroke animals underwent motor tests including the Horizontal Runway Elevated test (HRE), Grip Strength test (GST) and CatWalk™ XT. None of the animals had any health problems or complications following the procedures, and no animals were excluded from the tests, except for groups S1 and S1 + m, which had a short duration between general anesthesia and euthanasia, making it impractical to perform motor tests [17]. Using the GST test, we were able to analyze the strength of the front paws in stroke rats. Two variables were measured: the "peak pull force", which represents the maximum strength of the animal, and the "time of peak pull force", which represents average time in which the animal reached the maximum strength of the front paws. The variables at each time point were treated as multiple measures. Some of the variables did not have a normal distribution within the groups (Shapiro-Wilk test, $p > 0.05$); therefore, an ANOVA test was used [56,57]. The analysis of variance for the "peak pull force" variable for the groups showed a statistically significant difference between the S2 and S2 + m groups (ANOVA, $p < 0.026$). The results revealed no differences in the mean strength of animals among the studied groups before the procedure (which indicates a homogeneous starting point) and a negative effect of stroke induction. In each time point at which the measurement was taken was different from the others (Bonferroni *post hoc* test, $p < 0.001$; Figure 5a). For the "time of peak pull force" variable, the analysis was statistically significant (ANOVA, $p < 0.00001$). Each time peak at which the maximum power was reached was different from the other (Bonferroni *post hoc* test, $p < 0.001$). The animals from the group without minocycline lost some strength after FCI induction already on the first day. They also had lower levels of strength in their forelimbs. Therefore, they reached their peak strength within a very short time compared to the animals treated with minocycline. (Figure 5b).

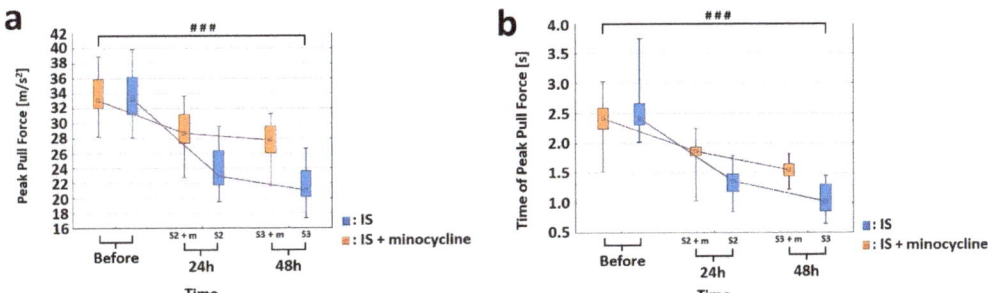

Figure 5. Effect of minocycline on the strength level of the front paws after prothrombotic stroke induction in rats: Grip Strength test. Administration of minocycline after stroke increased front paw strength relative to animals without minocycline. (**a**) For the "peak pull force" variable, the analysis of variance showed statistically significant differences in the mean values of the variable between the S2 vs. S2 + m groups (ANOVA, $p = 0.0254$) and as a function of time (ANOVA, $p = 0.0000$). The interaction between these two factors, group and time, was significant (ANOVA, $p = 0.0000$). The comparison showed that each time point at which the measurement was made differed from the other (The Bonferroni *post hoc* test, $p < 0.001$), where ### $p < 0.001$ for comparison of groups without versus groups with the administration of minocycline. (**b**) For the "time of peak pull force" variable, the analysis was significant for the two factors "group" (ANOVA, $p = 0.00001$) and "time" (ANOVA, $p = 0.0000$), as well as for the interaction between these two factors (ANOVA, $p = 0.00000$). The comparison showed that each peak time at which the maximum power was reached was different from the other (Bonferroni *post hoc* test, $p < 0.001$), where ### $p < 0.001$ for the comparison of groups without versus groups with the administration of minocycline.

The Horizontal Runway Elevated (HRE) test was performed to assess the effect of minocycline on motor performance in rats after FCI. Specifically, this test allowed us to evaluate the walking speed and the accuracy of beam crossing. To analyze changes in the motility of animals, all the experimental groups were compared based on the following two variables: "sum of errors" (number of paw slips) and "mean time of passage" through the beam. The comparison was carried out from the day before the induction of ischemic stroke (D6) until the day of euthanasia (DX). After four days of training (D2–D5), the rats always traversed the beam flawlessly on D5 (Figure 6a). In addition, during the HRE test, a dynamic learning process was observed in rats, with the acquisition of flawless motor skills on the beam followed by a rapid decline in motor skills after FCI induction. Following stroke, the administration of minocycline resulted in a reduction in the number of errors made by rats at both 24 h and 48 h post-stroke induction compared to those not receiving minocycline. Additionally, both the time elapsed since stroke induction and the use of minocycline had a statistically significant effect on the number of errors made by rats in the HRE test (ANOVA, $p = 0.0309$; Figure 6a). For the variable "mean time of passage", the analysis revealed that this variable was affected by training (D2-D5), the time elapsed since FCI induction, and the administration of minocycline (ANOVA, $p < 0.05$; Figure 6b). The animals that did not receive minocycline had a higher mean time of passage than the animals treated with minocycline. Moreover, the administration of minocycline resulted in a statistically significant reduction in the time needed to cross the beam in rats both 24 h and 48 h following FCI (Bonferroni *post hoc* test, $p < 0.05$; Figure 6b).

In order to assess the effect of minocycline on various gait parameters, CatWalk™ XT system (CWT) was used. CWT allowed us to assess the effect of ischemic stroke on locomotor functions and detect possible improvements induced by minocycline administration. The gait efficiency was assessed based on the nine most commonly used parameters: "Base of Support", "Print area", "Intensity", "Duty cycle", "Max area of contact", "Stride length", "Support time", "Swing speed", and the "Regularity Index". Given that the stroke focus was on the left motor cortex of the brain, gait analysis was only performed on the front right paw (RF) and hind right paw (RH). The "Swing Speed" variable allowed us to measure the speed of paw in the air. For this variable, the analysis of variance showed a statistically significant decrease in the RF and RH movement speed in rats after FCI induction. The animals treated with minocycline had a statistically significantly faster swing rate in air than the untreated animals at each time point (Figure 7a,b). For the "Stride length" variable, the analysis of variance revealed a statistically significant effect of both stroke induction and minocycline administration on the RF stride length. Following stroke, the animals not receiving minocycline made an approximately 1.5 cm shorter step compared to those treated with minocycline 48 h after FCI. The analysis of variance for the RH showed a statistically significant effect of both stroke induction and minocycline on the RH stride length. The post-stroke animals without minocycline had an approximately 3.0 cm shorter RF stride at 48 h compared to animals treated with minocycline (Figure 7c,d).

With respect to the "Regular Index" variable, the analysis of variance showed a statistically significant effect of minocycline on the level of step regularity. Animals without minocycline after the FCI challenge had a decrease in step regularity compared to animals treated with minocycline (Figure 8a). The "Duty cycle" (%) variable represents the ratio of stand time to step cycle (Duty cycle = stand time/step cycle). Stand time (s) was calculated by the duration of contact with the walkway of a specific paw. Step cycle (s) was calculated by the duration of two consecutive initial contacts of a specific paw (step cycle = stand time + swing time). Regarding this variable, the analysis of variance for the RF showed a statistically significant effect of stroke induction, substance, and time interval. Similarly, for the RH, the ANOVA demonstrated a statistically significant effect of stroke induction, substance, and time interval. Animals without minocycline had a higher "Duty cycle" ratio than animals receiving minocycline (Figure 8b,c). Concerning the other variables "Base of Support", "Print paw area", "Intensity of paw contact", "Max area of paw contact", and "Support time" the analysis of variance revealed no statistically significant differences.

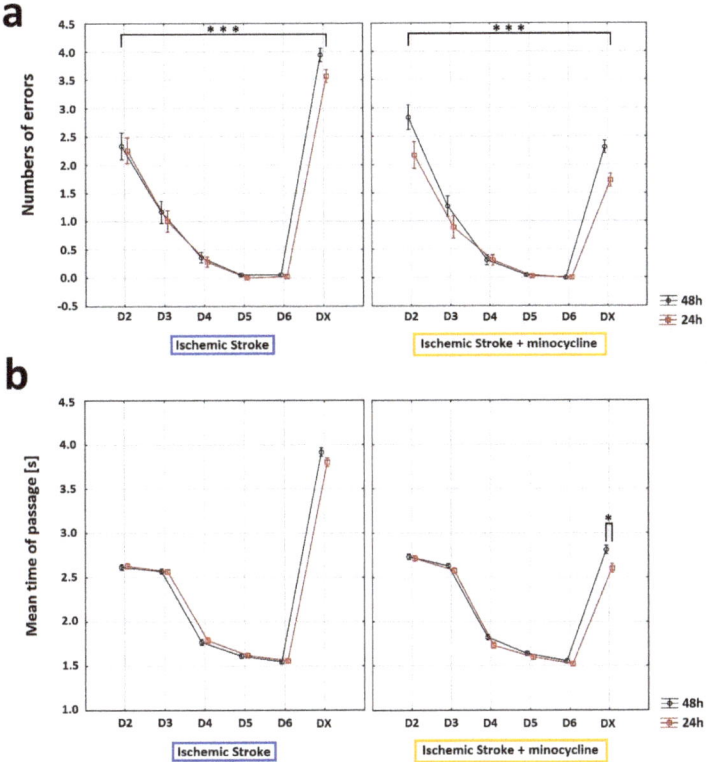

Figure 6. Influence of minocycline on the speed of passage and the number of errors after induction of prothrombotic stroke in rats: Horizontal runway elevated test (HRE). The administration of minocycline after stroke increased the speed of passage through the beam and reduced the number of errors made. (**a**) Concerning the "sum of errors", an analysis of variance was performed: "beam passage time" (ANOVA, $p = 0.0009$) and "minocycline" (ANOVA, $p = 0.009$) influenced the number of errors made by the rats. Moreover, the interaction between "minocycline" and "beam passage time" showed a statistically significant result (ANOVA, $p = 0.0000$). The "beam passage time" interaction with groups (pre-stroke vs. 24 h post FCI vs. 48 h post FCI) also reached a statistically significant result (ANOVA, $p = 0.0309$). Training days (D2–D5) and testing days (D6 and DX) differed significantly in terms of the average number of errors (ANOVA, $p = 0.0000$). Interactions between "minocycline" over time were statistically significant (ANOVA, $p = 0.0000$), as well as the beam passage time interaction between groups (pre-stroke vs. 24 h post FCI vs. 48 h post FCI; Bonferroni *post hoc* test, $p < 0.05$), where *** $p < 0.001$ for intragroup comparisons. (**b**) With respect to the "mean time of passage", the analysis of "mean time of passage" was performed. The variable was affected by training (D2–D5), time elapsed since FCI induction (24 h post-induction or 48 h post-induction), and minocycline administration (ANOVA, $p < 0.05$). The animals without minocycline had a higher mean time of passage. In the case of the animals with minocycline, time played a role—the animals passed the beam slower 48 h after the procedure than after 24 h (Bonferroni *post hoc* test, $p < 0.05$). The administration of minocycline resulted in a statistically significant reduction in the time needed for minocyclinetreated rats to pass the beam both 24 h and 48 h after FCI compared to the animals without minocycline (the Bonferroni *post hoc* test, $p < 0.05$); where * $p < 0.05$ for intragroup comparisons.

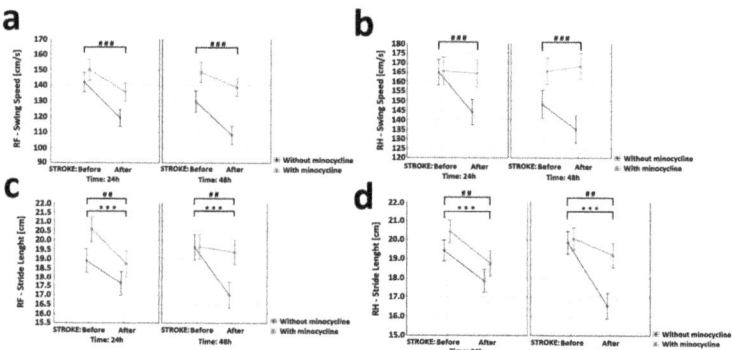

Figure 7. Effect of minocycline on gait speed and stride length in rats after ischemic stroke: CatWalk XT. Selected gait parameters improved after minocycline administration for both the right front (RF) and right hind (RH) paws. For the variable "Swing speed" (**a,b**) the analysis showed a decrease in RF (ANOVA, $p = 0.0003$) and RH (ANOVA, $p = 0.001$) movement speed after FCI induction. The animals receiving minocycline had a statistically significantly faster swing speed than animals without minocycline in each time group (ANOVA, $p = 0.0001$). Concerning the "Stride length" variable (**c,d**), the analysis revealed the effect of both stroke induction (ANOVA, $p = 0.003$) and minocycline (ANOVA, $p = 0.008$) on the RF stride length. Following FCI, animals without minocycline made an approximately 1.5 cm shorter step compared to animals with minocycline 48 h following FCI. The analysis of variance for RH showed the effect of both stroke induction (ANOVA, $p = 0.0000$) and minocycline (ANOVA, $p = 0.009$) on RH stride length. Following FCI, the animals without minocycline had an approximately 3.0 cm shorter RF stride compared to the animals with minocycline 48 h following FCI, where *** $p < 0.001$ for intragroup comparisons and ## $p < 0.01$, ### $p < 0.001$ for the comparison of groups with and without the administration of minocycline.

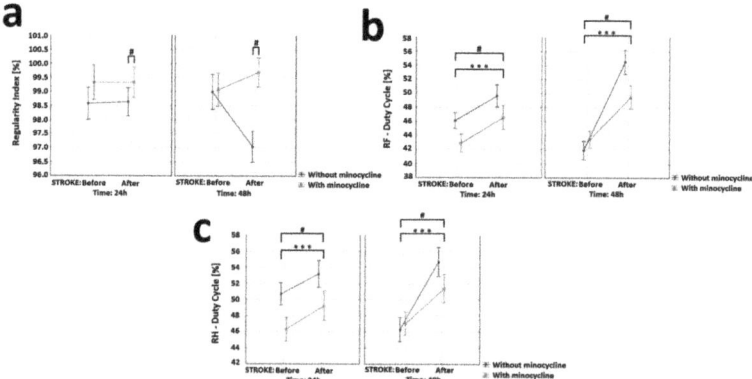

Figure 8. Effect of minocycline on gait regularity and step interval in rats after ischemic stroke induction: CatWalk XT. Selected gait parameters improved after minocycline administration for both the right front (RF) and right hind (RH) paws. Regarding the "Regular Index" variable (**a**), the analysis showed the effect of minocycline on the level of steps regularity (ANOVA, $p = 0.013$). Groups S2 and S3 displayed a decrease in step regularity after FCI compared to animals given minocycline (S2 + m and S3 + m). With respect to the "Duty cycle" variable (**b,c**), the analysis of the RF showed the effect of stroke induction (ANOVA, $p = 0.00000$), minocycline (ANOVA, $p = 0.0307$), and time interval (ANOVA, $p = 0.006$) on this parameter. For the RH, the results showed the effect of stroke induction (ANOVA, $p = 0.000057$), minocycline (ANOVA, $p = 0.03589$), and time interval (ANOVA, $p = 0.00751$) on this parameter, where *** $p < 0.001$ for intragroup comparisons, and # $p < 0.05$ for the comparison of groups with and without administration of minocycline.

3. Discussion

Overall, the results obtained in our research show that early administration of minocycline after ischemic stroke inhibits the enlargement of the necrotic area. At the molecular level, this event is associated with an increase in the content of both HSP70 protein and the RNA-binding protein HuR, and a decrease in the amount of TNFα in the peri-infarct tissue. Importantly, minocycline administration also produced an improvement in certain motor parameters following FCI.

Specifically, using Nissl staining, we assessed the volume, width, and depth of the necrotic focus. In our study, the stroke focus covered 5.5–7.0% of the brain volume, which is similar to that observed in humans [19]. In our study, the stroke focus covered 5.5–7.0% of the brain volume, which is similar to that observed in humans. This similarity enhances the translational potential of the results obtained using this animal model for the development of new therapies for humans. The volume of the stroke focus in rats progressed significantly 12 h after the induction of ischemic stroke and reached its maximum volume after 24 h, followed by a decrease after 48 h. This dynamic pattern of changes in the area affected by ischemic stroke aligns with other studies [14,58]. In the groups that received a single dose of minocycline, we observed statistically significant reductions in the infarct volume, width, and depth of the necrotic focus, with particularly remarkable improvement found in 12-week-old male rats. Reduced infarct volume after the administration of minocycline has also been observed in other studies using various animal models of ischemic stroke (i.e., FCI and middle cerebral artery occlusion (MCAO)) [14,31,33,59–62].

Accumulating evidence indicates that inflammation may play a key role in the pathogenesis of stroke, making it an interesting target for therapeutic interventions. Ischemic stroke is accompanied by inflammation, which is associated with elevated levels of pro-inflammatory cytokines, chemokines, and peripheral blood leukocytes (e.g., neutrophils, monocytes, T lymphocytes) observed in these areas [14,28,63–68]. The development of inflammation and the infiltration of pro-inflammatory cells (e.g., monocytes) are considered to be one of the phenomena responsible for increasing the area of secondary damage [69]. Notably, studies on animal models of ischemic stroke have demonstrated that minocycline has some anti-inflammatory properties [35,61,62,70,71] that inhibit the expression of pro-inflammatory cytokines and reduce brain damage [72,73]. Within this context, several investigations have documented that neuronal ischemia increases the expression of TNFα as early as 1 h after the onset of ischemia in the MCAO model [74,75]. Furthermore, Kondo et al. and Meng et al. demonstrated that the expression of TNFα in cells other than neurons (i.e., microglia and astrocytes) becomes visible more than 24 h after the onset of a stroke [37,76]. Considering that inflammatory processes stimulate neuroprotective effects if they persist for a short time but cause neurodegenerative processes if they persist for a longer time [28], we also examined the time course of TNFα expression in neurons located in the peri-stroke tissue. Using double labeling with TNFα and the neuronal marker NeuN, we were observed TNFα expression in neurons as early as 12 h after the induction of ischemic stroke. Similarly, Li et al. and Yang et al. showed that within 6–12 h from the onset of symptoms, an increasing amount of TNFα was detected in the blood of human patients and in the cerebral tissues of rats following stroke [77,78]. We used Western blotting to assess the amount of TNFα protein in the peri-stroke tissue, which supported the immunohistochemistry results. The data analysis showed a statistically significant decrease in TNFα levels in the groups receiving minocycline. Consistent with these findings, other authors have also noted a decrease in TNFα content after the administration of minocycline in animal models of ischemic stroke [33,71,79]. In particular, Yang et al. showed that a single dose of minocycline given immediately after the start of reperfusion significantly inhibits microglial activation after 48 h, indicating that early administration of minocycline after stroke can reduce inflammation levels [79]. Therefore, our results may be related to the inhibitory effect of minocycline on the inflammatory response in the acute phase of stroke. As mentioned earlier, HSP70 protein regulates inflammation both intracellularly, where it appears to play an anti-inflammatory role, and extracellularly, where it may enhance immune responses. We found that under homeostatic conditions, as also reported in other studies [80,81], HSP70 levels are low. Using NeuN-HSP70 double labeling, we observed changes in the number of HSP70-positive neurons in the peri-infarct tissue as early as 12 h after stroke induction. Most importantly, HSP70 expression was statistically significantly higher in the groups receiving minocycline compared to the groups without minocycline. The Western blotting data supported the results of immunohistology, demonstrating a statistically significant difference in HSP70 protein expression on the second day after stroke induction between the minocycline-treated groups and the untreated animals. Consistently, other authors have also reported an increase in the amount of HSP70 after ischemic stroke [80–83], suggesting that minocycline itself is likely responsible for the increase in HSP70 protein levels in the peri-stroke tissue [84,85].

Given that both HSP70 and TNF-α transcripts are targeted by HuR [45,50], we also determined the level of HuR protein in the peri-stroke tissue in order to examine the direct effect of minocycline on this RNA-stabilizing protein. Using NeuN-HuR double immunolabeling, we conducted analyses comparing the groups without minocycline to the groups with minocycline, which revealed a statistically significant increase in the number of neurons in the minocycline-treated groups. Furthermore, in the group without minocycline administration, the number of HuR-positive cells already decreased dramatically 24 h after the stroke, indicating the developing of inflammation in the peri-stroke tissue. Western blotting data analysis confirmed a statistically significantly higher HuR protein expression in the minocycline-treated group compared to the untreated group 48 h after FCI induction. These results suggest that following FCI, this RNA-binding protein promotes a protective response by shifting its binding towards HSP70 instead of TNFα. Notably, at 48 h, we observed a concomitant increase in HSP70 protein content and a decrease in TNFα expression. Similarly, Jamison et al. demonstrated a correlation between HuR and HSP70 protein levels following ischemic stroke, highlighting the functional importance of the correlation between HuR and the concomitant appearance of HSP70 in the same neurons [51]. Hence, our results suggest that HuR protein may play a role in modulating inflammation mitigate some secondary damage in the aftermath of stroke. Given that low-level inflammation has a protective effect on neurons while chronic high-level inflammation is detrimental [86–89], determining the exact role of HuR protein in the inflammation process may contribute to the improvement of new post-stroke therapies, especially in the context of neuronal protection.

In the present study, we also assess whether the positive biochemical and morphological changes observed under the influence of minocycline would translate into improved motor functions. In this regard, we would like to emphasize that our improved and minimally invasive animal model of ischemic stroke allows for motor tests to be performed after FCI [17]. The data from selected tests showed positive changes in gait, balance level, speed of movement, and leg strength. Specifically, the results obtained from the GST indicate that minocycline-treated animals achieved a statistically significant higher level of maximum paw strength duration and reached the maximum strength later compared to the untreated animals at each time point. In this respect, Soliman et al. also used GST in the MCAO model of ischemic stroke and demonstrated a statistically significant improvement in the animals treated with minocycline [31]. Using the HRE test, we examined the effect of minocycline on the speed of movement along the beam and the number of errors during the transition in stroke rats. The animals that did not receive minocycline were characterized by a statistically significantly higher number of errors (paw slipping off the beam during the transition) both 24 h and 48 h after FCI induction. We also document that, after FCI, the administration of minocycline resulted in a statistically significant reduction in the time needed by rats to cross the beam at each time point. In this regard, Soliman et al. along with Li et al., using the HRE test in the MCAO model, also demonstrated that the administration of minocycline improved the motor function of animals [31,90]. Using the CWT, we explored whether there was an improvement in gait parameters in the animals receiving minocycline after FCI. For the following gait parameters: stride length, duty cycle, swing speed, and regularity index, we observed statistically significant improvements in favor of minocycline administration. The animals receiving minocycline had a statistically significantly faster swing rate, longer strides, increased step regularity, and lower standing time to step cycle ratios compared to the untreated animals. All the motor tests used allowed us to observe even very subtle improvements in many parameters of gait, balance, and fitness in the acute phase of ischemic stroke in the rats treated with minocycline. It is worth emphasizing that these tests are much more accurate than neurological scales and provide objective changes in the parameters. In conclusion, our results indicate that motor tests are a valuable tool to verify whether positive changes, both biochemical and morphological, translate into improved motor efficiency after ischemic stroke. Improved motor performance is one of the goals of therapy after ischemic stroke in humans. Therefore, the use of these approaches can strongly improve the translation of therapies from animal models to patients with ischemic stroke [91–93].

4. Materials and Methods

4.1. Animals

Experimental protocols were approved by the Local Bioethics Committee at the Medical University of Silesia, Katowice, Poland, and were consistent with international guidelines on the ethical use of animals. All rats were bred in the Department for Experimental Medicine, Medical University of Silesia in Katowice, Poland. Throughout the entire study, the animals were housed in a temperature-controlled and humidity-controlled room with a 12 h light/dark cycle. They had ad libitum access to water and standard rat chow. From the 5th week of the animals' life until the start of the study, routine behaviors were implemented according to our protocol (see our previous publication [17]), resulting in a significant stress reduction in the animals.

Ninety-six male Long-Evans (LE) rats weighing 223–239 g were used. The rats were randomly divided into six experimental groups (Figure 1). Groups S1 (n = 14), S2 (n = 14), and S3 (n = 14) consisted of animals without minocycline administration, and the time between ischemic stroke induction and euthanasia was 12 h, 24 h, and 48 h, respectively. Groups S1 + m (n = 14), S2 + m (n = 14), and S3 + m (n = 14) consisted of animals with minocycline administration, and the time elapsed between ischemic stroke induction and euthanasia (DX) was equal to 12 h, 24 h, and 48 h, respectively. The Control group (n = 12) used in this study consisted of animals that did not undergo any procedures. For this animal model of ischemic stroke, in accordance with the 3R principles and our previous results, only one control group was created [17]. In order to verify motor deficits and the relative effects of minocycline, all groups underwent the Horizontal Runway Elevated test, CatWalk™ XT, and Grip Strength test both before the induction of ischemic stroke and on the euthanasia day.

4.2. Animal Model

A full and detailed description of the ischemic model used in the present study is available in our previous publication [17]. During the stroke induction surgery, the animals were placed under general anesthesia induced by intraperitoneal administration of xylazine hydrochloride (10 mg/kg of body weight) and ketamine hydrochloride (100 mg/kg of body weight). The infarct was created in the posterior motor cortex (the spot was marked with the coordinates 0.5 mm anterior to bregma and 3.0 mm laterally from the centerline). The center was determined using an optical fiber with a 5 mm diameter. A non-transparent mask was used to protect the remaining skull areas from the laser light. The skull was irradiated with white light at a wavelength of 560 nm and 3200 K [94] (KL2500, LCD SCHOTT, Mainz, Germany). The irradiation lasted for 15 min. The dye injection took place during the first minute of irradiation. Specifically, a Bengal Rose (BR) solution (20 mg of BR in 1 mL of PBS (Sigma-Aldrich, St. Louis, MO, USA)) was slowly injected at a dose of 1 mL/kg of body weight through a pre-inserted polyethylene catheter into the tail vein (*lateral caudal vein*) of each rat. After the irradiation was finished, the optical fiber was removed and the incisions were sutured with skin sutures.

4.3. Treatment with Minocycline

Rats in groups S1 + m, S2 + m, and S3 + m received a single dose of minocycline (Sigma-Aldrich, St. Louis, MO, USA) at 1 mg/kg body weight, dissolved in 1 mL 0.9% NaCl, administered intravenously 10 min after the ischemic stroke induction. The chosen single dose [32,79,95] of minocycline was based on previous studies that reported neuroprotection in the ischemic stroke model under similar conditions. Based on the reports obtained after a single dose in our experience, we decided to administer the lowest possible dose of 1 mg/kg body weight. This allows for the design of further in-depth studies, with the possibility of modulating the dose volume or changing the frequency of minocycline administration to the animals. Animals in groups S1, S2, and S3 received the same volume of saline intravenously.

4.4. Horizontal Runway Elevated Test

In this study, motor deficits resulting from the induction of ischemic stroke in rats were tested using the horizontal runway elevated (HRE) test. The HRE test is commonly used in animal models to evaluate forelimb and hindlimb function and coordination [96–99]. For each experimental group (n = 12–14), two variables were measured: the sum of the average number of errors made and the average time taken to pass through the slat. The HRE test consisted of an elevated ladder apparatus and a camera (GoPro Hero 8, San Mateo, CA, USA). The camera was necessary to register the animals' passage over the beam. The recorded videos were needed for a quantitative and qualitative analysis of the rats' gait. The HRE test used in this study was constructed by our team [17]. Successful completion of the HRE test required six runs for each animal: three runs from cage A to cage B, and three runs from cage B to cage A. The rats began by crossing the slat from cage A to cage B. This action was repeated in the opposite direction until the sixth successful passage. The final run concluded in cage A for all rats. The HRE test was divided into two phases: the training phase (D2–D5) and the official passage phase (D6–DX). After the training period, during the official passage phase, all rats performed one official pre-stroke passage on the stroke induction day (D6), and one official passage post-stroke on the day of euthanasia (DX).

4.5. Grip Strength Test

The forelimb Grip Strength test (GST) was performed using an electronic digital force gauge grip-strength meter (47200, UGO Basil, Gemonio, VA, Italy). The use of the GST following ischemic stroke is consistent with previous publications [100–103]. For each experimental group (n = 12–14), two variables were measured: the peak force exerted by the animal while gripping the sensor bar and the time of peak force. The back part of the rat's body was gently held and pulled back until its front paw loosened its grip on the sensor, and the maximum grip strength was automatically recorded. GST was performed three times on the day of ischemic stroke induction (D6) and three times after the ischemic stroke induction, on the euthanasia day (DX). The duration of the GST was 5 s; if the rat did not pull/hold the sensor within that time, the measurement was not recorded, and the animal was excluded.

4.6. CatWalk™ XT

An automated quantitative gait analysis system was used to assess rat motor function and coordination: CatWalk™ XT (CWT; Noldus, Wageningen, The Netherlands). Each test group consisted of the same number of rats (n = 10). The CWT system has a unique application in the study of strokes [104,105]. The CWT assessment was conducted in a quiet and darkened room. When rats made contact with the glass plate, the light signals from their paws were reflected and transformed into digital messages by a video camera. The performance of the CWT was divided into two phases: the training phase (5 days long; D1–D5) and the official passage phase (2 days long; D6–DX). After the training days, during the official passage phase, all rats performed one official pre-stroke passage on the stroke induction day (D6) and one official passage post-stroke on the day of euthanasia (DX). The five-day training phase helped to minimize stress in rats and ensure the performance of three consecutive uninterrupted runs [90,106]. A correctly performed CWT assessment consisted of three undisturbed runs for each rat [90]. A series of gait statistics were automatically generated when the system identified and marked each footprint. The statistics included the following parameters: "Base of Support", "Print paw area", "Intensity of paw contact", "Max area of paw contact", "Support time", "Duty cycle"," Stride length", "Swing speed", and "Regularity Index" [90,106–109].

4.7. Histological Analysis

Histological evaluation required the collection of brain tissues from each experimental group (n = 6) and the Control group (n = 6) in accordance with the assigned time interval between the induction of ischemic stroke and euthanasia. The rats were anesthetized and transcardially perfused with 4% paraformaldehyde. The fixed brains were then removed and postfixed in a paraformaldehyde solution overnight at 4 °C. Subsequently, the brains were dehydrated, embedded in paraffin, and sectioned using a microtome (Leica Microsystems, Mannheim, Germany) into coronal planes (-2.50 mm to -2.90 mm from bregma) with 7 μm-thick slices. The distance between each of the 10 sections used per animal was 50 μm.

4.7.1. Nissl Staining

The preparations were stained with 1 g/L cresyl violet dye (Sigma-Aldrich, St. Louis, MO, USA) in water, following the classical Nissl staining protocol with our own modifications [17,110]. Images of the peri-infarct cortex area in the ipsilateral hemisphere and a reference calibration slide were acquired using a digital camera (Olympus OM-D E-M10 Mark IV, Tokyo, Japan). The area of the infarct in each section, identified by pale staining, was measured using the ImageJ 1.43 software (Madison, WI, USA) [111]. The same software was also used to calculate the infarct volume, width, and depth of each brain.

4.7.2. Immunohistochemistry

Immunohistochemistry assay was used to measure the levels of HuR, TNFα, and HSP70 proteins expression in paraffin-embedded brain tissue slides. The tissue slices were blocked with 0.1% Triton X-100 (Sigma-Aldrich) and 10% serum (goat normal serum, Vector Labs). The sections were then incubated overnight at 4 °C with primary antibodies against HuR, NeuN, TNFα, and HSP70 (Table 1). The primary antibodies were followed by the following fluorochrome-conjugated secondary antibodies: goat anti-mouse Alexa Fluor® 488 (green Alexa; Cambridge, UK) and goat anti-rabbit Alexa Fluor® 594 (red Alexa; Cambridge, UK), which were incubated for 1h at room temperature. Finally, the sections were mounted on slides using a DAPI-containing medium. To initially characterize the changes in the brain tissue after FCI in ipsilateral hemisphere, images were obtained from double-immunolabeled sections of HuR-NeuN, TNFα-NeuN and HSP70-NeuN. Five regions of interest (ROIs) were incorporated, as shown in Figure 2a. These included ROIs at the lateral and medial edges of the infarct and more distant sites in the contralateral cerebral cortex. The immuno-positive cells were counted in the field of view from the ROI areas: Ipsi1, Ipsi2, Ipsi3, Cont4, and Cont5. The variables "nNeuN", "nX", and "relative X" (n = number of immunohistochemically positive cells in the field of view; X—double HuR+NeuN, TNFα+NeuN, or HSP70+NeuN immuno-positive cells from the tested protein in the field of view) were calculated. We also calculated the relative value from the growth: "relative X"(%) = nX/(nX + nNeuN). The sections of double-immunolabeled ROIs were captured and analyzed under a fluorescence microscope (Olympus BX43, Tokyo, Japan) using cellSens Standard software (Olympus) and processed with ImageJ 1.43usoftware. The ROIs with size of 500 × 500 μm were analyzed.

Table 1. Table of the antibodies used in the experiments.

Antibody	Abbreviation	Type	Company	Catalog Number	Dilution	Order
HuR/ELAV1	HuR	mouse monoclonal	Santa Cruz Biotechnology	sc-5261	for IHCP we used 1:1000	primary antibodies
Neuronal Marker	NeuN	rabbit monoclonal	Abcam	ab177487	for IHCP we used 1:1000	primary antibodies
Anti-TNFα	TNFα	mouse monoclonal	Santa Cruz Biotechnology	sc-52746	for IHCP we used 1:1000	primary antibodies
Anti-Hsp70	HSP70	mouse monoclonal	Abcam	ab2787S	for IHCP we used 1:500	primary antibodies
HuR/ELAV1	HuR	mouse monoclonal	Santa Cruz Biotechnology	sc-5261	for WB we used 1:1000	primary antibodies
Anti-TNFα	TNFα	rabbit monoclonal	Abcam	ab205587	for WB we uded 1:500	primary antibodies
HSC70/HSP70	HSP70	mouse monoclonal	Santa Cruz Biotechnology	sc-24	for WB we uded 1:500	primary antibodies
Anti-α-Tubulin	α-Tubulin	mouse monoclonal	Sigma-Aldrich	T0198	for WB we udes 1:1000	primary antibodies
Goat anti-mouse Alexa Fluor® 488	green Alexa	goat anti-mouse IgG	Abcam	ab150113	for IHCP we used 1:500	secondary antibodies
Goat anti-rabbit Alexa Fluor® 594	red Alexa	goat anti-rabbit IgG	Abcam	ab150080	for IHCP we used 1:500	secondary antibodies
Goat anti-mouse IgG-HRP	anti mouse	goat anti-mouse IgG	Sigma-Aldrich	A4416	for WB we used 1:3000	secondary antibodies
Goat anti-rabbit IgG-HRP	anti rabbit	goat anti-rabbit IgG	Merck Millipore	AP156P	for WB we used 1:3000	secondary antibodies

4.8. Western Blotting

Samples were collected from all the experimental groups (n = 6) and the Control group (n = 5) to determine proteins expression using the Western blot technique. The rats were sacrificed by decapitation and their brains were immediately removed from the skulls. The area containing the infarct, along with approximately 1.0 mm of the surrounding tissue, was dissected for analysis. For each rat, the material was collected using a biopsy punch of the same size. The tissue samples were immediately frozen on dry ice and stored in a freezer at −80 °C. Protein levels were measured using the Bradford method. Bovine albumin was used as an internal standard. The proteins were diluted in 2x SDS protein gel loading solution, boiled for 5 min, and separated on a 12% SDS-PAGE gel. HuR, TNFα and HSP70 antibodies were according to the instructions provided in each datasheet (Table 1). The nitrocellulose membrane signals were detected using chemiluminescence. The same membranes were re-probed with an α-tubulin antibody and used to normalize the data. Densitometric values obtained with the ImageJ image-processing program were subjected to statistical analysis for the Western blot data.

4.9. Statistical Analysis

The statistical analysis was performed using Statistica 13.1 software (Dell, Austin, TX, USA). The significance level was set at $p = 0.05$. Descriptive statistics of the studied variables in groups were presented, and tests examining the normality of distribution were carried out when appropriate (Shapiro-Wilk test $p > 0.05$). Additionally, Levene's test was performed to assess the homogeneity of variance. Based on these results, parametric (ANOVA) or non-parametric tests (Kruskal-Wallis, U Mann-Whitney) were selected, and when statistically significant results were obtained, appropriate post hoc tests (Bonferroni's and Dunn's) were carried out. The values are presented in charts as the mean ± standard deviations for variables analyzed with parametric tests, and as medians along with the quartile range (IQR) for variables analyzed with non-parametric tests.

5. Conclusions

Severe cerebral ischemia leads to neuronal damage and death in the ischemic area. Several previous studies have suggested that minocycline protects neurons from damage caused by cerebral ischemia. Our study confirmed that the administration of minocycline increases the viability of neurons and reduces neurodegeneration caused by ischemia. The effects of minocycline led to a significant reduction in the infarct volume after ischemia. Minocycline also affected selected parameters of inflammation: it reduced the content of TNFα in the peristroke tissue, while increasing the levels of HSP70 and HuR proteins in the same area. After ischemic stroke, minocycline could play an important role in modulating inflammation, particularly at the level the stability and/or translation of target mRNAs. The results show that the minocycline influences the level of ubiquitously expressed HuR protein (RNA-binding protein). The increase in the level of HuR protein translates into the improvement of molecular and motor parameters after ischemic stroke. Therefore, the role of the HuR protein in modulating inflammation may be important, although further in-depth research is required. Motor tests have demonstrated that the reduction in inflammation parameters and the decrease in the area of brain tissue damage after the administration of minocycline directly translates into a better motor performance. Therapies based on targeting inflammation appear to be a very interesting and effective approach in post-ischemic stroke therapy available to most patients. We believe that understanding both the cellular and molecular changes in the brain throughout all phases of ischemic stroke is essential for developing the most effective therapies capable of counteracting the negative effects of this devastating process.

Supplementary Materials: The supporting information can be downloaded at: https://www.mdpi.com/article/10.3390/ijms24119446/s1.

Author Contributions: Conceptualization, K.P. and H.J.-S.; methodology, K.P., K.B. and F.F.; software, N.M. and D.G.d.C.; validation, K.P. and J.J.B.; formal analysis, K.P., H.J.-S. and F.F.; investigation, A.P. and N.M.; resources, A.G. and D.G.d.C.; data curation, K.P.; writing—original draft preparation, K.P.; writing—review and editing, A.P., H.J.-S., J.J.B. and K.B.; visualization, A.G., K.B. and F.F.; supervision, K.P. and A.P.; project administration, K.P.; funding acquisition, K.P. and H.J.-S. All authors have read and agreed to the published version of the manuscript.

Funding: This research was supported by the research funds from the Department of Physiology at the Medical University of Silesia in Katowice, Poland (No. PCN-1-088/K/1/O) and the research funds for PhD students from the Medical University of Silesia in Katowice, Poland (No. KNW-2-O09/D/9/N).

Institutional Review Board Statement: All experimental procedures were approved by the Local Bioethics Committee for Experiments on Animals in Katowice, Poland (approvals No. 77/2018 on 12 July 2018 and No. 63/2019 on 24 July 2019). No human subjects or tissue were utilized in this study.

Informed Consent Statement: Not applicable.

Data Availability Statement: The dataset used and/or analyzed during this study is available from the corresponding author upon reasonable request.

Acknowledgments: We would like to acknowledge the employees of the Department for Experimental Medicine at the Medical University of Silesia for their support throughout the experiment and for providing us with the opportunity to conduct our research at the center.

Conflicts of Interest: The authors declare no conflict of interest.

Abbreviations

BR	the Bengal Rose
CWT	CatWalk™ XT
D1–D4	days of training
D6	days of photothrombotic ischemic stroke induction
DX	day of euthanasia
FCI	focal cerebral ischemia
GST	forelimb Grip Strength test
HRE	horizontal runway elevated test
HSP70	70 kilodalton heat shock proteins
HuR	human antigen R protein
IQR	the quartile range
IL-6	interleukin 6
LE	Long-Evans rats
MCAO	Middle Cerebral Artery Occlusion
PBS	phosphate-buffered saline
TNFα	tumor necrosis factor alpha
RBP	RNA-binding proteins
RH	right hind paw
ROI	region of interesting
RF	right front paw

References

1. Tsao, C.W.; Aday, A.W.; Almarzooq, Z.I.; Alonso, A.; Beaton, A.Z.; Bittencourt, M.S.; Boehme, A.K.; Buxton, A.E.; Carson, A.P.; Commodore-Mensah, Y.; et al. Heart Disease and Stroke Statistics—2022 Update: A Report from the American Heart Association. *Circulation* **2022**, *145*, e153–e639, Erratum in *Circulation* **2022**, *146*, e141. [CrossRef] [PubMed]
2. Bai, S.; Lu, X.; Pan, Q.; Wang, B.; Pong U, K.; Yang, Y.; Wang, H.; Lin, S.; Feng, L.; Wang, Y.; et al. Cranial Bone Transport Promotes Angiogenesis, Neurogenesis, and Modulates Meningeal Lymphatic Function in Middle Cerebral Artery Occlusion Rats. *Stroke* **2022**, *53*, 1373–1385. [CrossRef] [PubMed]
3. Feigin, V.L.; Stark, B.A.; Johnson, C.O.; Roth, G.A.; Bisignano, C.; Abady, G.G.; Abbasifard, M.; Abbasi-Kangevari, M.; Abd-Allah, F.; Abedi, V.; et al. Global, Regional, and National Burden of Stroke and Its Risk Factors, 1990–2019: A Systematic Analysis for the Global Burden of Disease Study 2019. *Lancet Neurol.* **2021**, *20*, 795–820. [CrossRef]
4. Donkor, E.S. Stroke in the 21st Century: A Snapshot of the Burden, Epidemiology, and Quality of Life. *Stroke Res. Treat.* **2018**, *2018*, 3238165.
5. Benjamin, E.J.; Virani, S.S.; Callaway, C.W.; Chamberlain, A.M.; Chang, A.R.; Cheng, S.; Chiuve, S.E.; Cushman, M.; Delling, F.N.; Deo, R.; et al. Heart Disease and Stroke Statistics—2018 Update: A Report from the American Heart Association. *Circulation* **2018**, *137*, E67–E492. [CrossRef]
6. Song, J.; Zhao, Y.; Yu, C.; Xu, J. DUSP14 Rescues Cerebral Ischemia/Reperfusion (IR) Injury by Reducing Inflammation and Apoptosis via the Activation of Nrf-2. *Biochem. Biophys. Res. Commun.* **2019**, *509*, 713–721. [CrossRef]
7. McMeekin, P.; White, P.; James, M.A.; Price, C.I.; Flynn, D.; Ford, G.A. Estimating the Number of UK Stroke Patients Eligible for Endovascular Thrombectomy. *Eur. Stroke J.* **2017**, *2*, 319–326. [CrossRef]
8. Kim, J.S. TPA Helpers in the Treatment of Acute Ischemic Stroke: Are They Ready for Clinical Use? *J. Stroke* **2019**, *21*, 160–174. [CrossRef]
9. Sun, M.S.; Jin, H.; Sun, X.; Huang, S.; Zhang, F.L.; Guo, Z.N.; Yang, Y. Free Radical Damage in Ischemia-Reperfusion Injury: An Obstacle in Acute Ischemic Stroke after Revascularization Therapy. *Oxid. Med. Cell. Longev.* **2018**, *2018*, 3804979. [CrossRef]
10. Dirnagl, U.; Iadecola, C.; Moskowitz, M.A. Pathobiology of Ischaemic Stroke: An Integrated View. *Trends Neurosci.* **1999**, *22*, 391–397. [CrossRef]
11. Fluri, F.; Schuhmann, M.K.; Kleinschnitz, C. Animal Models of Ischemic Stroke and Their Application in Clinical Research. *Drug Des. Dev. Ther.* **2015**, *9*, 3445–3454. [CrossRef]
12. Kurniawan, N.A.; Grimbergen, J.; Koopman, J.; Koenderink, G.H. Factor XIII Stiffens Fibrin Clots by Causing Fiber Compaction. *J. Thromb. Haemost.* **2014**, *12*, 1687–1696. [CrossRef] [PubMed]
13. Fagan, S.C.; Cronic, L.E.; Hess, D.C. Minocycline Development for Acute Ischemic Stroke. *Transl. Stroke Res.* **2011**, *2*, 202–208. [CrossRef] [PubMed]
14. Yew, W.P.; Djukic, N.D.; Jayaseelan, J.S.P.; Walker, F.R.; Roos, K.A.A.; Chataway, T.K.; Muyderman, H.; Sims, N.R. Early Treatment with Minocycline Following Stroke in Rats Improves Functional Recovery and Differentially Modifies Responses of Peri-Infarct Microglia and Astrocytes. *J. Neuroinflamm.* **2019**, *16*, 6. [CrossRef] [PubMed]
15. Schmidt, A.; Hoppen, M.; Strecker, J.K.; Diederich, K.; Schäbitz, W.R.; Schilling, M.; Minnerup, J. Photochemically Induced Ischemic Stroke in Rats. *Exp. Transl. Stroke Med.* **2012**, *4*, 13. [CrossRef] [PubMed]
16. Ostrova, I.V.; Kalabushev, S.N.; Ryzhkov, I.A.; Tsokolaeva, Z.I. A Novel Thromboplastin-Based Rat Model of Ischemic Stroke. *Brain Sci.* **2021**, *11*, 1475. [CrossRef]
17. Pawletko, K.; Jędrzejowska-Szypułka, H.; Bogus, K.; Pascale, A.; Fahmideh, F.; Marchesi, N.; Grajoszek, A.; Olakowska, E.; Barski, J.J. A Novel Improved Thromboembolism-Based Rat Stroke Model That Meets the Latest Standards in Preclinical Studies. *Brain Sci.* **2022**, *12*, 1671. [CrossRef]
18. Benowitz, L.I.; Carmichael, S.T. Promoting Axonal Rewiring to Improve Outcome after Stroke. *Neurobiol. Dis.* **2010**, *37*, 259–266. [CrossRef]
19. Uzdensky, A.B. Photothrombotic Stroke as a Model of Ischemic Stroke. *Transl. Stroke Res.* **2018**, *9*, 437–451. [CrossRef]
20. Lasek-Bal, A.; Jedrzejowska-Szypulka, H.; Student, S.; Warsz-Wianecka, A.; Zareba, K.; Puz, P.; Bal, W.; Pawletko, K.; Lewin-Kowalik, J. The Importance of Selected Markers of Inflammation and Blood-Brain Barrier Damage for Short-Term Ischemic Stroke Prognosis. *J. Physiol. Pharmacol.* **2019**, *70*, 209–217. [CrossRef]
21. Chen, Y.; Won, S.J.; Xu, Y.; Swanson, R.A. Targeting Microglial Activation in Stroke Therapy: Pharmacological Tools and Gender Effects. *Curr. Med. Chem.* **2014**, *21*, 2146–2155. [CrossRef]
22. Yang, C.; Hawkins, K.E.; Doré, S.; Candelario-Jalil, X.E. Neuroinflammatory Mechanisms of Blood-Brain Barrier Damage in Ischemic Stroke. *Am. J. Physiol. Cell Physiol.* **2019**, *316*, 135–153. [CrossRef]
23. Ramiro, L.; Simats, A.; García-Berrocoso, T.; Montaner, J. Inflammatory Molecules Might Become Both Biomarkers and Therapeutic Targets for Stroke Management. *Ther. Adv. Neurol. Disord.* **2018**, *11*, 1756286418789340. [CrossRef] [PubMed]
24. Parameswaran, N.; Patial, S. Tumor Necrosis Factor-α Signaling in Macrophages. *Crit. Rev. Eukaryot. Gene Expr.* **2010**, *20*, 87. [CrossRef] [PubMed]
25. Zhang, W.; Sato, K.; Hayashi, T.; Omori, N.; Nagano, I.; Kato, S.; Horiuchi, S.; Abe, K. Extension of Ischemic Therapeutic Time Window by a Free Radical Scavenger, Edaravone, Reperfused with TPA in Rat Brain. *Neurol. Res.* **2004**, *26*, 342–348. [CrossRef] [PubMed]

26. Cirillo, C.; Brihmat, N.; Castel-Lacanal, E.; Le Friec, A.; Barbieux-Guillot, M.; Raposo, N.; Pariente, J.; Viguier, A.; Simonetta-Moreau, M.; Albucher, J.F.; et al. Post-Stroke Remodeling Processes in Animal Models and Humans. *J. Cereb. Blood Flow Metab.* **2020**, *40*, 3–22. [CrossRef]
27. Ma, Y.; Wang, J.; Wang, Y.; Yang, G.Y. The Biphasic Function of Microglia in Ischemic Stroke. *Prog. Neurobiol.* **2017**, *157*, 247–272. [CrossRef]
28. Jayaraj, R.L.; Azimullah, S.; Beiram, R.; Jalal, F.Y.; Rosenberg, G.A. Neuroinflammation: Friend and Foe for Ischemic Stroke. *J. Neuroinflamm.* **2019**, *16*, 142. [CrossRef]
29. Alano, C.C.; Kauppinen, T.M.; Valls, A.V.; Swanson, R.A. Minocycline Inhibits Poly(ADP-Ribose) Polymerase-1 at Nanomolar Concentrations. *Proc. Natl. Acad. Sci. USA* **2006**, *103*, 9685–9690. [CrossRef]
30. Abbaszadeh, A.; Darabi, S.; Hasanvand, A.; Amini-Khoei, H.; Abbasnezhad, A.; Choghakhori, R.; Aaliehpour, A. Minocycline through Attenuation of Oxidative Stress and Inflammatory Response Reduces the Neuropathic Pain in a Rat Model of Chronic Constriction Injury. *Iran. J. Basic Med. Sci.* **2018**, *21*, 138–144. [CrossRef]
31. Soliman, S.; Ishrat, T.; Fouda, A.Y.; Patel, A.; Pillai, B.; Fagan, S.C. Sequential Therapy with Minocycline and Candesartan Improves Long-Term Recovery After Experimental Stroke. *Transl. Stroke Res.* **2015**, *6*, 309–322. [CrossRef] [PubMed]
32. Faheem, H.; Mansour, A.; Elkordy, A.; Rashad, S.; Shebl, M.; Madi, M.; Elwy, S.; Niizuma, K.; Tominaga, T. Neuroprotective Effects of Minocycline and Progesterone on White Matter Injury after Focal Cerebral Ischemia. *J. Clin. Neurosci.* **2019**, *64*, 206–213. [CrossRef] [PubMed]
33. Jin, Z.; Liang, J.; Wang, J.; Kolattukudy, P.E. MCP-Induced Protein 1 Mediates the Minocycline-Induced Neuroprotection against Cerebral Ischemia/Reperfusion Injury in Vitro and in Vivo. *J. Neuroinflamm.* **2015**, *12*, 39. [CrossRef]
34. Yrjänheikki, J.; Tikka, T.; Keinänen, R.; Goldsteins, G.; Chan, P.H.; Koistinaho, J. A Tetracycline Derivative, Minocycline, Reduces Inflammation and Protects against Focal Cerebral Ischemia with a Wide Therapeutic Window. *Proc. Natl. Acad. Sci. USA* **1999**, *96*, 13496–13500. [CrossRef] [PubMed]
35. Marques, B.L.; Carvalho, G.A.; Freitas, E.M.M.; Chiareli, R.A.; Barbosa, T.G.; Di Araújo, A.G.P.; Nogueira, Y.L.; Ribeiro, R.I.; Parreira, R.C.; Vieira, M.S.; et al. The Role of Neurogenesis in Neurorepair after Ischemic Stroke. *Semin. Cell Dev. Biol.* **2019**, *95*, 98–110. [CrossRef]
36. Stone, M.J.; Hayward, J.A.; Huang, C.; Huma, Z.E.; Sanchez, J. Mechanisms of Regulation of the Chemokine-Receptor Network. *Int. J. Mol. Sci.* **2017**, *18*, 342. [CrossRef]
37. Kondo, M.; Okazaki, H.; Nakayama, K.; Hohjoh, H.; Nakagawa, K.; Segi-Nishida, E.; Hasegawa, H. Characterization of Astrocytes in the Minocycline-Administered Mouse Photothrombotic Ischemic Stroke Model. *Neurochem. Res.* **2022**, *47*, 2839–2855. [CrossRef]
38. Offner, H.; Subramanian, S.; Parker, S.M.; Afentoulis, M.E.; Vandenbark, A.A.; Hurn, P.D. Experimental Stroke Induces Massive, Rapid Activation of the Peripheral Immune System. *J. Cereb. Blood Flow Metab.* **2006**, *26*, 654–665. [CrossRef]
39. Murakami, Y.; Saito, K.; Hara, A.; Zhu, Y.; Sudo, K.; Niwa, M.; Fujii, H.; Wada, H.; Ishiguro, H.; Mori, H.; et al. Increases in Tumor Necrosis Factor-α Following Transient Global Cerebral Ischemia Do Not Contribute to Neuron Death in Mouse Hippocampus. *J. Neurochem.* **2005**, *93*, 1616–1622. [CrossRef]
40. Van Molle, W.; Wielockx, B.; Mahieu, T.; Takada, M.; Taniguchi, T.; Sekikawa, K.; Libert, C. HSP70 Protects against TNF-Induced Lethal Inflammatory Shock. *Immunity* **2002**, *16*, 685–695. [CrossRef]
41. Zheng, Z.; Yenari, M.A. Post-Ischemic Inflammation: Molecular Mechanisms and Therapeutic Implications. *Neurol. Res.* **2004**, *26*, 884–892. [CrossRef]
42. Abdelmohsen, K.; Kuwano, Y.; Kim, H.H.; Gorospe, M. Posttranscriptional Gene Regulation by RNA-Binding Proteins during Oxidative Stress: Implications for Cellular Senescence. *Biol. Chem.* **2008**, *389*, 243–255. [CrossRef]
43. Kim, J.Y.; Han, Y.; Lee, J.E.; Yenari, M.A. The 70-KDa Heat Shock Protein (Hsp70) as a Therapeutic Target for Stroke. *Expert Opin. Ther. Targets* **2018**, *22*, 191–199. [CrossRef]
44. Giffard, R.G.; Yenari, M.A. Many Mechanisms for Hsp70 Protection from Cerebral Ischemia. *J. Neurosurg. Anesthesiol.* **2003**, *16*, 53–61. [CrossRef]
45. Pascale, A.; Govoni, S. The Complex World of Post-Transcriptional Mechanisms: Is Their Deregulation a Common Link for Diseases? Focus on ELAV-like RNA-Binding Proteins. *Cell. Mol. Life Sci.* **2012**, *69*, 501–517. [CrossRef]
46. Yi, J.; Chang, N.; Liu, X.; Guo, G.; Xue, L.; Tong, T.; Gorospe, M.; Wang, W. Reduced Nuclear Export of HuR MRNA by HuR Is Linked to the Loss of HuR in Replicative Senescence. *Nucleic Acids Res.* **2009**, *38*, 1547–1558. [CrossRef] [PubMed]
47. Doller, A.; Akool, E.-S.; Huwiler, A.; Müller, R.; Radeke, H.H.; Pfeilschifter, J.; Eberhardt, W. Posttranslational Modification of the AU-Rich Element Binding Protein HuR by Protein Kinase Cδ Elicits Angiotensin II-Induced Stabilization and Nuclear Export of Cyclooxygenase 2 MRNA. *Mol. Cell. Biol.* **2008**, *28*, 2608–2625. [CrossRef] [PubMed]
48. Gallouzi, I.-E.; Brennan, C.M.; Stenberg, M.G.; Swanson, M.S.; Eversole, A.; Maizels, N.; Steitz, J.A. HuR Binding to Cytoplasmic MRNA Is Perturbed by Heat Shock. *Proc. Natl. Acad. Sci. USA* **2000**, *97*, 3073–3078. [CrossRef]
49. Gallouzi, I.-E.; Brennan, C.M.; Steitz, J.A. Protein Ligands Mediate the CRM1-Dependent Export of HuR in Response to Heat Shock. *RNA* **2001**, *7*, 1348–1361. [CrossRef] [PubMed]
50. Amadio, M.; Scapagnini, G.; Laforenza, U.; Intrieri, M.; Romeo, L.; Govoni, S.; Pascale, A. Post-Transcriptional Regulation of HSP70 Expression Following Oxidative Stress in SH-SY5Y Cells: The Potential Involvement of the RNA-Binding Protein HuR. *Curr. Pharm. Des.* **2008**, *14*, 2651–2658. [CrossRef] [PubMed]

51. Jamison, J.T.; Kayali, F.; Rudolph, J.; Marshall, M.; Kimball, S.R.; Degracia, D.J. Persistent Redistribution of Poly-Adenylated MRNAs Correlates with Translation Arrest and Cell Death Following Global Brain Ischemia and Reperfusion. *Neuroscience* **2008**, *154*, 504–520. [CrossRef] [PubMed]
52. Wang, J.G.; Collinge, M.; Ramgolam, V.; Ayalon, O.; Fan, X.C.; Pardi, R.; Bender, J.R. LFA-1-Dependent HuR Nuclear Export and Cytokine MRNA Stabilization in T Cell Activation. *J. Immunol.* **2006**, *176*, 2105–2113. [CrossRef]
53. Sung, S.C.; Kim, K.; Lee, K.A.; Choi, K.H.; Kim, S.M.; Son, Y.H.; Moon, Y.S.; Eo, S.K.; Rhim, B.Y. 7-Ketocholesterol Upregulates Interleukin-6 via Mechanisms That Are Distinct from Those of Tumor Necrosis Factor-α, in Vascular Smooth Muscle Cells. *J. Vasc. Res.* **2008**, *46*, 36–44. [CrossRef] [PubMed]
54. Grammatikakis, I.; Abdelmohsen, K.; Gorospe, M. Posttranslational Control of HuR Function. *Wiley Interdiscip. Rev. RNA* **2017**, *8*, e1372. [CrossRef]
55. Srikantan, S.; Gorospe, M. HuR Function in Disease. *Front. Biosci. Landmark Ed.* **2012**, *17*, 189. [CrossRef] [PubMed]
56. Schmider, E.; Ziegler, M.; Danay, E.; Beyer, L.; Bühner, M. Is It Really Robust? Reinvestigating the Robustness of ANOVA against Violations of the Normal Distribution Assumption. *Methodology* **2010**, *6*, 147–151. [CrossRef]
57. Blanca, M.J.; Alarcón, R.; Arnau, J.; Bono, R.; Bendayan, R. Datos No Normales: ¿es El ANOVA Una Opción Válida? *Psicothema* **2017**, *29*, 552–557. [CrossRef]
58. Liu, N.W.; Ke, C.C.; Zhao, Y.; Chen, Y.A.; Chan, K.C.; Tan, D.T.W.; Lee, J.S.; Chen, Y.Y.; Hsu, T.W.; Hsieh, Y.J.; et al. Evolutional Characterization of Photochemically Induced Stroke in Rats: A Multimodality Imaging and Molecular Biological Study. *Transl. Stroke Res.* **2017**, *8*, 244–256. [CrossRef] [PubMed]
59. Lu, Y.; Zhou, M.; Li, Y.; Li, Y.; Hua, Y.; Fan, Y. Minocycline Promotes Functional Recovery in Ischemic Stroke by Modulating Microglia Polarization through STAT1/STAT6 Pathways. *Biochem. Pharmacol.* **2021**, *186*, 114464. [CrossRef]
60. Tanaka, M.; Ishihara, Y.; Mizuno, S.; Ishida, A.; Vogel, C.F.; Tsuji, M.; Yamazaki, T.; Itoh, K. Progression of Vasogenic Edema Induced by Activated Microglia under Permanent Middle Cerebral Artery Occlusion. *Biochem. Biophys. Res. Commun.* **2018**, *496*, 582–587. [CrossRef]
61. Lu, Y.; Xiao, G.; Luo, W. Minocycline Suppresses NLRP3 Inflammasome Activation in Experimental Ischemic Stroke. *Neuroimmunomodulation* **2017**, *23*, 230–238. [CrossRef] [PubMed]
62. Park, S.I.; Park, S.K.; Jang, K.S.; Han, Y.M.; Kim, C.H.; Oh, S.J. Preischemic Neuroprotective Effect of Minocycline and Sodium Ozagrel on Transient Cerebral Ischemic Rat Model. *Brain Res.* **2015**, *1599*, 85–92. [CrossRef] [PubMed]
63. Lakhan, S.E.; Kirchgessner, A.; Hofer, M. Inflammatory Mechanisms in Ischemic Stroke: Therapeutic Approaches. *J. Transl. Med.* **2009**, *7*, 97. [CrossRef] [PubMed]
64. Dugue, R.; Nath, M.; Dugue, A.; Barone, F.C. Roles of Pro- and Anti-Inflammatory Cytokines in Traumatic Brain Injury and Acute Ischemic Stroke. In *Mechanisms of Neuroinflammation*; IntechOpen: London, UK, 2017.
65. Maida, C.D.; Norrito, R.L.; Daidone, M.; Tuttolomondo, A.; Pinto, A. Neuroinflammatory Mechanisms in Ischemic Stroke: Focus on Cardioembolic Stroke, Background, and Therapeutic Approaches. *Int. J. Mol. Sci.* **2020**, *21*, 6454. [CrossRef] [PubMed]
66. Jin, R.; Yang, G.; Li, G. Inflammatory Mechanisms in Ischemic Stroke: Role of Inflammatory Cells. *J. Leukoc. Biol.* **2010**, *87*, 779–789. [CrossRef] [PubMed]
67. Ceulemans, A.G.; Zgavc, T.; Kooijman, R.; Hachimi-Idrissi, S.; Sarre, S.; Michotte, Y. The Dual Role of the Neuroinflammatory Response after Ischemic Stroke: Modulatory Effects of Hypothermia. *J. Neuroinflamm.* **2010**, *7*, 74. [CrossRef] [PubMed]
68. Xu, H.; Tan, G.; Zhang, S.; Zhu, H.; Liu, F.; Huang, C.; Zhang, F.; Wang, Z. Minocycline Reduces Reactive Gliosis in the Rat Model of Hydrocephalus. *BMC Neurosci.* **2012**, *13*, 148. [CrossRef]
69. Emerich, D.F.; Dean, R.L.; Bartus, R.T. The Role of Leukocytes Following Cerebral Ischemia: Pathogenic Variable or Bystander Reaction to Emerging Infarct? *Exp. Neurol.* **2002**, *173*, 168–181. [CrossRef]
70. Camargos, Q.M.; Silva, B.C.; Silva, D.G.; de Brito Toscano, E.C.; da Silva Oliveira, B.; Bellozi, P.M.Q.; de Oliveira Jardim, B.L.; Vieira, É.L.M.; de Oliveira, A.C.P.; Sousa, L.P.; et al. Minocycline Treatment Prevents Depression and Anxiety-like Behaviors and Promotes Neuroprotection after Experimental Ischemic Stroke. *Brain Res. Bull.* **2020**, *155*, 1–10. [CrossRef]
71. Naderi, Y.; Sabetkasaei, M.; Parvardeh, S.; Zanjani, T.M. Neuroprotective Effects of Pretreatment with Minocycline on Memory Impairment Following Cerebral Ischemia in Rats. *Behav. Pharmacol.* **2017**, *28*, 214–222. [CrossRef]
72. Pfau, M.L.; Russo, S.J. Neuroinflammation Regulates Cognitive Impairment in Socially Defeated Mice. *Trends Neurosci.* **2016**, *39*, 353–355. [CrossRef] [PubMed]
73. Chen, Y.; Yi, Q.; Liu, G.; Shen, X.; Xuan, L.; Tian, Y. Cerebral White Matter Injury and Damage to Myelin Sheath Following Whole-Brain Ischemia. *Brain Res.* **2013**, *1495*, 11–17. [CrossRef] [PubMed]
74. Liu, T.; Clark, R.K.; McDonnell, P.C.; Young, P.R.; White, R.F.; Barone, F.C.; Feuerstein, G.Z. Tumor necrosis factor-alpha expression in ischemic neurons. *Stroke* **1994**, *25*, 1481–1488. [CrossRef]
75. Botchkina, G.I.; Meistrell, M.E.; Botchkina, I.L.; Tracey, K.J. Expression of TNF and TNF Receptors (P55 and P75) in the Rat Brain after Focal Cerebral Ischemia. *Mol. Med.* **1997**, *3*, 765–781. [CrossRef] [PubMed]
76. Meng, H.; Zhao, H.; Cao, X.; Hao, J.; Zhang, H.; Liu, Y.; Zhu, M.; Fan, L.; Weng, L.; Qian, L.; et al. Double-Negative T Cells Remarkably Promote Neuroinflammation after Ischemic Stroke. *Proc. Natl. Acad. Sci. USA* **2019**, *116*, 5558–5563. [CrossRef] [PubMed]
77. Sotgiu, S.; Zanda, B.; Marchetti, B.; Fois, M.L.; Arru, G.; Pes, G.M.; Salaris, F.S.; Arru, A.; Pirisi, A.; Rosati, G. Inflammatory Biomarkers in Blood of Patients with Acute Brain Ischemia. *Eur. J. Neurol.* **2006**, *13*, 505–513. [CrossRef]

78. Li, J.; Hao, M.; Liu, M.; Wang, J.; Gao, D.; Han, S.; Yu, D. Transcutaneous Electrical Acupoint Stimulation Pretreatment Alleviates Cerebral Ischemia–Reperfusion Injury in Rats by Modulating Microglia Polarization and Neuroinflammation Through Nrf2/HO-1 Signaling Pathway. *Neurochem. Res.* **2023**, *48*, 862–873. [CrossRef]
79. Yang, Y.; Salayandia, V.M.; Thompson, J.F.; Yang, L.Y.; Estrada, E.Y.; Yang, Y. Attenuation of Acute Stroke Injury in Rat Brain by Minocycline Promotes Blood-Brain Barrier Remodeling and Alternative Microglia/Macrophage Activation during Recovery. *J. Neuroinflamm.* **2015**, *12*, 26. [CrossRef] [PubMed]
80. Biagioni, F.; Mastroiacovo, F.; Lenzi, P.; Puglisi-Allegra, S.; Busceti, C.L.; Ryskalin, L.; Ferese, R.; Bucci, D.; Frati, A.; Nicoletti, F.; et al. The Autophagy-Related Organelle Autophagoproteasome Is Suppressed within Ischemic Penumbra. *Int. J. Mol. Sci.* **2021**, *22*, 10364. [CrossRef]
81. Liu, F.; Lu, Z.; Li, Z.; Wang, S.; Zhuang, L.; Hong, M.; Huang, K. Electroacupuncture Improves Cerebral Ischemic Injury by Enhancing the Epo-Jak2-Stat5 Pathway in Rats. *Neuropsychiatr. Dis. Treat.* **2021**, *17*, 2489–2498. [CrossRef]
82. Kim, H.J.; Wei, Y.; Wojtkiewicz, G.R.; Lee, J.Y.; Moskowitz, M.A.; Chen, J.W. Reducing Myeloperoxidase Activity Decreases Inflammation and Increases Cellular Protection in Ischemic Stroke. *J. Cereb. Blood Flow Metab.* **2019**, *39*, 1864–1877. [CrossRef] [PubMed]
83. Yao, X.; Yang, W.; Ren, Z.; Zhang, H.; Shi, D.; Li, Y.; Yu, Z.; Guo, Q.; Yang, G.; Gu, Y.; et al. Neuroprotective and Angiogenesis Effects of Levetiracetam Following Ischemic Stroke in Rats. *Front. Pharmacol.* **2021**, *12*, 638209. [CrossRef] [PubMed]
84. Shi, W.; Pu, J.; Wang, Z.; Wang, R.; Guo, Z.; Liu, C.; Sun, J.; Gao, L.; Zhou, R. Effects of Minocycline on the Expression of NGF and HSP70 and Its Neuroprotection Role Following Intracerebral Hemorrhage in Rats. *J. Biomed. Res.* **2011**, *25*, 292–298.
85. Shi, W.; Wang, Z.; Pu, J.; Wang, R.; Guo, Z.; Liu, C.; Sun, J.; Gao, L.; Zhou, R. Changes of Blood-Brain Barrier Permeability Following Intracerebral Hemorrhage and the Therapeutic Effect of Minocycline in Rats. In *Early Brain Injury or Cerebral Vasospasm*; Acta Neurochirurgica, Supplementum; Springer: Wien, Austria, 2011; Volume 110, pp. 61–67.
86. Bollaerts, I.; Van Houcke, J.; Andries, L.; De Groef, L.; Moons, L. Neuroinflammation as Fuel for Axonal Regeneration in the Injured Vertebrate Central Nervous System. *Mediat. Inflamm.* **2017**, *2017*, 9478542. [CrossRef] [PubMed]
87. Rauf, A.; Badoni, H.; Abu-Izneid, T.; Olatunde, A.; Rahman, M.M.; Painuli, S.; Semwal, P.; Wilairatana, P.; Mubarak, M.S. Neuroinflammatory Markers: Key Indicators in the Pathology of Neurodegenerative Diseases. *Molecules* **2022**, *27*, 3194. [CrossRef]
88. Kempuraj, D.; Thangavel, R.; Selvakumar, G.P.; Zaheer, S.; Ahmed, M.E.; Raikwar, S.P.; Zahoor, H.; Saeed, D.; Natteru, P.A.; Iyer, S.; et al. Brain and Peripheral Atypical Inflammatory Mediators Potentiate Neuroinflammation and Neurodegeneration. *Front. Cell. Neurosci.* **2017**, *11*, 216. [CrossRef]
89. Lucas, S.M.; Rothwell, N.J.; Gibson, R.M. The Role of Inflammation in CNS Injury and Disease. *Br. J. Pharmacol.* **2006**, *147*, S232–S240. [CrossRef]
90. Li, S.; Hua, X.; Zheng, M.; Wu, J.; Ma, Z.; Xing, X.; Ma, J.; Zhang, J.; Shan, C.; Xu, J. PLXNA2 Knockdown Promotes M2 Microglia Polarization through MTOR/STAT3 Signaling to Improve Functional Recovery in Rats after Cerebral Ischemia/Reperfusion Injury. *Exp. Neurol.* **2021**, *346*, 113854. [CrossRef]
91. Jickling, G.C.; Sharp, F.R. Improving the Translation of Animal Ischemic Stroke Studies to Humans. *Metab. Brain Dis.* **2015**, *30*, 461–467. [CrossRef]
92. Narayan, S.K.; Cherian, S.G.; Phaniti, P.B.; Chidambaram, S.B.; Vasanthi, A.H.R.; Arumugam, M. Preclinical Animal Studies in Ischemic Stroke: Challenges and Some Solutions. *Anim. Model. Exp. Med.* **2021**, *4*, 104–115. [CrossRef]
93. Boboc, I.K.S.; Rotaru-Zavaleanu, A.D.; Calina, D.; Albu, C.V.; Catalin, B.; Turcu-Stiolica, A. A Preclinical Systematic Review and Meta-Analysis of Behavior Testing in Mice Models of Ischemic Stroke. *Life* **2023**, *13*, 567. [CrossRef]
94. Watson, B.D.; Dietrich, W.D.; Busto, R.; Wachtel, M.S.; Ginsberg, M.D. Induction of Reproducible Brain Infarction by Photochemically Initiated Thrombosis. *Ann. Neurol.* **1985**, *17*, 497–504. [CrossRef]
95. Hoda, N.; Fagan, S.C.; Khan, M.B.; Vaibhav, K.; Chaudhary, A.; Wang, P.; Dhandapani, K.M.; Waller, J.L.; Hess, D.C. A 2 × 2 Factorial Design for the Combination Therapy of Minocycline and Remote Ischemic Perconditioning: Efficacy in a Preclinical Trial in Murine Thromboembolic Stroke Model. *Exp. Transl. Stroke Med.* **2014**, *6*, 10. [CrossRef]
96. Metz, G.A.; Whishaw, I.Q. The Ladder Rung Walking Task: A Scoring System and Its Practical Application. *J. Vis. Exp.* **2009**, *28*, e1204. [CrossRef]
97. Metz, G.A.; Whishaw, I.Q. Cortical and Subcortical Lesions Impair Skilled Walking in the Ladder Rung Walking Test: A New Task to Evaluate Fore- and Hindlimb Stepping, Placing, and Co-Ordination. *J. Neurosci. Methods* **2002**, *115*, 169–179. [CrossRef] [PubMed]
98. Alaverdashvili, M.; Moon, S.K.; Beckman, C.D.; Virag, A.; Whishaw, I.Q. Acute but Not Chronic Differences in Skilled Reaching for Food Following Motor Cortex Devascularization vs. Photothrombotic Stroke in the Rat. *Neuroscience* **2008**, *157*, 297–308. [CrossRef]
99. Qian, H.Z.; Zhang, H.; Yin, L.L.; Zhang, J.J. Postischemic Housing Environment on Cerebral Metabolism and Neuron Apoptosis after Focal Cerebral Ischemia in Rats. *Curr. Med. Sci.* **2018**, *38*, 656–665. [CrossRef] [PubMed]
100. Ishrat, T.; Pillai, B.; Soliman, S.; Fouda, A.Y.; Kozak, A.; Johnson, M.H.; Ergul, A.; Fagan, S.C. Low-Dose Candesartan Enhances Molecular Mediators of Neuroplasticity and Subsequent Functional Recovery After Ischemic Stroke in Rats. *Mol. Neurobiol.* **2015**, *51*, 1542–1553. [CrossRef] [PubMed]
101. Kaushik, P.; Ali, M.; Tabassum, H.; Parvez, S. Post-Ischemic Administration of Dopamine D2 Receptor Agonist Reduces Cell Death by Activating Mitochondrial Pathway Following Ischemic Stroke. *Life Sci.* **2020**, *261*, 118349. [CrossRef]

102. Li, C.; Sun, R.; Chen, J.; Hong, J.; Sun, J.; Zeng, Y.; Zhang, X.; Dou, Z.; Wen, H. Different Training Patterns at Recovery Stage Improve Cognitive Function in Ischemic Stroke Rats through Regulation of the Axonal Growth Inhibitor Pathway. *Behav. Brain Res.* **2022**, *421*, 113730. [CrossRef]
103. Zhang, T.; Wu, C.; Yang, X.; Liu, Y.; Yang, H.; Yuan, L.; Liu, Y.; Sun, S.; Yang, J. Pseudoginsenoside-F11 Protects against Transient Cerebral Ischemia Injury in Rats Involving Repressing Calcium Overload. *Neuroscience* **2019**, *411*, 86–104. [CrossRef] [PubMed]
104. Wang, Y.; Bontempi, B.; Hong, S.M.; Mehta, K.; Weinstein, P.R.; Abrams, G.M.; Liu, J. A Comprehensive Analysis of Gait Impairment after Experimental Stroke and the Therapeutic Effect of Environmental Enrichment in Rats. *J. Cereb. Blood Flow Metab.* **2008**, *28*, 1936–1950. [CrossRef] [PubMed]
105. Encarnacion, A.; Horie, N.; Keren-Gill, H.; Bliss, T.M.; Steinberg, G.K.; Shamloo, M. Long-Term Behavioral Assessment of Function in an Experimental Model for Ischemic Stroke. *J. Neurosci. Methods* **2011**, *196*, 247–257. [CrossRef]
106. Fan, Q.Y.; Liu, J.J.; Zhang, G.L.; Wu, H.Q.; Zhang, R.; Zhan, S.Q.; Liu, N. Inhibition of SNK-SPAR Signaling Pathway Promotes the Restoration of Motor Function in a Rat Model of Ischemic Stroke. *J. Cell. Biochem.* **2018**, *119*, 1093–1110. [CrossRef]
107. Wu, J.; Lin, B.; Liu, W.; Huang, J.; Shang, G.; Lin, Y.; Wang, L.; Chen, L.; Tao, J. Roles of Electro-Acupuncture in Glucose Metabolism as Assessed by 18F-FDG/PET Imaging and AMPKα Phosphorylation in Rats with Ischemic Stroke. *Int. J. Mol. Med.* **2017**, *40*, 875–882. [CrossRef] [PubMed]
108. Orgah, J.O.; Ren, J.; Liu, X.; Orgah, E.A.; Gao, X.M.; Zhu, Y. Danhong Injection Facilitates Recovery of Post-Stroke Motion Deficit via Parkin-Enhanced Mitochondrial Function. *Restor. Neurol. Neurosci.* **2019**, *37*, 375–395. [CrossRef] [PubMed]
109. Yang, L.; Lei, J.F.; Ouyang, J.Y.; Li, M.Z.; Zhan, Y.; Feng, X.F.; Lu, Y.; Li, M.C.; Wang, L.; Zou, H.Y.; et al. Effect of Neurorepair for Motor Functional Recovery Enhanced by Total Saponins from Trillium Tschonoskii Maxim. Treatment in a Rat Model of Focal Ischemia. *Front. Pharmacol.* **2021**, *12*, 763181. [CrossRef]
110. de Prisco, N.; Chemiakine, A.; Lee, W.; Botta, S.; Gennarino, V.A. Protocol to Assess the Effect of Disease-Driving Variants on Mouse Brain Morphology and Primary Hippocampal Neurons. *STAR Protoc.* **2022**, *3*, 101244. [CrossRef]
111. Schroeder, A.B.; Dobson, E.T.A.; Rueden, C.T.; Tomancak, P.; Jug, F.; Eliceiri, K.W. The ImageJ Ecosystem: Open-Source Software for Image Visualization, Processing, and Analysis. *Protein Sci.* **2021**, *30*, 234–249. [CrossRef]

Disclaimer/Publisher's Note: The statements, opinions and data contained in all publications are solely those of the individual author(s) and contributor(s) and not of MDPI and/or the editor(s). MDPI and/or the editor(s) disclaim responsibility for any injury to people or property resulting from any ideas, methods, instructions or products referred to in the content.

Hypothesis

The Labyrinthine Landscape of APP Processing: State of the Art and Possible Novel Soluble APP-Related Molecular Players in Traumatic Brain Injury and Neurodegeneration

Mirco Masi [1], Fabrizio Biundo [2], André Fiou [3], Marco Racchi [3,*], Alessia Pascale [3,†] and Erica Buoso [3,4,†]

1. Computational and Chemical Biology, Italian Institute of Technology, Via Morego 30, 16163 Genova, Italy; masi.mirco1994@gmail.com
2. Department of Developmental and Molecular Biology, Albert Einstein College of Medicine, 1300 Morris Park Ave, Bronx, NY 10461, USA; fabrizio.biundo@einsteinmed.edu
3. Department of Drug Sciences, Pharmacology Section, University of Pavia, Via Taramelli 12/14, 27100 Pavia, Italy; alessia.pascale@unipv.it (A.P.); buoso.erica@gmail.com (E.B.)
4. Department of Pharmacology and Experimental Therapeutics, Boston University School of Medicine, Boston, MA 02118, USA
* Correspondence: racchi@unipv.it
† These authors contributed equally to this work.

Abstract: Amyloid Precursor Protein (APP) and its cleavage processes have been widely investigated in the past, in particular in the context of Alzheimer's Disease (AD). Evidence of an increased expression of APP and its amyloidogenic-related cleavage enzymes, β-secretase 1 (*BACE1*) and γ-secretase, at the hit axon terminals following Traumatic Brain Injury (TBI), firstly suggested a correlation between TBI and AD. Indeed, mild and severe TBI have been recognised as influential risk factors for different neurodegenerative diseases, including AD. In the present work, we describe the state of the art of APP proteolytic processing, underlining the different roles of its cleavage fragments in both physiological and pathological contexts. Considering the neuroprotective role of the soluble APP alpha (sAPPα) fragment, we hypothesised that sAPPα could modulate the expression of genes of interest for AD and TBI. Hence, we present preliminary experiments addressing sAPPα-mediated regulation of *BACE1*, Isthmin 2 (*ISM2*), Tetraspanin-3 (*TSPAN3*) and the Vascular Endothelial Growth Factor (*VEGFA*), each discussed from a biological and pharmacological point of view in AD and TBI. We finally propose a neuroprotective interaction network, in which the Receptor for Activated C Kinase 1 (RACK1) and the signalling cascade of PKCβII/nELAV/VEGF play hub roles, suggesting that vasculogenic-targeting therapies could be a feasible approach for vascular-related brain injuries typical of AD and TBI.

Keywords: *BACE1*; *TSPAN3*; *VEGF*; *ISM2*; ELAV; secretase; PKC; RACK1

1. Introduction

Alzheimer's Disease (AD) is a chronic neurodegenerative disease characterised by a progressive impairment of cognitive functions ultimately resulting in dementia. Many hypotheses for AD development have been proposed, including the formation of twisted fibres of Tau proteins inside neurons called Neurofibrillary Tangles (NFTs), ribosomal impairment and the RNA-binding protein cascade hypothesis [1,2]. However, one of the most accredited theories suggests the abnormal deposition of Amyloid β (Aβ) protein oligomers in neuronal intracellular space as one of the main pathology drivers [3]. Aβ is a 4 kDa peptide derived from the cleavage of its precursor, the Amyloid Precursor Protein (APP), whose role in the pathogenesis and progression of AD has been intensively investigated [4]. Neuropathologic markers like NFTs and senile plaques composed of Aβ aggregates histopathologically characterise the brain tissue of AD patients [5]. In this regard, the AD amyloid hypothesis focuses on the toxic role of the excessive formation of Aβ, which tends to accumulate into extracellular senile plaques, directly responsible for AD pathogenesis. Accordingly, the excessive formation of Aβ derives either from an increased production of Aβ after APP processing or from its reduced elimination [3]. Mutations in *APP* gene, located on chromosome 21, have played an important role to understand AD aetiology, although APP mutations accounted only for a small fraction of all AD cases. Further studies reported mutations also in different APP processing-related genes, including Beta-site APP Cleaving Enzyme 1 (*BACE1*, that codes for β-secretase 1), the structural components of the γ-secretase complex *PSEN1* and *PSEN2* (located on chromosome 14 and 1 and coding for Presenilin 1 (PS1) and PS2, respectively) and other genes belonging to the γ-secretase complex [3]. In addition, the ε4 polymorphism in the *APOE* gene (coding for apolipoprotein E, which modulates Aβ oligomerisation into fibrils leading to senile plaques formation) is associated with an increased risk of late-onset AD [6] and represents a major susceptibility risk factor for AD [7].

Observational epidemiological studies suggested a series of additional environmental influences that can be either protective or risk factors for AD. Among the protective factors, anti-inflammatory and anti-oxidant influences associated with increased brain neurogenesis and Brain-Derived Neurotrophic Factor (BDNF) production promote a healthier brain aging [8,9], while a history of cancer appears to be beneficial at reducing the likelihood of AD development [10]. Environmental risk factors for AD include depression [11,12], cardiovascular and metabolic status and history of head injury [13]. In this regard, Traumatic Brain Injury (TBI) has been suggested to trigger a deleterious cascade of secondary damage, leading to neuroinflammation, persistent neurological and cognitive impairment, and ultimately dementia [14,15]. Both mild and severe TBI are influential risk factors for different delayed-onset neurodegenerative diseases, including AD [16,17]. Following TBI with axonal transection, APP, β-secretase 1 and γ-secretase (the enzymes that contribute to APP cleavage towards Aβ formation) show an increased expression particularly prominent at the hit axon terminals [18–20]. This leads to an increased Aβ production and deposition at the axon bulbs and strengthens the correlation between TBI and increased risk for AD.

APP and the implications of its processing are important not only for neurodegeneration, particularly for AD, but also for TBI. Hence, the aim of this work is to present the state of the art of APP proteolytic processing, highlighting the different roles of its cleavage fragments in both physiological and pathological contexts, with a particular focus on the soluble APP fragments. In addition, we aim to discuss specific genes of interest for AD and TBI, and regulated by soluble APP peptides emerged from our preliminary in vitro data here presented from a biological and pharmacological point of view.

2. Amyloid Precursor Protein: Structure, Expression and Processing

2.1. APP Structure, Expression, Trafficking and Modification

2.1.1. APP Structure and Expression

The human *APP* gene, which is mapped to chromosome 21q21.3, spans 290,586 bp and consists of 18 exons. As a result of alternative splicing, the generation of multiple *APP* mRNA isoforms allows the production of different APP proteins with a number of amino acids ranging from 365 to 770 residues (APP365–APP770) [4] (Figure 1a). The highly conserved APP family consists of APP, the homologous APP-Like Protein 1 (APLP1) and APLP2, which are single-pass integral membrane proteins that feature a bulky N-terminal extracellular domain, an intramembrane domain and a small, intracellular C-terminal tail characterised by a sequence identity highly conserved among the three APP family members. However, APP is the only member of the family characterised by the presence of an Aβ domain [21]. The glycosylated N-terminal portion is relatively conserved among the different APP family members and the different APP isoforms and contains: the Signal Peptide (SP) sequence, the cysteine-rich globular domain (E1), the Extension Domain (ED), the Acidic Domain (AcD), a helix-rich domain (E2) and part of the Aβ domain, [4]. The E1 domain features a Heparin-Binding Site (HBS) (that confers APP its neuroprotective effects [22]) and a Metal-Binding Motif (MBM) with Cu^+ and Zn^{2+} binding sites (ZnBS and CuBS, respectively). Specific splicing variants feature additional domains, e.g., the Kunitz Protease Inhibitor (KPI) after the AcD domain and the OX-2 antigen domain after the KPI domain, while others lack these particular regions [4]. The E2 domain features six α-helices that form a coiled-coil structure, an HBS and a Collagen Binding Site (CBS). Importantly, the short cytoplasmic C-terminal domain contains the conserved YENPTY motif important for the protein–protein interactions (Figure 1b). Both APP N-terminal and C-terminal portions are involved in different cellular mechanisms (reviewed in [23]) and appear to participate in several signalling pathways as APP full-length and cleavage fragments. In the Central Nervous System (CNS), APP works as a cell surface receptor and is correlated with neurite growth, neuronal adhesion and axonogenesis [24]. However, increasing evidence suggests that both APP and its cleavage fragments play important roles also in peripheral tissues, where their abnormal expression, location and cleavage have been linked to the development of metabolic diseases (reviewed in [23]). Regarding APP isoforms, different splicing variants exhibit a tissue-specific expression and, among the brain-specific APP splicing variants, APP695 is the most abundant isoform expressed in the brain [25], although APP751 and APP770 are the main coding proteins of Aβ peptide [4]. Among the different APP family members, APLP1 expression is restricted to neurons and, while APLP2 and APP are highly brain-enriched and their expression has been found also in several peripheral tissues. While APP and APLP2 appear to be functionally redundant, the solely CNS-expressed APLP1 may have distinct roles as part of the synaptic network (reviewed in [26]). Indeed, recent findings point at APLP1 functions in neuronal morphology [27], synaptic plasticity [28,29], dendritic spine maintenance [30] and even as a possible biomarker of AD progression [31].

2.1.2. APP Trafficking and Post-Translational Modifications (PTMs)

After its synthesis, APP is firstly translocated to the Endoplasmic Reticulum (ER) upon the removal of its SP sequence, then it transits the ER/ER-Golgi Intermediate Compartment (ERGIC) to locate into the Golgi apparatus and the Trans-Golgi Network (TGN). Although the majority of APP localises in the Golgi apparatus and TGN, a small fraction of the nascent APP is translocated to the plasma membrane, where either α-secretase mediates its non-amyloidogenic cleavage or its C-terminal YENPTY motif mediates its internalisation into endosomes [32]. Internalised APP then traffics through the endo-lysosome pathway (mostly for APP degradation or, to a less extent, for its recycling to the plasma membrane or TGN), secretory pathway and recycling pathway. APP trafficking is strictly correlated with its processing, since α-secretase mainly resides in the plasma membrane, while β-secretase 1 locates in endosomes and lysosomes [32]. In the secretory pathway, APP can undergo different PTMs that influence its residency and trafficking, ultimately affecting the production of the different APP fragments. In this regard, each of APP PTMs here presented have different effects on Aβ generation (reviewed in [32]) and abnormal APP PTMs and alterations of its trafficking have been reported in AD patients [32].

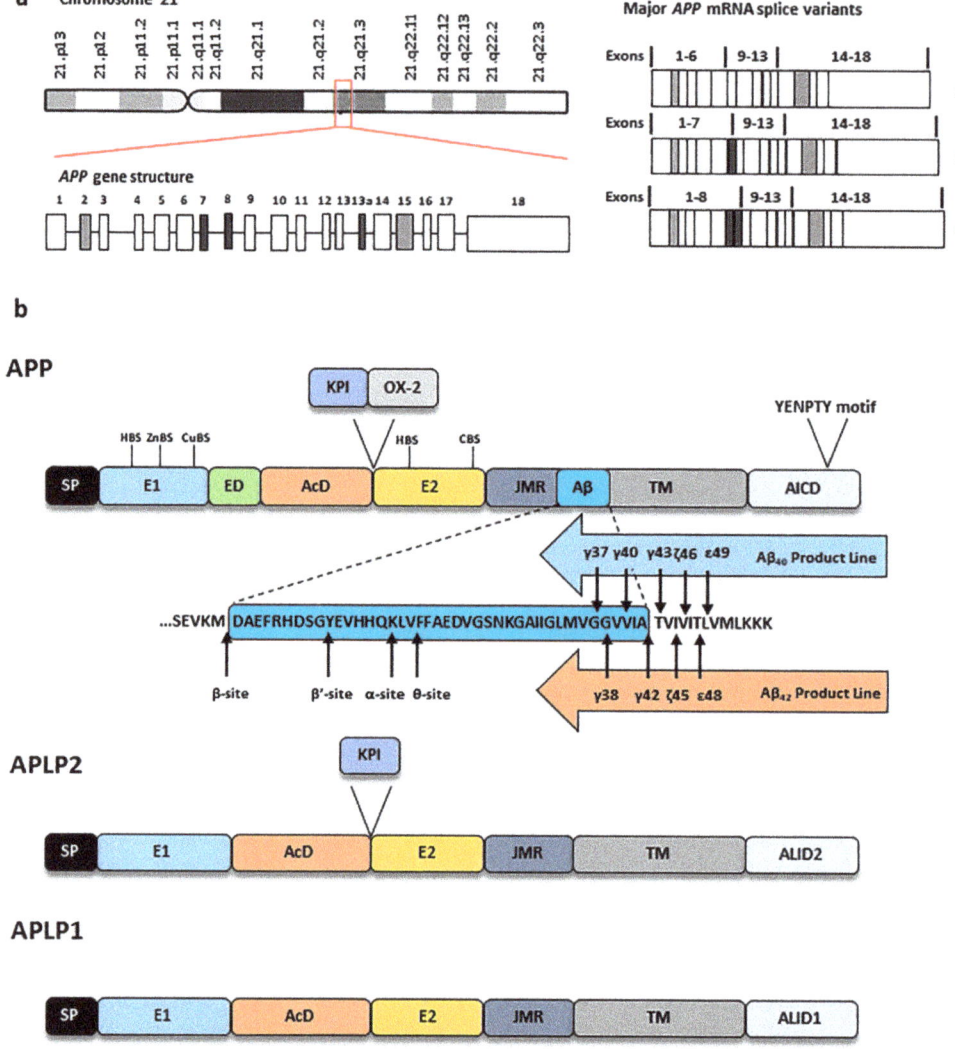

Figure 1. APP gene, mRNA and protein structure. (**a**) Structure of *APP* gene and mRNA. *APP* gene, located on chromosome 21q21.3, features 18 exons. Alternative splicing of exons 7 and 8 (*dark grey*) leads to the expression of APP695, 751 and 770 major isoforms, while differential splicing of exons 2 and 15 (*light grey*) generates APP639 and L-APP, respectively. (**b**) Structure of the three APP protein family members APP, APLP1 and APLP2. From the N-terminus to the C-terminus, APP features the cysteine-rich E1 domain (with Heparin-Binding Site (HBS), a Zinc-Binding Site (ZnBS) and Copper-Binding Site (CuBS)), the Extension Domain (ED), the Acidic Domain (AcD), the helix-rich E2 domain (with a second HBS and a Collagen-Binding Site (CBS)), the Juxtamembrane Region (JMR), the Aβ sequence, the Transmembrane Domain (TM) and APP Intracellular Domain (AICD) which contains a YENPTY sorting motif. APP751 and APP770 contain the additional Kunitz Protease Inhibitor (KPI) domain and an OX-2 antigen domain. Amino-acid sequence of Aβ region is shown along with the different secretases cleavage sites as well as the Aβ product lines. Both APLP1 and APLP2 lack Aβ sequence and present the APLP-intracellular domain 1 (ALID1) and ALID2, respectively. APLP2 features a KPI domain similarly to some APP isoforms.

- Glycosylation and phosphorylation

Upon its translocation into the ER, APP is N-glycosylated at N467 and N496 by the Oligosaccharyl Transferase (OST) complex forming immature APP, while APP O-glycosylation at multiple sites (T291, T292, T353, T576, S606, S611, T616, T634, T635, S662 and S680 found in cell cultures and human Cerebrospinal Fluid (CSF)) occurs in Golgi apparatus to allow APP maturation and its localisation in TGN and the plasma membrane [32]. APP PTMs and the interplay between APP classical O-GalNAcylation and O-GlcNAcylation (i.e., the addition of a single β-N-acetylglucosamine) at serine and threonine residues is pivotal for APP trafficking. Its N-glycosylation is essential for APP sorting from the Golgi apparatus to the plasma membrane as well as for its transport to the axonal synaptic membrane [32]. APP O-GlcNAcylation favours its trafficking from the TGN to the plasma membrane while inhibiting its endocytosis. Indeed, alterations of this APP O-glycosylation is crucial for the regulation of APP processing and Aβ production [33].

APP can undergo phosphorylation at two sites in the ectodomain (S198, S206) and eight sites in the cytoplasmic domain (Y653, Y682, Y687, S655, S675, T654, T668, T686) [32]. These PTMs are mainly catalysed by Protein Kinase C (PKC) (on S655, mainly detected in the mature APP), Ca^{2+}/Calmodulin-dependent Protein Kinase II and APP kinase I (on S655 and T654), Glycogen Synthase Kinase 3 beta (GSK-3β), Cyclin-Dependent Kinase 1 (CDK1), CDK5, Stress-Activated Protein Kinase 1 beta (SAPK1β), Dual-specificity Tyrosine phosphorylation-Regulated Kinase 1A (DYRK1A) and c-Jun N-terminal protein Kinase (JNK) (on T668 mainly detected in immature APP and occurring in the ER) [32]. APP phosphorylation is required for its trafficking as demonstrated by mutagenesis experiments [32].

- Palmitoylation, ubiquitination, SUMOylation and sulphation

The two palmitoyl acyltransferases DHHC-7 and DHHC-21 catalyse APP palmitoylation at C186 and C187 in the ER. APP palmitoylation is pivotal for the regulation of its trafficking, maturation, localisation to lipid rafts and its interactions with other proteins as demonstrated by double mutagenesis experiments on the involved cysteine residues [34]. Regarding ubiquitination, different ubiquitin-activating enzymes (E1), ubiquitin-conjugating enzymes (E2) and ubiquitin ligases (E3) act in concert to catalyse APP ubiquitination at residues K649–651 and K688 located in its ectodomain to regulate maturation, degradation and protein–protein interactions. This process is required for APP sorting and trafficking, especially to the endosomal compartment, as observed in hippocampal neurons [35]. Conversely, APP ubiquitination mediated by F-Box/LRR-repeat protein 2 (FBXL2) inhibits its endocytosis, increases its exposure to the plasma membrane and decreases its presence in lipid rafts [36]. Similarly to ubiquitination, SUMOylation (i.e., the covalent addition of Small Ubiquitin-like Modifier (SUMO) SUMO-1, -2 and -3) is catalysed by SUMO E1, E2 and E3 at APP K587 and K595 to regulate its functions [37]. Finally, APP sulphation (common PTM for cell surface proteins) at Y217 and Y262 residue occurs in the late Golgi compartment and has been hypothesised to be implicated in APP trafficking and degradation, although APP sulphation sites and functions still need to be completely elucidated [32].

2.2. APP Processing

As previously mentioned, APP can undergo different cleavage mechanisms that differentially produce several smaller peptides. Notably, APP cleavage processing involves a canonical and a non-canonical pathway. APP canonical cleavage processing includes two different proteolytic mechanisms, i.e., the non-amyloidogenic and the amyloidogenic pathways, that differently cleave APP via α-, β-, and γ-secretases and release different proteolytic products. Rather than a single α-secretase, several A Disintegrin And Metalloprotease (ADAM) family members, in particular ADAM9, ADAM10 and ADAM17 (also known as Tumour necrosis factor α-Converting Enzyme, TACE) are involved in APP cleavage [21,38]. In addition, unlike α-secretase, β-secretase 1 is a single transmembrane aspartyl protease. Finally, γ-secretase is a high molecular weight complex that consists of PS1 and/or PS2, Presenilin Enhancer 2 (PEN2), Anterior Pharynx defective 1 (APH1) and Nicastrin (NCSTN, also known as APH2) [39]. On the other hand, APP non-canonical cleavage includes different soluble and membrane-bound secretases whose mechanisms and their actual contribution to AD are still under investigation.

2.2.1. APP Canonical Cleavage: Amyloidogenic and Non-Amyloidogenic Pathways

In the amyloidogenic pathway, APP is firstly cut by β-secretase 1 in endosomes at the N-terminal side of the Aβ sequence (termed β-site, M671-D672). This produces an externally released, N-terminally truncated APP form termed soluble APPβ (sAPPβ) and the membrane-associated C-terminal fragment (C99 or β-CTF), which remains associated to the endosomal system (Figure 2a, right green panel). A second, less prominent β-secretase 1 cleavage site (termed β'-site, Y681-E682) located 10 residues to the C-terminus of APP leads to the generation of β'-CTF (or C89), whose further cleavage results in the production of the N-terminally truncated $A\beta_{11-x}$ [40]. sAPPβ can undergo a further cleavage at APP286 residue to produce N-APP [41], a 35 kDa peptide reported to bind death receptor 6 (DR6, also known as Tumour Necrosis Factor Receptor Superfamily member 21, TNFRSF21) thus triggering apoptosis and axon pruning, but also neuronal death and possibly AD development [42,43]. The β-CTF fragment is then cleaved into two additional peptides, i.e., APP Intracellular Domain (AICD) and Aβ peptides, by the γ-secretase complex. $AICD_{50}$ (composed of 50 residues) is the dominant fragment, although other species (i.e., $AICD_{48}$, $AICD_{51}$ and $AICD_{53}$) have also been identified and demonstrated to result from additional γ-secretase-mediated cleavages. In contrast, in the non-amyloidogenic pathway, APP is firstly cut by α-secretase between K687-L688 (termed α-site) in the plasma membrane, cleaving APP within the Aβ sequence and thereby preventing Aβ formation. This proteolytic cleavage produces soluble APPα (sAPPα), a secreted peptide released into the extracellular space, and the membrane-associated C-terminal fragment (C83 or α-CTF) [44]. From this remaining peptide, two additional peptides, i.e., AICD and the 3 kDa product p3, are generated after its cytoplasmatic cleavage by the γ-secretase complex (Figure 2a, left blue panel). Even though they share a similar peptide sequence, AICD produced in these two proteolytic pathways appear to have distinct functions. AICD produced through the non-amyloidogenic pathway undergo a rapid cytoplasmatic degradation through the endolysosomal system [45] and by the Insulin-Degrading Enzyme (IDE, a large zinc-binding protease of the M16 metalloprotease family) [46,47]. In contrast, AICD generated via the amyloidogenic pathway bind the Fe65 adaptor protein and translocate into the nucleus, where they associate with Tip60 to form the ATF complex [48]. The ATF complex acts as a transcription factor and regulates the expression of different APP-related genes, including *APP* itself (its own precursor), *BACE1*, *GSK3B* (coding for GSK-3β) and *MME* (coding for the Aβ-degrading enzyme Neprilysin, also known as Membrane Metallo-Endopeptidase (MME), Neutral Endopeptidase (NEP), cluster of differentiation 10 (CD10), and Common Acute Lymphoblastic Leukaemia Antigen (CALLA)) among the others [49–51].

The two APP homologues APLP1 and APLP2 are similarly processed by the same secretases, producing the intracellular fragments APLP-Intracellular Domain 1 (ALID1) and ALID2, respectively [52]. Similarly to AICD, ALID1 and ALID2 have been proposed to play a functional role as transcriptional regulators [53], although the validity of these speculations is still controversial due to the lack of adequate animal models.

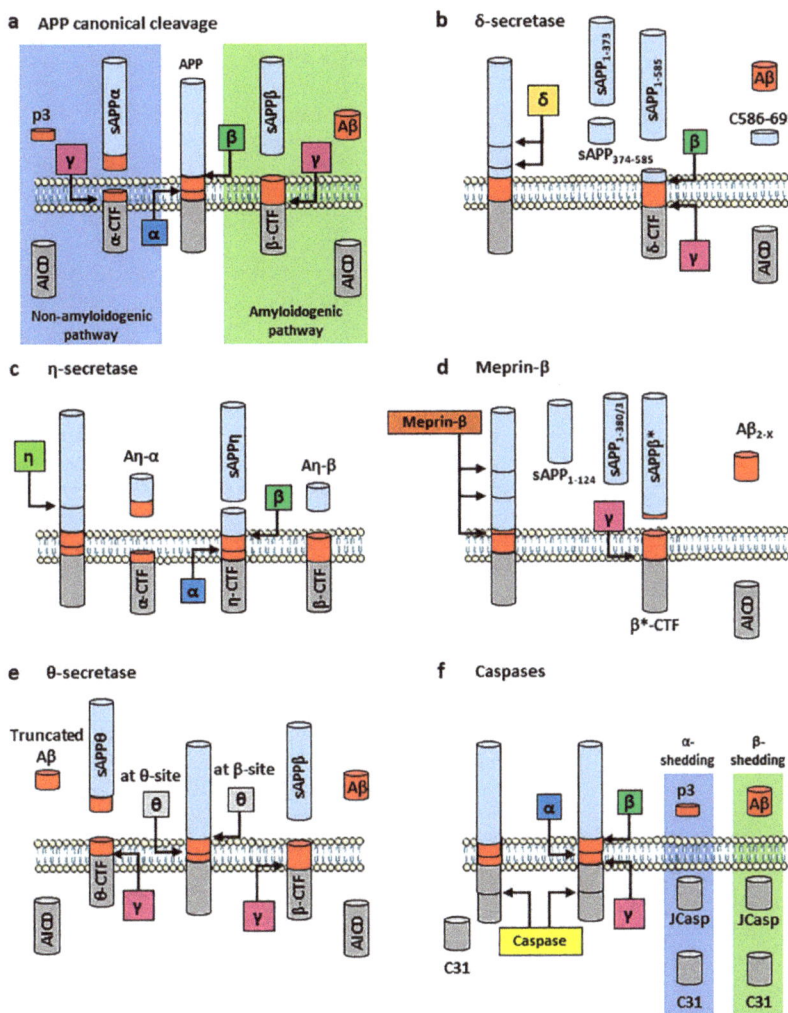

Figure 2. Schematic overview of APP-processing pathways. (**a**) APP canonical proteolytic processing. In the canonical cleavage, APP is either processed in the non-amyloidogenic pathway, where the sequential cleavage by α-secretase (ADAM10) (*blue square*) and the γ-secretase complex (*purple square*) produces sAPPα and p3, or in the amyloidogenic pathway, where the sequential cleavage by β-secretase 1 (*green square*) or Cathepsin B and the γ-secretase complex liberates sAPPβ and Aβ. While α-produced AICD are rapidly degraded in the cytoplasm, β-generated AICD form the transcriptional factor ATF complex together with Fe65 and Tip60, that translocates into the nucleus to up-regulate APP-related genes (see text for details). (**b–f**) APP non-canonical proteolytic processing. (**b**) APP processing mediated by δ-secretase (*orange square*) releases three soluble APP fragments (sAPP$_{1-585}$, sAPP$_{1-373}$, and sAPP$_{374-585}$) and δ-CTF, which is further processed by β- and γ-secretases, releasing Aβ, AICD and the C586-695 fragment. (**c**) η-secretase (*light green square*) releases sAPPη and η-CTF, which is further processed by either α- or β-secretase 1, releasing Aη-α or Aη-β respectively; the remaining CTFs are cleaved by the γ-secretase complex, releasing p3 and AICD, or Aβ and AICD respectively. (**d**) Meprin-β (*brown rectangle*) produces sAPPβ* (similar to sAPPβ) and two shorter soluble fragments (sAPP$_{1-124}$ and sAPP$_{1-380/3}$), while the remaining β*-CTF is processed by the γ-secretase complex, releasing AICD and Aβ$_{2-X}$. (**e**) θ-secretase (*grey square*) can either cleave APP at

the θ-site, releasing sAPPθ and a θ-CTF that is further processed by the γ-secretase complex releasing AICD and a truncated form of Aβ, or act as a conditional β-secretase. (**f**) Caspase-3, -6 and -8 (*yellow rectangle*) cleave within APP Intracellular Domain, releasing C31 while, after the sequential cleavage operated by the γ-secretase complex, the small peptide JCasp is released in the cytoplasm.

The γ-secretase complex can operate different proteolytic cleavages in the CTFs produced by both amyloidogenic and non-amyloidogenic pathways. The proteolytic cleavage operated by γ-secretase can be further separated in the sequentially occurring γ-, ζ-, and ε-cleavage sites (five γ-sites, two ζ-sites and two ε-sites) [54] (Figure 1b). This is particularly important for the generation of Aβ species, since the diverse possible cleavages exerted by γ-secretase result in the production of different Aβ peptides. After β-secretase 1-mediated APP cleavage, β-CTFs are processed through ε-cleavage, either producing $A\beta_{49}$ and $AICD_{50-99}$ or $A\beta_{48}$ and $AICD_{49-99}$. Within the $A\beta_{40}$ product line, $A\beta_{49}$ is cleaved at the ζ-site to $A\beta_{46}$ and at γ-sites to $A\beta_{43}$, $A\beta_{40}$ and $A\beta_{37}$ via a tripeptide trimming. On the other hand, within the $A\beta_{42}$ product line, $A\beta_{48}$ is cleaved at the ζ-site to $A\beta_{45}$ and at γ-sites to $A\beta_{42}$ and $A\beta_{38}$ via a tetrapeptide trimming [55]. A balanced generation and elimination of Aβ peptide products occurs in the healthy brain and the length of Aβ species found in CSF ranges from 37 to 43 amino acids [56]. However, in AD brain, Aβ peptides are more prone to aggregation into toxic amyloid oligomers—that eventually evolve in protofibrils and fibrils—via different assembly processes, affecting neuronal function and synaptic activity ultimately leading to synapse loss and impaired cerebral capillary blood flow [57]. The production ratio $A\beta_{42}/A\beta_{40}$ is around 1 to 9 but, due to its enhanced hydrophobicity, $A\beta_{42}$ has a stronger aggregation ability and is more toxic than $A\beta_{40}$. Indeed, $A\beta_{42}$ is the major amyloid plaques component, although $A\beta_{43}$ was also reported in the human AD brain amyloid deposition [23,56].

2.2.2. APP Non-Canonical Cleavage

Although its canonical cleavage has been thoroughly investigated in the past, the complete APP processing involves an increasing number of additional secretases—globally referred to as APP non-canonical cleavage—able to proteolytically cleave APP in both the ectodomain and the intracellular domain, recently identified also in vivo [58].

- δ-secretase

δ-secretase (also known as Asparagine Endopeptidase (AEP) and Legumain) is a soluble, pH-controlled lysosomal cysteine protease, previously linked to AD due to its ability to proteolytically cleave Tau [59] and recently reported to participate in APP ectodomain processing [60]. δ-secretase has been shown to cut APP between N373-E374 and N585-I586 both in vitro and in vivo, producing three soluble fragments ($sAPP_{1-373}$, $sAPP_{1-585}$ and $sAPP_{374-585}$) and the membrane-bound C-terminal fragment (δ-CTF), which is then processed by β- and γ-secretases, resulting in Aβ and AICD release [60] (Figure 2b). Increased δ-secretase expression and activity were reported in aged mice and in the brains of AD patients. On the other hand, its knock-out (KO) resulted in decreased Aβ production, dendritic spine and synapse loss, as well as behavioural impairments, protecting against memory deficits in two different AD mice models (i.e., 5 × FAD and APP/PS-1) [60]. In addition, the δ-secretase-generated APP C586–695 fragment has been shown to directly bind the inflammation-related CCAAT/Enhancer Binding Protein beta (C/EBPβ) transcription factor, eliciting its nuclear translocation and enhancing its transcriptional activity. This resulted in the induced transcription and expression of *APP*, *MAPT* (coding for the microtubule-associated protein Tau), *LGMN* (coding for δ-secretase) and inflammatory cytokines, escalating AD-related gene expression and pathogenesis and resulting in AD pathology and cognitive disorder [61]. These results suggest a role for δ-secretase in AD, although further studies are required to confirm and elucidate its contribution to AD and to consider δ-secretase as a potential drug target.

- η-secretase

η-secretase (also known as Membrane-type 5-Matrix Metalloproteinase, MT5-MMP, and MMP-24) is a glycosylated transmembrane proteinase and Zn^{2+}-dependent MMP, intracellularly activated by the Ca^{2+}-dependent proprotein convertase furin and primarily expressed in neural cells [62]. η-secretase has been shown to contribute to both physiologic and pathologic processes in the nervous system and its co-localisation with senile plaques suggested its possible involvement in AD pathogenesis [62]. η-secretase cleaves APP between N504-M505, producing a N-terminal soluble 95 kDa fragment (sAPP95 or sAPPη) and the membrane-bound C-terminal fragment (η-CTF or C191) [63,64]. η-CTF is then cut by α- or β-secretase, releasing the soluble fragments Aη-α or Aη-β, respectively, while the remaining CTF is then cleaved by the γ-secretase complex, producing p3 and AICD or Aβ and AICD, respectively [63,64] (Figure 2c). In addition to proteolytically cleave APP and release Aβ both in vitro and in vivo [65,66], η-secretase has been shown to contribute to the production of proteolytic fragments able to induce synaptic dysfunction [63,64]. Notably, η-secretase KO in 5xFAD mice led to a significant reduction of Aβ plaque deposition in the brain, along with preserved hippocampal function and improved spatial memory [63]. These observations indicate a potentially important role for η-secretase in AD context, although further investigations to confirm its pathophysiologic implications are required.

- Meprin-β

Meprin-β is a Zn^{2+} metalloprotease that acts as β-secretase 1 and competes with it [67], proteolytically cleaving within APP β-site M596-D597 as well as in the adjacent sites (D597-A598 and A598-E599) [68]. However, unlike for β-secretase 1, this APP cleavage takes place at the cell surface, indicating a direct competition with α-secretase in vivo [67]. Meprin-β proteolytic cleavage produces a fragment similar to sAPPβ (sAPPβ*) and two shorter soluble fragments ($sAPP_{1-380/3}$ and $sAPP_{1-124}$), while the remaining membrane-bound CTF (β*-CTF) undergoes a γ-secretase-mediated cleavage releasing $A\beta_{2-x}$ and AICD (Figure 2d). However, $A\beta_{2-x}$ abundance in the brain is severalfold lower compared to $A\beta_{42}$ species [67], indicating that meprin-β possible contribution to AD pathogenesis needs further investigation. Moreover, meprin-β KO resulted in an increased production of sAPPβ, altering the $A\beta_{2-40}/A\beta_{1-40}$ ratio [67]. In addition to the β-site, meprin-β can cleave APP in three further sites, between A124-D125 (resulting in the production of the 11 kDa fragment p11), E380-T381 and G383-D384 [69]. Therefore, it has been proposed that meprin-β can process APP by proteolytically cleaving in these different sites depending on APP subcellular localisation (soluble meprin-β releases the N-terminal APP fragments, while membrane-bound meprin-β cleaves at APP β-site) [70].

- θ-secretase

θ-secretase (also known as β-secretase 2, encoded by BACE2) is a BACE1 homologue located on chromosome 21q22.2-q22.3. θ-secretase-mediated APP cleavage releases the soluble N-terminal fragment sAPPθ and the membrane-bound C-terminal fragment (θ-CTF or C80), which is further cleaved by the γ-secretase complex, producing AICD and truncated Aβ (Figure 2e). By performing a proteolytic cleavage at APP θ-site F690-F691, downstream of the α-site, θ-secretase cleaves APP within the Aβ domain, abolishing Aβ production [71]. For this reason, it is considered as a possible therapeutic target to prevent the disease progression. Its relevance in AD has been suggested not only for its role as θ-secretase but also as a conditional β-secretase capable of processing APP at β-site, although APP Juxtamembrane Region (JMR) normally inhibits this activity. An increased binding of clusterin protein to JMR and the presence of JMR-disrupting mutations have been found in aged mouse brain, which correlated to an enhanced θ-secretase β-cleavage during aging. In this regard, both clusterin-JMR binding and JMR mutations prevent APP θ-cleavage, favouring β-cleavage of nascent APP and worsening AD symptoms [72]. Indeed, θ-secretase has been reported to be dysregulated in AD and this dysregulation has been hypothesised to be mediated by proteasomal and lysosomal impairments observed in AD [73]. However, since θ-secretase regulation has been less investigated compared to β-secretase 1, further studies are needed to elucidate its contribution to AD as well as putative drug target.

- Other secretases

The identification of additional Aβ peptides—both N-terminally truncated (e.g., Aβ$_{5-X}$) and N-terminally extended [74,75]—and APP N-terminal fragments (e.g., N-APP$_{18-286}$ fragment) [76,77] in human CSF suggests that APP could be proteolytically cleaved by additional secretases. Different caspases—namely caspase-3, caspase-6 and caspase-8 (reviewed in [58])—can mediate APP C-terminal domain cleavage at D664. This cleavage releases a membrane bound N-terminal fragment (APP-Ncas) and the C-terminal 31 residues-long fragment (APP-Ccas or C31) in the cytoplasm [64], which plays a role in neuronal apoptosis [58]. Notably, after α- or β-secretase 1 cut, the resulting CTF undergoes a combined cleavage by γ-secretase and caspase, releasing p3 or Aβ, respectively, in the extracellular space and the small intracellular peptide JCasp (Figure 2f), which interacts with and sequesters proteins involved in the vesicle-release machinery [78]. Moreover, the Rhomboid-like protein-4 (RHBDL4) is mainly located in the ER and belongs to the five-member family of intramembrane proteinases rhomboids (the secretory pathway-located RHBDL1-4 and the mitochondrial Presenilin Associated Rhomboid Like (PARL)). RHBDL4 cleaves APP ectodomain at multiple sites, generating ~70 kDa different N-terminal and C-terminal fragments with unknown functions. RHBDL4-mediated APP cleavage is negatively regulated by cholesterol and decreases Aβ$_{38}$, Aβ$_{40}$ and Aβ$_{42}$ levels, although these in vitro observations still need to be validated for their relevance regarding AD pathogenesis [79]. Finally, Cathepsin B is a lysosomal cysteine protease proposed as a putative β-secretase and whose role in Aβ pathology is still debated due to conflicting evidence [80–82]. Cathepsin B cleaves APP at the A673-E674 site, producing the Aβ peptides Aβ$_{3-X}$ or Aβ$_{11-X}$, whose N-terminal glutamate residue undergoes a glutaminyl cyclase-mediated cyclisation to release N-terminally truncated pyro-glutamylated Aβ peptides (pE-Aβ) [83].

2.3. APP and Its Processing in TBI

An increased expression of APP, β-secretase 1 and γ-secretase components, accompanied by increased Aβ production and deposition, were observed at the hit axonal terminals after both mild and severe TBI [18–20], hinting at a possible correlation between TBI history and AD development. Epidemiological evidence highlighted that even remote TBI history may anticipate AD onset trajectory, with greater Aβ deposition accompanied by cortical thinning [84]. Indeed, an elevated accumulation of Aβ peptides—in particular the Aβ$_{42}$ species—in peripheral blood was reported among patients with a history of TBI with impaired cognition [85]. Moreover, Aβ persistency in the blood of both mild and severe TBI patients even months after the injury incident [86] clearly indicates a correlation between TBI, Aβ production and presence of symptoms. In this regard, TBI activates C/EBPβ transcription factor, leading to increased δ-secretase expression and activity, mediating AD pathogenesis by promoting Aβ production as well as Tau hyperphosphorylation (Figure 3a). This results in neurotoxicity and neuroinflammation [87,88], which is also exacerbated in the presence of a defective BDNF and TrkB neurotrophic signalling [89]. KO of *CTSB* gene that codes for Cathepsin B—involved in the production of Aβ peptides relevant for AD—resulted in the amelioration of brain dysfunctions in both AD and TBI contexts, improving behavioural deficits and neuropathology in both diseases [90]. Moreover, caspase-3-mediated APP processing has been observed in axons undergoing traumatic axonal injury after TBI, co-localising with Aβ formation and suggesting that non-canonical APP processing pathways may have an important role in TBI and future AD development [91]. Although the precise mechanism that links TBI with APP alterations and Aβ production has still to be completely elucidated, an epigenetic and a physical components have been proposed. In this regard, TBI has been reported to induce a differential CpG methylation of different genes related to neurodegeneration, among which *APP* and *MAPT* were top differentially methylated CpG sites [92]. As for the physical component, the inertial loading stress to the head causes a dynamic mechanical shearing within the brain, leading to a deformation of the brain tissue that damages long-tract structures like axons and blood vessels [93]. Notably, APP is transported through a fast axoplasmic transport and accumulates in proximity of the axonal injury site [93]. Hence, the TBI-induced distortion of the axonal cytoskeleton impairs normal transport and triggers APP cleavage in the injured region, disrupting APP axonal transport and leading to Aβ generation and alteration of neuronal homeostasis [94] (Figure 3b).

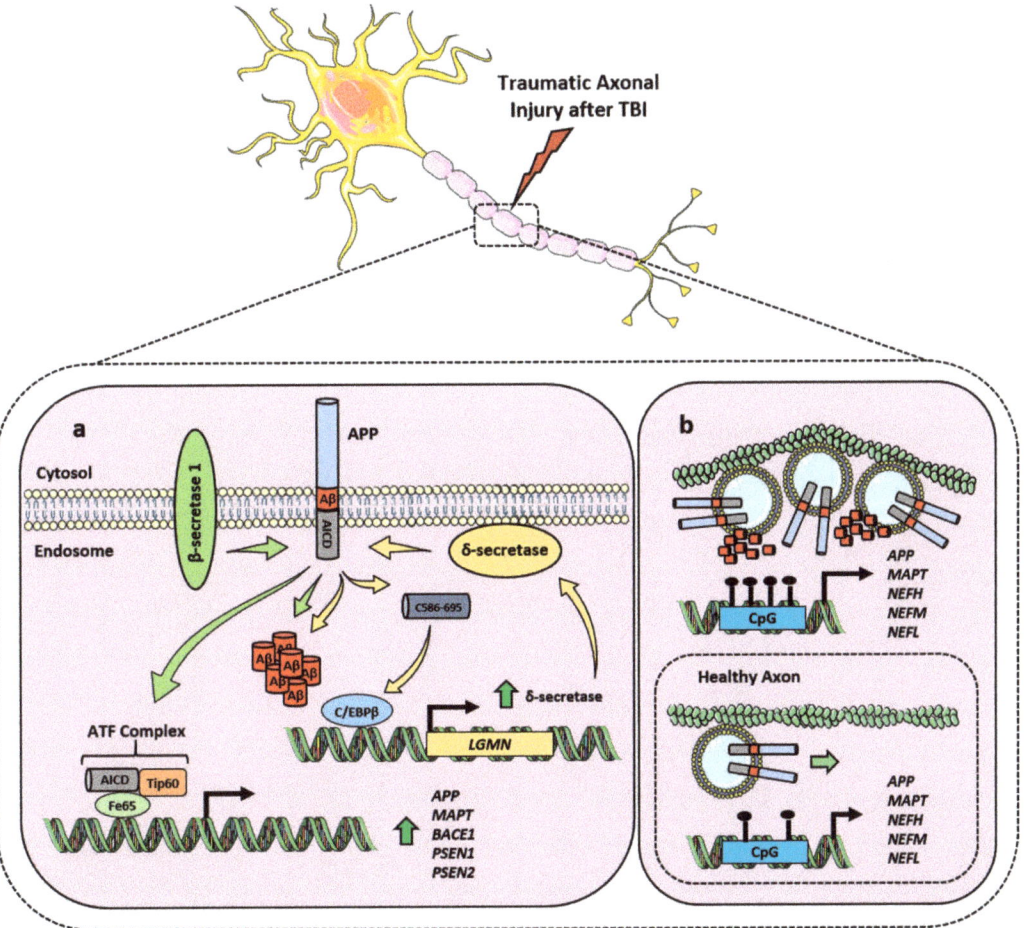

Figure 3. Alteration of APP processing after TBI. (**a**) Acute axonal damage after TBI induces the expression of APP, β-secretase 1 and γ-secretase components PS1 and PS2 (*dark green arrow*), as well as an increased Aβ generation and deposition. In addition, TBI triggers C/EBPβ activation, which induces the expression of δ-secretase (*dark green arrow*) that, in turn, cleaves APP forming Aβ and the C586–695 peptide that activates C/EBPβ. This suggests the establishment of a deleterious vicious loop possibly correlated to AD development. (**b**) Epigenetic and mechanical components of TBI-triggered APP processing alterations. After TBI, a differential CpG methylation of *APP*, *MAPT*, Neurofilament Heavy (*NEFH*), Neurofilament Medium (*NEFM*) and Neurofilament Light (*NEFL*) is observed [92]. Moreover, the induced axonal cytoskeleton distortion impairs the fast-axonal transport of APP (*light green arrow*), which accumulates in proximity of the axonal injury site, resulting in Aβ deposition.

3. Physiological and Pathological Roles of APP and Its Cleavage Fragments

Although it has been reported to act as a cell surface receptor to facilitate cell adhesion and regulate synapse formation and cell division, APP has been shown to exhibit both neuroprotective and neurotoxic effects [4]. However, both in vitro and in vivo models employed to investigate APP processing pathways and their contribution to AD and TBI pathologies rely on its over-expression or down-regulation. For these reasons, addressing the precise physiological roles of non-cleaved APP is rather challenging. In addition, most literature data focused their studies on Aβ or other APP fragments and the possible existence of compensatory mechanisms of APLP1 and APLP2 further complicate its investigation [4]. Despite these experimental caveats, full-length APP and its cleavage fragments have been widely studied in the past decades, thus generating an increasing amount of data that contributes to extricate this complex landscape in both physiological and pathological contexts. Hence, for a more functional presentation of their effects reported in literature, properties of the different proteolytic fragments generated from APP processing pathway here treated, as well as full-length APP functions, are presented in Table 1.

Table 1. APP proteolytic fragments and their reported functions.

APP Processing	APP Fragment	Cell Line/Model	Characteristics and Functions	Ref.
-	APP full-length	PC12 pheochromocytoma cells; APP- B103 cells; embryonic carcinoma P19 and NT2 cell lines; NB-1 neuroblastoma cell line; SK-N-MC cells (human neuroblastoma cell line); rat hippocampal neurons; in vivo (hAPP751 or hAPP695 over-expressing mice, APP−/− mice, Down's Syndrome (DS) Ts65Dn and 1YeY mice)	Acting as cell surface receptor; involved in neuronal adhesion and iron transport; promotes cell division, neurite outgrowth, axonogenesis, synapse formation and maintenance and synaptic plasticity; neuroprotective role against Aβ and glutamate toxicity	[58]
		Human Embryonic Stem Cells (hESCs)	Induction of stem cells neural differentiation	[95]
	sAPPβ	Rat hippocampal cells	100-fold less active neurotrophic effects compared to sAPPα in protecting hippocampal neurons against excitotoxicity, Aβ-induced toxicity, and glucose deprivation	[96]
		Sprague–Dawley rats brain slices	No marked changes in Long-Term Potentiation (LTP) compared to sAPPα	[97]
		N9 cells (myc-immortalized murine microglial cell line),	Stimulation of microglia activation through MAP kinase signaling pathways (i.e., ERKs, p38 kinase, JNKs) and NF-κB activity; production of proinflammatory and neurotoxic products (e.g., iNOS, IL-1β, ROS)	[98,99]
	N-APP	E13 rat dorsal spinal cord explant; mouse sensory and motor neuron explants; dissociated sensory neuron cultures; In vivo (DR6 KO, Bax KO and p75NTR KO mice)	Interaction with DR6 to recruit caspase-3 and caspase-6 (in cell bodies and axons respectively) and triggering of axonal pruning, but also neuronal death and AD development	[42,43]
		Neuro-2a cells (neuroblast cell line); in vivo (mouse)	LTP disruption	[100]
Canonical— Amyloidogenic	β-CTF (C99)	In vivo (APP−/− and APP+/− mice)	Synaptotoxicity induction and spine density reduction	[101]
		In vivo (3xTgAD with PS1M146V, βAPPswe and TauP301L transgenes); APP695-H4 cells (human glioma cell line)	Early pathological accumulation and learning and memory deficits	[102,103]
		PC12 cells (pheochromocytoma cell line); SK-N-MC cells (human neuroblastoma cell line); rat neuronal cultures; transgenic mouse models	Selective neurotoxicity, cortical atrophy, loss of hippocampal granule cells, astrogliosis, Aβ and APP immunoreactivity, impaired working memory, neocortical and hippocampal neurodegeneration and gliosis	[104–107]
	β'-CTF (C89)	-	Unknown physiologic and pathologic properties	-
	Aβ	PC12 pheochromocytoma cells; APP- B103 cells; embryonic carcinoma P19 and NT2 cell lines; NB-1 neuroblastoma cell line; SK-N-MC cells (human neuroblastoma cell line); rat hippocampal neurons; in vivo (hAPP751 or hAPP695 over-expressing mice, APP−/− mice, Down's Syndrome (DS) Ts65Dn and 1Ye Y mice)	Major APP metabolic fragment involved in AD development and progression - Aβ40 reported to act as transcription factor; involved in cholesterol transport and kinase activation; promotes neurogenesis and neurite outgrowth; exerts neuroprotective effects against oxidative stress; inhibits Aβ42 oligomerisation; interacts with extracellular matrix components (e.g., laminin and fibronectin) to promote neurite proliferation. - Aβ42 inhibits LTP and synaptic transmission; enhances Long-Term Depression (LTD); reduces synaptic spine density; promotes synaptic injury and cognitive impairment	[58]
	AICD	SH-SY5Y cells wild type (wt) and APP/APPswe); Mouse Embryonic Fibroblasts (MEF) and mouse brains (wt, PS1/2−/−, APP/APLP2−/− and APPΔCT15)	Transcriptional regulation, together with Tip60 and Fe65 and forming the AFT complex, of APP and AD-related genes	[108,109]
		Differentiated PC12 cells; rat primary cortical neurons	Induction of neurotoxicity by up-regulating the expression of GSK-3β and activating p53	[110,111]
		AICD-transfected Jurkat cells	Apoptosis induction through Fas-Associated protein with Death Domain (FADD)-induced programmed cell death	[112]

Table 1. Cont.

APP Processing	APP Fragment	Cell Line/Model	Characteristics and Functions	Ref.
Canonical—Non-amyloidogenic	sAPPα	SH-SY5Y cells; B103 cells; rat primary cortical neurons; murine hippocampal neurons; MEFs; in vivo (wt and APP$^{-/-}$ mice)	Induction of Akt neuronal cell survival-correlated pathway; facilitation of normal neurophysiological functions (e.g., memory functions) and promotion of neurite outgrowth	[113–115]
		In vivo (wt, APP$_{swe}$/PS1$_{\Delta E9}$ and APP$^{-/-}$ mice)	Neuroprotective effect against synaptic dysfunction and TBI	[116,117]
		In vivo (APP$^{-/-}$ and APLP2$^{-/-}$ mice); Sprague–Dawley rats brain slices	Contribution to the regulation of synaptic plasticity and LTP induction	[97,118]
	α-CTF (C83)	In vivo (APP$^{-/-}$ and APP$^{+/-}$ mice)	Induction of synaptotoxicity and reduction of spine density	[101]
		CHO cells	Indirect promotion of survival by lowering C99 levels	[119]
		In vitro assay: HEK293-APP cells	Hypothesised to be a γ-secretase inhibitor	[120]
	p3	In vitro assay: APP$^{-/-}$ MEFs; human cortical neurons	Induction of neuronal excitotoxicity by contributing to the formation of Ca^{2+}-permeable ion channels	[121]
		AD brain human samples	Accumulation in amyloid plaques	[122]
		Differentiated THP-1 cells (human monocyte line); MG7 cells (microglia cell line); D30 (murine astrocyte line); U373 cells (human astrocyte line)	Induction of apoptosis, inflammatory responses and neurotoxic effects by producing proinflammatory cytokines (e.g., Interleukin (IL)-1α, IL-1β, IL-6, Tumour Necrosis Factor-α (TNF-α), chemokine MCP-1)	[123]
Non-canonical—δ-secretase	sAPP$_{1-373}$ sAPP$_{1-585}$ sAPP$_{374-585}$	GFP-APP- and GST-APP-HEK293 cells; primary cultured neurons; in vivo (wt and AEP$^{-/-}$ 5xFAD and APP/PS1 mice)	sAPP$_{1-373}$, but not sAPP$_{1-585}$ nor sAPP$_{374-585}$, exhibited neurotoxic properties	[60]
	δ-CTF	AD brain human samples	Accumulation in brain lysates from AD patients	[60]
Non-canonical—η-secretase	sAPPη (sAPP95) η-CTF (C191)	Mouse hippocampal cultures; acute hippocampal slices; in vivo (Thy1-GCaMP6 mice)	Binding to the γ-Aminobutyric Acid (GABA) receptor and modulation of GABAergic neurotransmission	[124]
		In vivo (5xFAD MT5-MMP$^{-/-}$ mice); AD brain human samples	Accumulation in the surrounding of amyloid plaques in dystrophic neurites of transgenic mice and AD patients and contribution to cognitive decline	[63,64]
		In vitro assay: SH-SY5Y/APP$_{751}$ cells; H4/APP$_{751}$ human neuroglioma cells	Processed by Cathepsin L, although its physiological role has not been investigated	[125]
	Aη-α Aη-β	Murine hippocampal neurons and brain slices; human CSF	Both detected in mouse brain homogenates and human CSF (5-fold higher levels than Aβ); Aη-α, but not Aη-β inhibited LTP, suppressed neuronal activity and resides in the halo of the amyloid plaque.	[64]
Non-canonical—Meprin-β	sAPP$_{1-380/3}$ sAPP$_{1-124}$	-	*Unknown physiologic and pathologic properties*	-
	CTF	-	*Unknown physiologic and pathologic properties*	-
	Aβ$_{2-x}$	In vivo (APP$_{swe}$-based mouse models); AD patient brain samples	Increased potential to aggregate compared to Aβ$_{1-x}$ peptides	[126]
	p11	Differentiated SH-SY5Y cells; in vivo (wt, APP$^{-/-}$ and APLP2$^{-/-}$ C57BL6j × 129/Sv mice); AD brain human samples	Increased production detected during neuronal differentiation	[127]
Non-canonical—θ-secretase	sAPPθ	-	*Unknown physiologic and pathologic properties*	-
	θ-CTF (C80)	-	*Unknown physiologic and pathologic properties*	-
	APP-Ncas	-	*Unknown physiologic and pathologic properties*	-
Non-canonical Caspases	APP-Ccas (C31)	Neuro-2a cells; AD brain human samples	Synaptic dysfunction, neuronal apoptosis and death; APP-dependent toxicity	[128]
	JCasp	Primary neuronal cultures	Induction of neuronal apoptosis by transducing a tyrosine-dependent signalling	[129]

Table 1. Cont.

APP Processing	APP Fragment	Cell Line/Model	Characteristics and Functions	Ref.
Non-canonical—Cathepsin B	$A\beta_{3-x}$ $A\beta_{11-x}$ (pE-$A\beta$)	In vitro assay; HEK293, 20E2, 2EB2, HAW and BAW cell lines; human AD brain samples	High aggregation propensity, cellular toxicity, disruption of LTP and proposed as predominant $A\beta$ peptide species in AD brain patients	[38]
	$A\beta_{4-x}$ $A\beta_{5-x}$	In vivo (APP_{swe} mouse models); AD patient brain samples	Increased potential to aggregate compared to $A\beta_{1-x}$ peptides	[126]
	N-APP_{18-286}	neonatal C57BL/6 × SJL mice hippocampal cultures	Binding an unknown neuronal receptor and increase of phosphatidylinositol phosphate levels	[77]
Other secretases	APP_{1-119} APP_{1-121} APP_{1-122} APP_{1-123} APP_{1-126}	Human CSF	~12 kDa sAPP fragments reported by mass spectrometry analyses with unknown physiologic or pathologic properties	[76]
	17–28 kDa APP N-Terminal Fragments	SH-SY5Y cells with HSV-1-mediated APP expression; rat cortical neuronal cultures	Generated through a developmentally regulated PKC-related APP processing pathway independent of α-secretase or β-secretase 1, with a putative important role in APP physiological function	[127,130]

The literature data reported that α-secretase-mediated APP processing occurs via constitutive pathways in response to physiological processes in neuronal circuits and to nervous system injury like TBI, specifically through multiple receptor-mediated activation of signal transduction pathways, among which PKC plays a pivotal role [131,132]. As reported in Table 1, several studies suggested sAPPα involvement in neuroprotective mechanisms, such as synaptic plasticity, synaptogenesis and neurite outgrowth as well as neurotrophic actions [133]. It is well known that the dysregulation of APP processing and metabolism is correlated to neurological disorders not limited to AD, but also Down's Syndrome (DS), Fragile X Syndrome and Autism, in which increased sAPPα levels contributed to an excessive induction and stimulation of brain growth signals during development [134–136]. Conversely, reductions of constitutive and regulated release of sAPPα and decreased sAPPα levels have been reported in the CSF of AD patients [137–139]. Therefore, a loss of sAPPα neuroprotective and neurotrophic functions could be involved in the decreased neuronal plasticity and the increased neuronal susceptibility to cellular stress observed in aging and neurodegeneration. Experimental evidence suggests that sAPPα neuroprotective actions are correlated with effects on ion channel function followed by late transcription-dependent events [140], as well as pleiotropic effects on cell survival via the PI3K/Akt/NF-κB pathway as we previously demonstrated [141]. In this context, a deeper understanding of the sAPPα-correlated modulation of genes of interest for both AD and TBI could be significant in terms of basic research and future pharmacologic intervention [142].

4. Results

4.1. Neuron-Related Differential sAPPα-Mediated Gene Regulation In Vitro

Experiments on sAPPα-treated SH-SH5Y cells—which are widely used as preliminary in vitro models for both AD and TBI preclinical investigations [143,144]—resulted in the activation of MAPK-related pathway (Figure 4a–c) in line with literature data [145], and consequently in the differential modulation of the expression of different genes at mRNA level, as reported in Table 2. Genes of our interest (bold and highlighted in Table 2) were then validated through quantitative PCR (qPCR).

Table 2. In vitro sAPPα-mediated differentially regulated genes obtained from the differential display analysis performed on SH-SY5Y neuroblastoma cells (*green highlight* = up-regulated genes of interest; *orange highlight* = down-regulated genes of interest).

Gene	Accession Number	Location	Encoded Protein	sAPPα-Mediated Regulation
TSPAN3	**NM_198902.3**	**15q24.3**	**Tetraspanin-3**	**Up-regulated**
ISM2	**NM_199296**	**14q24.3**	**Isthmin 2**	**Up-regulated**
MNAT1	AY165512.1	14q23.1	MNAT1 component of CDK activating kinase	Up-regulated
HSPA8	NM_153201.4	11q24.1	Heat Shock Protein Family A (Hsp70) Member 8	Up-regulated
SOX11	AB028641.1	2p25.2	SRY-Box Transcription Factor 11	Up-regulated
USE1	AB097050.1	19p13.11	Unconventional SNARE in the ER 1	Up-regulated
KALRN	NM_007064.5	3q21.1-q21.2	Kalirin RhoGEF kinase	Up-regulated
MAP3K5	NM_005923	6q23.3	Mitogen-Activated Protein Kinase Kinase Kinase 5	Up-regulated
PTGES3	NM_006601.7	12q13.3; 12	Prostaglandin E Synthase 3	Up-regulated

Table 2. Cont.

Gene	Accession Number	Location	Encoded Protein	sAPPα-Mediated Regulation
BACE1	BC065492.1	11q23.3	β-secretase 1	Down-regulated
VEGFA	AF022375.1	6p21.1	Vascular Endothelial Growth Factor A	Down-regulated
RBM8A	NM_005105.5	1q21.1	RNA Binding Motif Protein 8A	Down-regulated
SLC27A3	BC003654.2	1q21.3	Solute Carrier Family 27 Member 3	Down-regulated
METTL21A	BC009462.1	2q33.3	Methyltransferase 21A, HSPA Lysine	Down-regulated
RPS28	NM_001031.5	19p13.2	Ribosomal Protein S28	Down-regulated
RPL24	NM_000986.4	3q12.3	Ribosomal Protein L24	Down-regulated
UBE3A	NM_130839.5	15q11.2	Ubiquitin Protein Ligase E3A	Down-regulated
QDPR	BC000576.2	4p15.32	Quinoid Dihydropteridine Reductase	Down-regulated
MTX1	BC001906.1	1q22	Metaxin 1	Down-regulated
COMMD1	NM_152516.4	2p15	Copper Metabolism Domain Containing 1	Down-regulated
PSMC6	NM_002806.5	14q22.1	Proteasome 26S Subunit, ATPase 6	Down-regulated

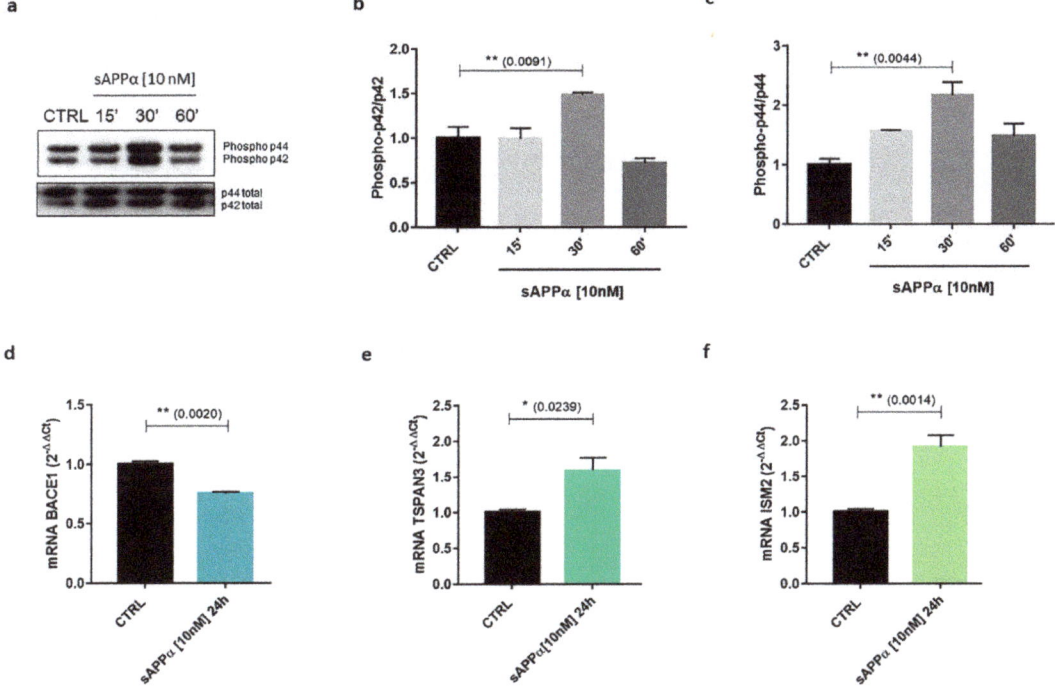

Figure 4. Effects of sAPPα treatment on early MAPK activation and *BACE1*, *TSPAN3* and *ISM2* transcriptional regulation. Human neuroblastoma SH-SY5Y cells were cultured and treated with 10 nM sAPPα for 15, 30 or 60 min (**a–c**) or for 24 h (**d–f**) as previously detailed [141]. Western blot analysis and qPCR were performed as previously reported [141]. (**a–c**) Evaluation of early MAPK activation. The image is a representative Western blot. Phosphorylation of p42 and p44 was normalised to their respective total p42 and p44 levels. (**d–f**) Evaluation of sAPPα-mediated transcriptional regulation on

BACE1, *TSPAN3* and *ISM2*. mRNA levels were evaluated by qPCR (endogenous reference, *RPL6*). Results are expressed as mean ± SEM, n = 3 independent experiments. Statistical analysis was performed with one-way ANOVA followed by Dunnett's multiple comparison test (**b**,**c**) or with Student's *t*-test (**d–f**) with * $p < 0.05$ and ** $p < 0.01$ vs. control (CTRL). Statistical significance is detailed in the respective figure panel.

We performed preliminary experiments on four sAPPα-modulated target genes, (i.e., *BACE1*, *TSPAN3*, *VEGFA* and *ISM2*) with potential correlations with sAPPα neuroprotective actions. Then, we discussed these genes in light of sAPPα neuroprotective actions aiming to unravel possible novel cytosolic- and membrane-related molecular players interesting for AD and TBI contexts [141,142]. Other sAPPα modulated genes are presented in Table 3 with their putative or reported roles in AD and TBI.

Table 3. Reported involvement in AD and TBI of sAPPα-correlated up- and down-regulated genes here not investigated.

Gene	Reported Correlation with AD/TBI	Ref.
HSPA8	Decreased in AD patients' samples and possible molecular biomarker for prognosis among HSP70 family in AD; part of the alcohol-sensitive protein networks modulated by AD-associated proteins that exacerbate neural and behavioural pathology upon alcohol drinking; potential drug target for preventing protein misfolding aggregation and cell death in AD and other neurodegenerative pathologies	[146–148]
SOX11	Hypothesised to participate in the modulation of neuron plasticity in the dentate gyrus of the hippocampus; involved in the early attempts of axon regeneration and neuronal survival; modulates peripheral nerve regeneration in adult mice and BDNF expression in an exon promoter-specific manner; favours endogenous neurogenesis and locomotor recovery in mice spinal cord injury	[149–153]
USE1	Involved in ER morphology maintenance and in the regulation of ER stress-induced neuronal apoptosis	[154]
KALRN	Key role in synaptic plasticity and in dendritic arbours and spines formation; proposed as possible therapeutic target for pharmacological intervention for synapse dysregulation; its deficit contributes to AD-related cognitive decline and memory loss; prevents dendritic spine dysgenesis induced by Aβ oligomers	[155–157]
MAP3K5	Neuroprotective action against apoptosis as part of the Notch1/ASK1/p38 MAPK signalling pathway; neuroprotective role against oxidative stress; involved in neuronal death after its IRE1α-mediated recruitment upon ER stress and UPR	[158–160]
RBM8A	Potential contribution to AD pathophysiological changes by regulating components of key complexes in autophagy	[161]
SLC27A3	Highly expressed in in human neural stem cells and involved in early brain development	[162]
RPS28	Promotion of P-body assembly and hypothesised to be linked with neurodegeneration	[163,164]
UBE3A	Involved in synaptic function and plasticity; age-dependently decreased in AD mice models; possible critical player in AD pathogenesis and potential therapeutic target	[165,166]
COMMD1	Hypothesised to be involved in hypoxia-induced AD neurodegeneration and brain injury via its interaction with Hypoxia-Inducible Factor 1 alpha (HIF-1α)	[167]

4.2. BACE1

The human *BACE1* gene is located on chromosome 11q23.3 and encodes for β-secretase 1, the main APP degrading enzyme involved in the amyloidogenic pathway. Research on BACE1 has been historically focused on its role in AD development/Aβ production and its neuronal and non-neuronal roles, as well as its state of the art, have been recently and excellently reviewed [160]. *BACE1* is abundantly expressed in brain and pancreatic tissues, although its low expression is also detected in many other cell types and has been investigated in multiple pathological contexts [160]. Together with its homologue *BACE2*, *BACE1* encodes for a type 1 membrane protein part of the membrane-bound aspartyl proteases subfamily [168]. β-secretase 1 is a 501 residues pre-protein, whose structure features five domains: SP, Pro-Peptide (PP), Catalytic Domain (CD), Transmembrane Domain (TM) and the C-Terminal Region (CTR). The SP traffics BACE1 to the ER, where furin cleaves PP to form mature β-secretase 1, while the TM domain localises β-secretase 1 to the late Golgi and its post-transcriptional activation occurs in the trans-Golgi. Subsequently, β-secretase 1 proteolytically cleaves its substrates in endosomes while being membrane-bound [168]. Due to its involvement in APP amyloid cleavage processing, β-secretase 1 has a key role in controlling Aβ production. Noteworthy, sAPPα has been shown to act as a potent β-secretase 1 allosteric inhibitor [169], regulating APP processing and decreasing Aβ production [170]. Moreover, sAPPα could affect APP processing also by inducing a significant down-regulation of *BACE1* expression (Figure 4d). Therefore, these data suggest that restoring sAPPα levels or enhancing its association with β-secretase 1 in AD patients to rebalance the impaired APP processing could be potential strategies to ameliorate AD symptoms, as also indicated by sAPPα inhibitory effects on Tau phosphorylation [171].

4.3. TSPAN3

The human *TSPAN3* gene is located on chromosome 15q24.3 and encodes for Tetraspanin-3 (previously known as Oligodendrocyte-Specific Protein (OSP)/Claudin-11-Associated Protein, OAP1), a N-terminally glycosylated transmembrane protein [172] belonging to the Tetraspanin superfamily (also named Tetraspans or Transmembrane 4 Superfamily, TM4SF), which comprises 33 mammalian members [173]. Tetraspanins are evolutionarily conserved, glycosylated and palmitoylated transmembrane proteins, characterised by four TMs (with TM1, 3 and 4 containing polar residues), a short extracellular loop (EC1), a very short (4 residues) intracellular loop, a long extracellular loop (EC2) subdivided into a constant region (containing the A, B and E α-helices) and a variable region, and short (8–21 residues) N-terminal and C-terminal cytoplasmic regions [173]. Structurally, all tetraspanins present the CCG motif after the B helix and two conserved cysteine residues forming intramolecular disulphide bonds. Cysteine number varies among different tetraspanins, with members presenting two additional cysteines to seven or eight cysteine residues, forming both intramolecular and intermolecular disulphide bonds [173]. In addition to interact with a variety of transmembrane proteins—e.g., integrins, cell adhesion proteins, cytokines and Growth Factor (GF) receptors, membrane-bound enzymes—different tetraspanins can interact with each other via their TM domains, EC2 loop and the surrounding lipid composition. Acting in concert, they form an interaction network called "Tetraspanin Web" or Tetraspanin-Enriched Microdomains (TEMs), localising different membrane-bound molecular players in segregated microdomains in a tissue-specific fashion [174–177]. Tetraspanins have been reported to take part in the regulation of multiple biological processes, including cell adhesion, migration and proliferation, as well as regulation of immune responses, infection, cancer progression and nervous system development [173,178]. However, their supramolecular organisation and function at synapses is still being investigated [179–181]. Tetraspanin-3 presents six cysteine residues in the EC2 loop and was reported to interact with Integrin β1 and Claudin-11 to regulate oligodendrocyte proliferation and migration [172,182]. In addition to oligodendrocytes, Tetraspanin-3 is highly expressed also in astrocytes and neurons [172], where it interacts with Sphingosine-1-Phosphate Receptor 2 (S1PR2), regulating its clustering with its ligand Nogo-A to control cell spreading and neurite outgrowth inhibition [183]. Importantly, Tetraspanin-3 has been found highly expressed in human AD brains and demonstrated to act in concert with other tetraspanins to stabilise APP, ADAM10 and the γ-secretase complex in both the cell membrane and the endocytic pathway [184]. Since *TSPAN3* expression is positively regulated by sAPPα treatment (Figure 4e), altogether these data support the notion that sAPPα could also exert neuroprotective effects promoting the APP non-amyloidogenic pathway. Accordingly, as mentioned, sAPPα also induces a significant down-regulation of BACE1 expression, thus affecting Aβ formation.

4.4. ISM2

The human *ISM2* gene is located on chromosome 14q24.3 and encodes for Isthmin 2 (also known as Thrombospondin and AMOP containing Isthmin-like 1, TAIL1), which is present in three different isoforms [185]. Isthmin 2 belongs to the isthmin family, a group of secreted proteins [186] characterized by an N-terminal SP, a central Thrombospondin-1 (TSR1) domain and C-terminal Adhesion-associated domain in MUC4 and Other Proteins (AMOP) domain, as well as multiple sites of C-mannosylation and N-glycosilation [187]. The two different human isthmin genes, *ISM1* and *ISM2*, encode for secreted proteins of 50 and 64 kDa respectively. Isthmin 1 structure and functions have been investigated in different contexts, reporting both angiogenic and anti-angiogenic activities [188–190] as well as a pleiotropic role as adipokine [186,191], while Isthmin 2 is still poorly characterised. Isthmin 2 structure suggests a possible angiogenic activity, since, besides Isthmin 1, the only other proteins in the human genome that feature a C-terminal AMOP domain—namely, Mucin 4 Cell Surface Associated (MUC4) and Sushi Domain Vontaining 2 (SUSD2)—are important elements in angiogenesis [185]. However, the presence of the central TSR-1 domain in Isthmin 2 structure may indicate that, like Isthmin 1, can be both pro-angiogenic and anti-angiogenic [185]. In this regard, our cellular in vitro model shows that sAPPα significantly up-regulated *ISM2* expression (Figure 4f) suggesting a possible role in neuronal context. Interestingly, *ISM2* is mainly expressed in the placenta and has been associated with preeclampsia and choriocarcinoma [185]. However, multiple transcriptomic analyses revealed that *ISM2* is also highly expressed in the brain, in particular in the nucleus accumbens (part of the basal ganglia) [192]. Within this context, it should be emphasised that Deep Brain Stimulation (DBS) of the nucleus accumbens itself has been observed to enhance learning and cognitive functions after TBI [193,194]. Interestingly, electromagnetic stimulation of SH-SY5Y neuroblastoma cells resulted in the increased expression of ADAM10 and an enhanced sAPPα release [195], suggesting the existence of a positive feedback loop and hinting at a possible correlation with Isthmin 2 putative, yet to be demonstrated neuronal roles of interest for TBI.

4.5. VEGFA

The human *VEGFA* gene is located on chromosome 6p21.1 and encodes for the Vascular Endothelial Growth Factor A (VEGF-A or VEGF, previously known as Vascular Permeability Factor, VPF), a secreted and glycosylated protein member of a family including VEGF-B, VEGF-C and VEGF-D (implicated in lymphangiogenesis regulation), the virally encoded VEGF-E, VEGF-F (snake venom VEGF), Endocrine Gland-derived VEGF (EG-VEGF) and the Placental Growth Factor (PLGF) [196]. VEGF plays a variety of different roles with key functions in regulating vasculogenesis and angiogenesis in both homeostatic and pathological contexts—promotes growth of the vascular endothelium, participates in differentiation mechanisms, increases permeability and molecule transport, supports anti-apoptotic processes and contributes to blood and lymphatic vessels development [196]. As a consequence of *VEGF* mRNA alternative splicing, VEGF is present in different isoforms, namely $VEGF_{121}$ (highly diffusible), $VEGF_{145}$, $VEGF_{148}$, $VEGF_{165}$ (the most frequently expressed isoform), $VEGF_{183}$, $VEGF_{189}$ (extracellular matrix-bound isoform) and $VEGF_{206}$, and each isoform exhibits a differential heparin-binding ability [197]. VEGF family members can bind to three different receptors belonging to the tyrosine kinase receptor superfamily: VEGFR1 (Fms-like tyrosine kinase 1, Flt-1) and VEGFR2 (Kinase-insert Domain Receptor, KDR) are mainly expressed on vascular endothelial cells and are bound by VEGF-A/VEGF-B and VEGF-A/VEGF-E, respectively, while VEGFR3 (Flt-4) is expressed only on lymphatic endothelial cells and is therefore bound by VEGF-C and VEGF-D. VEGF-A heparin-binding isoforms and PLGF can also bind Neuropilin 1 (NRP-1) to increase their affinity for VEGFR2, while VEGF-C and VEGF-D can bind NRP-2 through a similar interaction involving VEGFR3 to regulate lymphangiogenesis [197]. From the N-terminus to the C-terminus, VEGFs present a SP sequence, the N-terminal portion, the dimerisation sites, VEGFR1 binding site, N-glycosylation site, VEGFR2 binding site, Plasmin Cleavage Sequence (PCS), multiple heparin-binding sites and the Neuropilin binding site. However, VEGFs and VEGF-Rs expression is not limited to endothelial cells, but they are also found in blood system cells, tumour cells and neurogenic cells [198]. VEGF has been shown to contribute to neuronal development and regeneration in the CNS [199,200] and to exert neuroprotective and neurorestorative effects [201]. In particular, VEGF has been recognised to promote neurogenesis, neuronal survival, proliferation and migration, as well as axonal growth and guidance. VEGF exerts its effects also in neuron-related cell types, by favouring glia survival, and glia and oligodendrocyte migration [202]. The modulation of VEGF expression has been suggested as a potential mechanism associated with AD development and its clinical deterioration [203] and VEGF was found lowly expressed in patients with AD [204]. In this regard, our preliminary in vitro observations showed that sAPPα could exert its neuroprotective effects through the regulation of VEGF expression (Figure 5a,b) specifically the pro-angiogenic isoforms $VEGF_{165}$ and $VEGF_{189}$ (Figure 5c). Within this context, as a consequence of alternative splicing, the 8-exon *VEGF* pre-mRNA is differentially spliced to form mRNAs encoding for the so-called $VEGF_{xxx}b$ isoforms [205]. The differential splice-acceptor-site selection in the 3′UTR within exon 8 results in the presence of two sub-exons, 8a and 8b, distinguishing an alternate family of VEGF termed $VEGF_{xxx}b$ (opposed to the canonical family $VEGF_{xxx}$), mainly formed by $VEGF_{121}b$, $VEGF_{145}b$, $VEGF_{165}b$, $VEGF_{183}b$, $VEGF_{189}b$ and $VEGF_{206}b$ [205]. All $VEGF_{xxx}$ family members feature the 8a sub-exon, while $VEGF_{xxx}b$ isoforms present the 8b sub-exon. The alternative C-terminal region allows $VEGF_{xxx}b$ family members to inhibit the pro-angiogenic, proliferative, migratory and vasodilatory properties of $VEGF_{xxx}$ proteins [205,206]. The observed sAPPα-mediated up-regulating effects on *VEGF* mRNA were due to a sAPPα-induced increased stability of *VEGF* mRNA (Figure 5d) mirrored by an increased VEGF release (Figure 5e).

An additional up-stream player in the regulation of VEGF expression is the PKCβII/ELAV (Embryonic Lethal Abnormal Vision) cascade [207–209]. ELAV are a small family of proteins, which includes the ubiquitously expressed ELAVL1 (also known as HuA and HuR) and the neuron-specific members neuronal ELAV (nELAV, namely HuB, HuC and HuD). These RNA binding proteins act post-transcriptionally to dictate the fate of several transcripts during their journey from the nucleus to the cytoplasm [210]. At brain level, nELAV proteins contribute to regulate neuronal differentiation and maintenance, and are involved in synaptic plasticity associated with learning and memory processes [211–214]. The amount of nELAV proteins was found significantly reduced, along with clinical dementia progression, in the hippocampi from AD patients, where it also negatively correlated with Aβ levels [215]. Further, the direct treatment of human SH-SY5Y cells with both $Aβ_{40}$ [216] and $Aβ_{42}$ [215] induces a strong decrease in nELAV content together with a reduction in ADAM10, the best characterised α-secretase involved in APP non-amyloidogenic pathway and sAPPα production. Noteworthily, sAPPα treatment resulted in the increased translocation of nELAV in the nucleus (Figure 6a) and cytoskeleton (Figure 6c,d), along with their concomitant decrease in the cytosol (Figure 6b). Notably, the cytoskeleton represents an important site of protein synthesis and, at this level, a parallel rise in PKCβII amount was also observed (Figure 6c–e) which is in line with PI3K/Akt activation [141]. This strongly suggests the implication of the PKCβII/nELAV cascade in the regulation of VEGF expression at neuronal level as well.

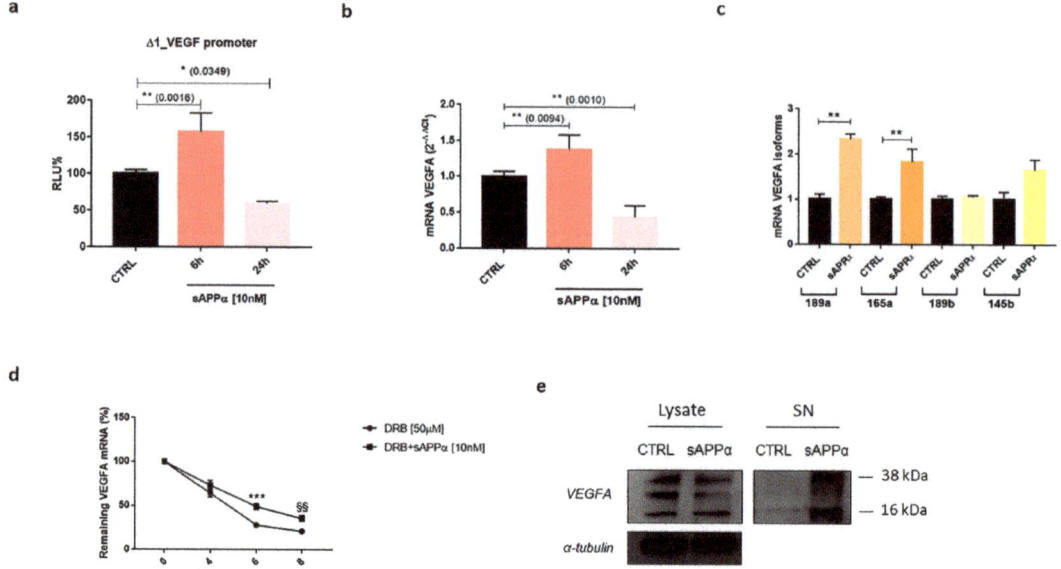

Figure 5. Effects of sAPPα treatment on VEGF expression. SH-SY5Y cells were treated with 10 nM sAPPα for 6 or 24 h. (**a**) SH-SY5Y cells transiently transfected with Δ1_VEGF luciferase-reporter plasmid and treated with sAPPα were lysed and luciferase activity was measured as previously described [141]. Luciferase activity is expressed as RLU% normalised to non-treated construct (set as 100%). (**b**,**c**) Evaluation of sAPPα-mediated *VEGFA* transcriptional regulation. mRNA levels were assessed by qPCR and normalised on *RPL6* (**b**) or the respective *VEGFA* isoform (employed primers described in [206]) (**c**). (**d**) Evaluation of sAPPα effects on *VEGFA* mRNA stability. SH-SY5Y cells were pre-treated with 50 μM DRB 53-85-0 (a classic RNA polymerase II inhibitor), then treated with 10 nM sAPPα for 0, 4, 6 or 8 h. RNA was extracted and reverse-transcribed as previously described [141]. mRNA levels were assessed by qPCR. Results are expressed as a percentage of the initial steady-state *VEGFA* mRNA levels. (**e**) Evaluation of VEGF protein levels in cell lysates and supernatants (SN). The image is a representative Western blot. Results are expressed as mean ± SEM, n = 3 independent experiments. Statistical analysis was performed with one-way ANOVA followed by Dunnett's multiple comparison test (**a**–**c**), with Bonferroni multiple comparison test (**d**) or Student's *t*-test (**e**) with * $p < 0.05$ and ** $p < 0.01$ vs. control (CTRL), *** $p < 0.001$ DRB vs. DRB + sAPPα (6 h) and §§ $p < 0.01$ DRB vs. DRB + sAPPα (8 h). Statistical significance is detailed in the respective figure panel.

The observed VEGF increase in human SH-SY5Y cells after sAPPα exposure is in line with data showing that VEGF is able to improve the cognitive decline in Tg2576 AD mouse model [217]. Besides the importance of this vascular factor in AD, Cerebrovascular Injury (CVI) is a recognised hallmark of TBI that affects function and integrity of the cerebrovascular system, contributing to neuronal dysfunction and neurodegeneration [218]. VEGF has been reported to mediate TBI amelioration [219], suggesting that new vasculogenic therapies targeting VEGF and its expression could be a feasible approach for vascular-related brain injuries typical of AD and TBI.

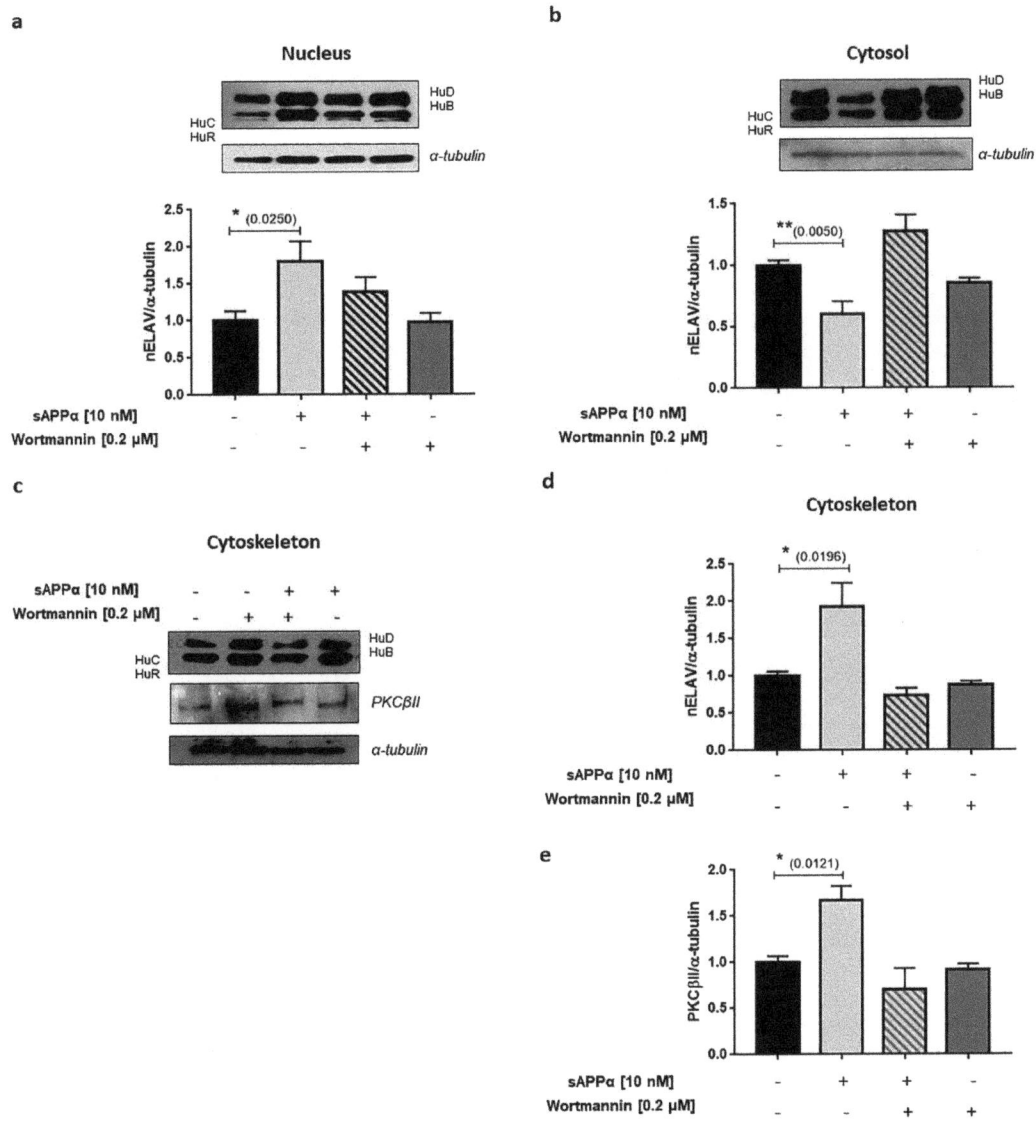

Figure 6. Evaluation of the PKCβII/nELAV/VEGF pathway in sAPPα-mediated effects on VEGF. (**a**–**e**) SH-SY5Y cells were treated with 10 nM sAPPα alone or in combination with 0.2 µM Wortmannin (an irreversible PI3K inhibitor). Subcellular fractionation was performed as previously described [141]. The image is a representative Western blot. nELAV protein levels were analysed in the nucleus (**a**), cytosol (**b**) and cytoskeleton (**c**,**d**) fractions. PKCβII protein levels were analysed in the cytoskeleton fraction (**c**,**e**). Protein levels were normalised to α-tubulin expression. Results are expressed as mean ± SEM, n = 3 independent experiments. Statistical analysis was performed with one-way ANOVA followed by Dunnett's multiple comparison test with * $p < 0.05$ and ** $p < 0.01$ vs. control (untreated cells). Statistical significance is detailed in the respective figure panel.

5. Discussion

The functions of APP and its cleavage fragments in the CNS have been extensively investigated in the past, especially for their relationship with AD. As a consequence of the increasingly aging population and the improvement of quality of life, the prevalence of AD and other neurodegenerative diseases is also increasing. In parallel, TBI has been effectively recognised as an important risk factor for the development of sporadic AD. Hence, it is of great significance to elucidate the role of APP and its cleavage peptides in these diseases. APP fragments produced through non-amyloidogenic pathways, particularly sAPPα, exert favourable effects in the CNS with important neuroprotective actions. Conversely, APP fragments generated via the amyloidogenic and non-canonical pathways have been demonstrated to have detrimental effects in the CNS. Indeed, amyloidogenic pathway-generated AICDs aggravate AD progression through positive feedback mechanisms by transcriptionally up-regulating *APP* and *BACE1* expression. Noteworthily, an increasing number of β-secretase 1 substrates has been reported together with the accumulation of neurotoxic APP fragments (e.g., η-CTF and Aη-α) upon β-secretase 1 genetic and pharmacological inhibition [64]. Consequently, specifically blocking β-secretase 1-mediated APP cleavage without affecting other substrates and ensuring that alternative neurotoxic APP fragments accumulation does not occur under the investigated therapeutic intervention will be mandatory for future research in this field. Therefore, pharmacological approaches aiming to reduce the production of detrimental APP fragments and, at the same time, to increase the generation of non-amyloidogenic pathways peptides could be feasible strategies for the prevention and treatment of AD, and may also provide new guidance for TBI treatment.

5.1. A Possible Therapeutic Intervention via sAPPα?

Since TBI has been proven as an important risk factor for AD, sAPPα modulatory activity on gene transcription may be of great interest for its neurotrophic effects. The ability of sAPPα not only to inhibit β-secretase 1 activity [169,170] but also to transcriptionally regulate *BACE1* mRNA expression may have important consequences on future β-secretase 1-targeting therapies aiming to reduce the production of amyloidogenic APP fragments. The sAPPα-mediated up-regulation of *TSPAN3* mRNA, together with its reported stabilising activity towards APP, ADAM10 and γ-secretase [184], suggest Tetraspanin-3 as a possible novel drug target to increase APP non-amyloidogenic processing. In addition, its importance for S1PR2/Nogo-A clustering and Nogo-A important role in AD pathogenesis due to its ability to modulate Aβ generation [220], further hints at Tetraspanin-3 as a possible important player in the sAPPα neuroprotective circuit. Although *ISM2* has not been investigated yet in neuronal context, the ability of sAPPα to mediate its up-regulation at mRNA level together with its elevated expression in the nucleus accumbens, important in TBI context [193,194], may suggest a possible role in sAPPα neuroprotective network and warrant further analyses. Finally, the early VEGF up-regulation and the late VEGF down-regulation mediated by sAPPα suggest a physiologic fine-tuning of its production in which isthmins may play a possible important role (although available data are limited to *ISM1* and cancer context [188,190]). Moreover, besides *VEGF*, *ADAM10* mRNA is also a target of PKC/nELAV pathway [216] and Aβ was shown to impair ADAM10 expression both in vitro and in AD hippocampi [215]. VEGF has been shown to improve the cognitive decline in Tg2576 AD mouse model by inducing *ADAM10* expression and decreasing *BACE1* production [217], thus suggesting the existence of a loop between APP cleavage fragments functions, PKC/nELAV/VEGF pathway and the potential protective functions of non-amyloidogenic sAPPα. These considerations may have possible important consequences in the dysregulated APP metabolism occurring in several conditions (e.g., from physiological aging and AD to brain injury response) [141] and point towards possible sAPPα-based therapeutic strategies. The neuroprotective, neurotrophic and neurogenic properties of sAPPα relevant against AD and TBI are mediated via the HBS located in APP E1 domain, within residues 96–110 [221]. In addition, the peptide APP derivative APP96–110 has been shown effective towards TBI following intravenous administration [222,223]. In this regard, recent studies both in vitro and in vivo reported that sAPPα acute administration in mice models or its chronic delivery through gene therapy effectively ameliorated both AD and TBI symptoms, further hinting at the proposed neurotrophic and neuroprotective roles of sAPPα [224,225].

5.2. A Putative Interaction Network for the Receptor for Activated C Kinase 1?

We previously demonstrated that sAPPα activates the PI3K/Akt/NF-κB pathway, influencing PKCβII signalling via the up-regulation of the Receptor for Activated C Kinase 1 (RACK1) [141]. RACK1 is a scaffold and ribosomal protein involved in a variety of molecular mechanisms, with crucial roles in both physiologic and pathologic conditions. RACK1 exerts its roles in several cellular contexts, including the immune system [226–235], cancer cells [236–240], intestinal homeostasis [241,242] and neurons [2,44,141,243–245]. In this regard, at a neuronal level, RACK1 has been reported to be required for point contact formation, axon outgrowth [246,247], dendritic arborisation [248], corticogenesis [249], synaptic plasticity, addiction, learning and memory by regulating N-methyl D-Aspartate (NMDA) receptor function [250], metabotropic glutamate receptor 1/5 (mGluR1/5)-triggered control of protein synthesis via its association with PKCβII [2], protection against oxidative stress [251] and BDNF expression [252–254]. Notably, reduced RACK1 levels were observed in both aged rat and human AD brains [255–257]. Aβ oligomers decrease RACK1 distribution in the membrane fraction of cortical neurons impairing PKC-mediated GABAergic transmission [258]. Moreover, RACK1 decreased levels have been also reported to induce Beclin-1-mediated autophagy in neurons [259]. In TBI context, RACK1 exerts neuroprotective effects via the activation of the Integrated Stress Response (ISR) pathway involving Inositol-Requiring Enzyme 1 (IRE1) and X-box Binding Protein 1 (XBP1) [260]. Although RACK1 has been initially discovered as the scaffold of different isoforms of activated PKC [231,245], literature data indicate that its interaction network is still increasing. Thanks to its β-propeller structure, RACK1 is able not only to interact with a broad range of binding partners, but also to participate in a variety of cellular mechanisms with potential implications also in neuronal context. Besides its well-known interaction with different PKC isoforms, RACK1 interacts directly or indirectly with genes/proteins here discussed or mentioned, including MAPK [261] and ADAM10 [262] via PKC signalling in neuronal context and VEGF via the PI3K/Akt/mTOR pathway [263–266], although these observations were limited to cancer cells. In addition, both RACK1 [2] and nELAV [267] are observed within stress granules, although their putative interaction has still to be demonstrated. Finally, despite the negative correlation between *ISM1*/Isthmin 1 and VEGF in cancer context [188,190], literature data correlating *ISM2*/Isthmin 2 with VEGF are still lacking, although a possible interaction could be hypothesised based on its pro- or anti-angiogenic properties. Therefore, the reported interactions among the different players presented in the previous sections and the possible existence of additional correlations—not yet demonstrated or investigated—indicate a possible important role played by VEGF and RACK1 in the construction of a sAPPα-related interaction network, with potential implications for neuroprotection (Figure 7).

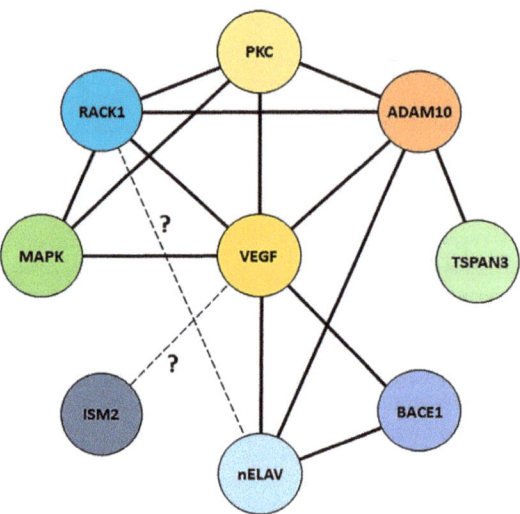

Figure 7. Putative sAPPα-related VEGF-RACK1 neuroprotective interaction network. RACK1 has been demonstrated to play pivotal roles in neuronal context and its modulation has been observed to be influenced by sAPPα treatment. Therefore, considering the reported and putative interactions among RACK1 and several players here discussed, it is possible to hypothesise a molecular network correlated to sAPPα and with potential implications in both AD and TBI context, from both a biological and pharmacological point of view (*bold lines* = protein-protein interactions or protein functional correlations reported in literature and cited in the text; *dash lines* = putative structural and/or functional protein correlations hypothesised based on available literature data).

6. Materials and Methods

6.1. Chemicals

Wortmannin (PubChem CID: 312145), sAPPα and the RNA polymerase II inhibitor 5,6-dichloro-1-beta-D-ribofuranosylbenzimidazole (DRB) (PubChem CID: 5894) were obtained from Sigma-Aldrich (St. Louis, MO, USA). Wortmannin and DRB were dissolved in DMSO at concentration of 100 mM and frozen in stock aliquots, then diluted at the concentration of use in culture medium. All reagents for cell culture were supplied by EuroClone (Milan, Italy). Mouse monoclonal anti-α-tubulin was purchased from Sigma-Aldrich. Rabbit polyclonal anti-PKCβII, rabbit polyclonal anti-VEGF and the anti-nELAV were obtained from Santa Cruz Biotechnology (Santa Cruz, CA, USA). Rabbit polyclonal anti-p42/44 MAPK and anti-phospho-p42/44 MAPK (Thr202/Tyr204) were purchased from Cell Signaling Technology, Inc. (Danvers, MA, USA). Host-specific peroxidase conjugated IgG secondary antibodies were purchased from Pierce (Rockford, IL, USA). Electrophoresis reagents were from Bio-Rad (Richmond, CA, USA).

6.2. Cell Culture and Treatments

Human neuroblastoma SH-SY5Y cells from the European Collection of Cell Cultures (ECACC No. 94030304) were cultured in 1:1 MEM-Ham's F-12 medium mixture supplemented with 10% Foetal Bovine Serum (FBS), 2 mM glutamine, 100 U/mL penicillin, 100 μM streptomycin, 1% non-essential amino acids. Cells were maintained at 37 °C in a humidified 5% CO_2 atmosphere. At 24 h before treatments, cells were cultured in medium without FBS and antibiotics. Subsequently, cells were treated with 10 nM sAPPα and/or Wortmannin 0.2 μM for different timings as reported in figure legends. When indicated, cells were exposed to 50 μM DRB [214] (or DMSO as vehicle control) for 1 h before sAPPα treatment.

6.3. Subcellular Fractionation

A total of 2×10^6 cells were seeded in 60 mm dishes and incubated in fresh serum-free medium for 24 h at 37 °C before treatments. After treatment, cells were washed with $1 \times$ PBS and homogenised 15 times using a Teflon glass homogeniser in fractionation buffer (0.32 M sucrose, 20 mM Tris-HCl pH 7.4, 2 mM EDTA, 10 mM EGTA, 50 mM β-mercaptoethanol, 0,3 mM phenylmethylsulfonyl difluoride, 20 µg/mL leupeptin). Homogenates were centrifuged at $3600 \times g$ for 5 min to the obtain the nuclear fraction; supernatants were centrifuged at $100,000 \times g$ for 30 min to separate cytosol and membrane fractions. The pelleted membrane fraction was sonicated in the same fractionation buffer supplemented with 0.2% (vol/vol) Triton X-100, incubated at 4 °C for 45 min and then centrifuged at $100,000 \times g$ for 30 min to separate membrane (supernatant) and cytoskeleton (pellet) fractions. Aliquots of the different fractions were assayed for protein quantification via the Bradford method.

6.4. Plasmid DNA Preparation, Transient Transfections and Luciferase Assays

Plasmids were purified with the HiSpeed® Plasmid Midi Kit (Qiagen, Valencia, CA, USA). DNA was quantified and assayed for purity using a DUR24 530UV/Vis Spectrophotometer (Beckman Coulter Inc., Fullerton, CA, USA). Transient transfections were carried out using Lipofectamine® 2000 (Invitrogen, Carlsbad, CA, USA) following manufacturer's instructions and performed in 24 multi-well culture plates. For each well, 7×10^5 cells were seeded in MEM-Ham's F-12 medium without FBS, antibiotics and supplemented with 1% L-glutamine. The pGL3-VEGF luciferase-reporter construct plasmid (indicated as Δ1_VEGF and obtained as indicated in literature [268,269]) was co-transfected with pRL-TK Renilla luciferase expressing vector to measure transfection efficiency (Promega, Madison, WI, USA). During transfection, SH-SY5Y cells were incubated at 37 °C in 5% CO_2 and then treated directly for with 10 nM sAPPα. Cells were then lysed with $1 \times$ Passive Lysis Buffer provided by Dual-Luciferase Reporter Assay System according to manufacturer's specifications (Promega, Madison, WI, USA). Luminescence was measured employing a 20/20n Luminometer (Turner BioSystems, Sunnyvale, CA, USA) with 10 s integration time.

6.5. qPCR

qPCR was carried out as previously described [270]. A total of 2×10^6 cells were seeded in 60 mm dishes and treated as described. Total RNA was extracted using RNeasyPlus Mini Kit (Qiagen, Valencia, CA, USA) following manufacturer's instructions. QuantiTect® reverse transcription kit and QuantiTect® SYBR Green PCR kit (Qiagen, Valencia, CA, USA) were used for cDNA synthesis and gene expression analysis following manufacturer's specifications. QuantiTect® primers for *BACE1*, *TSPAN3*, *ISM2*, *VEGFA* and *RPL6* were provided by Qiagen. Primers for *VEGFA* isoforms were purchased according to literature data [206]. *RPL6* was used as endogenous reference because it remained substantially stable in the 8 h time frame of the experiments with DRB [214]. Transcript quantification was performed via the $2^{(-\Delta\Delta Ct)}$ method.

6.6. mRNA Stability Analysis

The decay rate analysis of *VEGFA* mRNA was carried out as previously described [214]. 2×10^6 cells were seeded in 60 mm dishes, pre-treated with 50 µM DRB for 1 h and then treated with 10 nM sAPPα. Cells were collected at different time points (0, 4, 6 or 8 h). Total RNA was extracted and reversed transcribed as previously mentioned. Kinetic determination of *VEGFA* mRNA levels was assessed via qPCR as previously described [214]. *VEGFA* mRNA levels were normalised to *RPL6* mRNA levels and expressed as a percentage of the initial steady-state *VEGFA* mRNA levels.

6.7. Immunoblot

Immunoblot samples were prepared by mixing the cell lysate with 5× sample buffer (125 mM Tris-HCl pH 6.8, 4% SDS, 20% glycerol, 6% β-mercaptoethanol, 0.1% bromophenol) and denaturing at 95 °C for 5 min. Samples were electrophoresed into a 10% SDS-polyacrylamide gel under reducing conditions. Proteins were transferred to poly-vinylidene fluoride (PVDF) membrane (Amersham, Little Chalfont, UK), blocked in TBS-Tween 5% non-fat dry milk, and subsequently incubated with primary antibodies (mouse anti-α-tubulin, anti-nELAV, anti-p42/44 and anti-phospho-p42/44 1:1000, rabbit anti-PKCβII 1:300, rabbit anti-VEGF 1:150) diluted in TBS-Tween 5% non-fat dry milk. Immuno-reactivity was measured using host-specific secondary IgG peroxidase conjugated antibodies (1:5000 diluted) and ECL.

6.8. Densitometry and Statistics

Following immunoblot image acquisition through an AGFA scanner and analysis by means of the NIH IMAGE 1.47 program (Wayne Rasband, NIH, Research Services Branch, NIMH, Bethesda, MD, USA), the relative densities of the bands were expressed as arbitrary units and normalised to data obtained from control samples run under the same conditions. Data were analysed using the analysis of variance test followed, when significant, by an appropriate post hoc comparison test. A p value < 0.05 was considered significant. The data reported are expressed as mean ± SEM of at least three independent experiments.

7. Conclusions

The identification of further APP proteolytic cleavages in addition to the canonical α-, β-, and γ-secretases considerably complicates the whole APP biological frame. This raises important questions not only on the physiological role of APP full-length and its cleavage fragments, but also their possible pathological contributions in both AD and TBI contexts. Evidence shows that most non-canonical APP secretases, particularly δ- and η-secretases, increase Aβ production and generate neurotoxic fragments. Hence, investigating their actual contribution to AD development and progression may suggest possible future pharmacologic strategies also for TBI. Further research is required to fully understand the complexity of APP biology in health and disease. Among the different APP fragments, sAPPα neuroprotective effects have been addressed and studied in different research models, both in vitro and in vivo, strengthening the correlation between sAPPα modulating effects on gene transcription and its observed neuroprotective effects. Indeed, investigating sAPPα ability to modulate the expression of genes relevant for neuroprotection in both AD and TBI contexts may offer relevant and feasible approaches for future pharmacologic interventions.

Author Contributions: Conceptualization and methodology: M.M., F.B., M.R., A.P. and E.B. Investigation: performed the experiments M.M., F.B. and E.B. Formal analysis: M.M., F.B. and E.B. Writing—Original Draft: M.M., A.P. and E.B. Writing—Review and Editing: M.M., F.B., AF, M.R., A.P. and E.B. Visualization: M.M., F.B. and E.B. Critical discussion: M.M., F.B., A.F., M.R., A.P. and E.B. Project administration: F.B., M.R. and E.B. Supervision: F.B., M.R. and E.B. Funding acquisition: M.R. and A.P. All authors have read and agreed to the published version of the manuscript.

Funding: Research has been supported by Ministero dell'Istruzione, dell'Università e della Ricerca to Marco Racchi (PRIN2020, Project number 202039WMFP) and to Alessia Pascale (PRIN2020, Project number 2020FR7TCL).

Acknowledgments: The authors would like to thank SMART—Servier Medical ART (https://smart.servier.com/, accessed on 12 October 2022) used to perform Figures 2 and 3.

Conflicts of Interest: The authors declare no conflict of interests.

References

1. Wolozin, B.; Ivanov, P. Stress granules and neurodegeneration. *Nat. Rev. Neurosci.* **2019**, *20*, 649–666. [CrossRef]
2. Masi, M.; Attanzio, A.; Racchi, M.; Wolozin, B.; Borella, S.; Biundo, F.; Buoso, E. Proteostasis Deregulation in Neurodegeneration and Its Link with Stress Granules: Focus on the Scaffold and Ribosomal Protein RACK1. *Cells* **2022**, *11*, 2590. [CrossRef]
3. Hardy, J.; Selkoe, D.J. The amyloid hypothesis of Alzheimer's disease: Progress and problems on the road to therapeutics. *Science* **2002**, *297*, 353–356. [CrossRef] [PubMed]
4. Zheng, H.; Koo, E.H. Biology and pathophysiology of the amyloid precursor protein. *Mol. Neurodegener.* **2011**, *6*, 27. [CrossRef] [PubMed]
5. Racchi, M.; Mazzucchelli, M.; Porrello, E.; Lanni, C.; Govoni, S. Acetylcholinesterase inhibitors: Novel activities of old molecules. *Pharmacol. Res.* **2004**, *50*, 441–451. [CrossRef] [PubMed]
6. Strittmatter, W.J.; Saunders, A.M.; Schmechel, D.; Pericak-Vance, M.; Enghild, J.; Salvesen, G.S.; Roses, A.D. Apolipoprotein E: High-avidity binding to beta-amyloid and increased frequency of type 4 allele in late-onset familial Alzheimer disease. *Proc. Natl. Acad. Sci. USA* **1993**, *90*, 1977–1981. [CrossRef] [PubMed]
7. Farrer, L.A.; Cupples, L.A.; Haines, J.L.; Hyman, B.; Kukull, W.A.; Mayeux, R.; Myers, R.H.; Pericak-Vance, M.A.; Risch, N.; van Duijn, C.M. Effects of age, sex, and ethnicity on the association between apolipoprotein E genotype and Alzheimer disease. A meta-analysis. APOE and Alzheimer Disease Meta Analysis Consortium. *JAMA* **1997**, *278*, 1349–1356. [CrossRef]
8. Esiri, M.M. Ageing and the brain. *J. Pathol.* **2007**, *211*, 181–187. [CrossRef]
9. Mattson, M.P.; Maudsley, S.; Martin, B. BDNF and 5-HT: A dynamic duo in age-related neuronal plasticity and neurodegenerative disorders. *Trends Neurosci.* **2004**, *27*, 589–594. [CrossRef]
10. Lanni, C.; Masi, M.; Racchi, M.; Govoni, S. Cancer and Alzheimer's disease inverse relationship: An age-associated diverging derailment of shared pathways. *Mol. Psychiatry* **2021**, *26*, 280–295. [CrossRef]
11. Green, R.C.; Cupples, L.A.; Kurz, A.; Auerbach, S.; Go, R.; Sadovnick, D.; Duara, R.; Kukull, W.A.; Chui, H.; Edeki, T.; et al. Depression as a risk factor for Alzheimer disease: The MIRAGE Study. *Arch. Neurol.* **2003**, *60*, 753–759. [CrossRef] [PubMed]
12. Diniz, B.S.; Butters, M.A.; Albert, S.M.; Dew, M.A.; Reynolds, C.F., 3rd. Late-life depression and risk of vascular dementia and Alzheimer's disease: Systematic review and meta-analysis of community-based cohort studies. *Br. J. Psychiatry* **2013**, *202*, 329–335. [CrossRef]
13. Gorelick, P.B. Risk factors for vascular dementia and Alzheimer disease. *Stroke* **2004**, *35* (Suppl. S1), 2620–2622. [CrossRef]
14. Danna-Dos-Santos, A.; Mohapatra, S.; Santos, M.; Degani, A.M. Long-term effects of mild traumatic brain injuries to oculomotor tracking performances and reaction times to simple environmental stimuli. *Sci. Rep.* **2018**, *8*, 4583. [CrossRef] [PubMed]
15. De Freitas Cardoso, M.G.; Faleiro, R.M.; de Paula, J.J.; Kummer, A.; Caramelli, P.; Teixeira, A.L.; de Souza, L.C.; Miranda, A.S. Cognitive Impairment Following Acute Mild Traumatic Brain Injury. *Front. Neurol.* **2019**, *10*, 198. [CrossRef] [PubMed]
16. LoBue, C.; Wadsworth, H.; Wilmoth, K.; Clem, M.; Hart, J., Jr.; Womack, K.B.; Didehbani, N.; Lacritz, L.H.; Rossetti, H.C.; Cullum, C.M. Traumatic brain injury history is associated with earlier age of onset of Alzheimer disease. *Clin. Neuropsychol.* **2017**, *31*, 85–98. [CrossRef] [PubMed]
17. Iacono, D.; Raiciulescu, S.; Olsen, C.; Perl, D.P. Traumatic Brain Injury Exposure Lowers Age of Cognitive Decline in AD and Non-AD Conditions. *Front. Neurol.* **2021**, *12*, 573401. [CrossRef] [PubMed]
18. Van den Heuvel, C.; Blumbergs, P.C.; Finnie, J.W.; Manavis, J.; Jones, N.R.; Reilly, P.L.; Pereira, R.A. Upregulation of amyloid precursor protein messenger RNA in response to traumatic brain injury: An ovine head impact model. *Exp. Neurol.* **1999**, *159*, 441–450. [CrossRef]
19. Nadler, Y.; Alexandrovich, A.; Grigoriadis, N.; Hartmann, T.; Rao, K.S.; Shohami, E.; Stein, R. Increased expression of the gamma-secretase components presenilin-1 and nicastrin in activated astrocytes and microglia following traumatic brain injury. *Glia* **2008**, *56*, 552–567. [CrossRef]
20. Blasko, I.; Beer, R.; Bigl, M.; Apelt, J.; Franz, G.; Rudzki, D.; Ransmayr, G.; Kampfl, A.; Schliebs, R. Experimental traumatic brain injury in rats stimulates the expression, production and activity of Alzheimer's disease beta-secretase (BACE-1). *J. Neural. Transm.* **2004**, *111*, 523–536. [CrossRef]
21. Galvão, F., Jr.; Grokoski, K.C.; da Silva, B.B.; Lamers, M.L.; Siqueira, I.R. The amyloid precursor protein (APP) processing as a biological link between Alzheimer's disease and cancer. *Ageing Res. Rev.* **2019**, *49*, 83–91. [CrossRef]
22. Corrigan, F.; Pham, C.L.; Vink, R.; Blumbergs, P.C.; Masters, C.L.; van den Heuvel, C.; Cappai, R. The neuroprotective domains of the amyloid precursor protein, in traumatic brain injury, are located in the two growth factor domains. *Brain Res.* **2011**, *1378*, 137–143. [CrossRef] [PubMed]
23. Guo, Y.; Wang, Q.; Chen, S.; Xu, C. Functions of amyloid precursor protein in metabolic diseases. *Metabolism* **2021**, *115*, 154454. [CrossRef]
24. Baumkötter, F.; Schmidt, N.; Vargas, C.; Schilling, S.; Weber, R.; Wagner, K.; Fiedler, S.; Klug, W.; Radzimanowski, J.; Nickolaus, S.; et al. Amyloid precursor protein dimerization and synaptogenic function depend on copper binding to the growth factor-like domain. *J. Neurosci.* **2014**, *34*, 11159–11172. [CrossRef]
25. Sisodia, S.S.; Koo, E.H.; Hoffman, P.N.; Perry, G.; Price, D.L. Identification and transport of full-length amyloid precursor proteins in rat peripheral nervous system. *J. Neurosci.* **1993**, *13*, 3136–3142. [CrossRef] [PubMed]
26. Ludewig, S.; Korte, M. Novel Insights into the Physiological Function of the APP (Gene) Family and Its Proteolytic Fragments in Synaptic Plasticity. *Front. Mol. Neurosci.* **2017**, *9*, 161. [CrossRef]

27. Erdinger, S.; Amrein, I.; Back, M.; Ludewig, S.; Korte, M.; von Engelhardt, J.; Wolfer, D.P.; Müller, U.C. Lack of APLP1 leads to subtle alter-ations in neuronal morphology but does not affect learning and memory. *Front. Mol. Neurosci.* **2022**, *15*, 1028836. [CrossRef] [PubMed]
28. Lee, S.H.; Kang, J.; Ho, A.; Watanabe, H.; Bolshakov, V.Y.; Shen, J. APP Family Regulates Neuronal Excitability and Synaptic Plasticity but Not Neuronal Survival. *Neuron* **2020**, *108*, 676–690.e8. [CrossRef] [PubMed]
29. Onodera, W.; Asahi, T.; Sawamura, N. Rapid evolution of mammalian APLP1 as a synaptic adhesion molecule. *Sci. Rep.* **2021**, *11*, 11305. [CrossRef] [PubMed]
30. Schilling, S.; Mehr, A.; Ludewig, S.; Stephan, J.; Zimmermann, M.; August, A.; Strecker, P.; Korte, M.; Koo, E.H.; Müller, U.C.; et al. APLP1 Is a Synaptic Cell Adhesion Molecule, Supporting Maintenance of Dendritic Spines and Basal Synaptic Transmission. *J. Neurosci.* **2017**, *37*, 5345–5365. [CrossRef]
31. Lim, B.; Tsolaki, M.; Soosaipillai, A.; Brown, M.; Zilakaki, M.; Tagaraki, F.; Fotiou, D.; Koutsouraki, E.; Grosi, E.; Prassas, I.; et al. Liquid biopsy of cerebrospinal fluid identifies neuronal pentraxin receptor (NPTXR) as a biomarker of progression of Alz-heimer's disease. *Clin. Chem. Lab. Med.* **2019**, *57*, 1875–1881. [CrossRef] [PubMed]
32. Wang, X.; Zhou, X.; Li, G.; Zhang, Y.; Wu, Y.; Song, W. Modifications and Trafficking of APP in the Pathogenesis of Alzheimer's Disease. *Front. Mol. Neurosci.* **2017**, *10*, 294. [CrossRef] [PubMed]
33. Chun, Y.S.; Park, Y.; Oh, H.G.; Kim, T.W.; Yang, H.O.; Park, M.K.; Chung, S. O-GlcNAcylation promotes non-amyloidogenic processing of amyloid-? protein precursor via inhibition of endocytosis from the plasma membrane. *J. Alzheimers Dis.* **2015**, *44*, 261–275. [CrossRef]
34. Bhattacharyya, R.; Barren, C.; Kovacs, D.M. Palmitoylation of amyloid precursor protein regulates amyloidogenic processing in lipid rafts. *J. Neurosci.* **2013**, *33*, 11169–11183. [CrossRef] [PubMed]
35. Morel, E.; Chamoun, Z.; Lasiecka, Z.M.; Chan, R.B.; Williamson, R.L.; Vetanovetz, C.; Dall'Armi, C.; Simoes, S.; Point Du Jour, K.S.; McCabe, B.D.; et al. Phosphatidylinositol-3-phosphate regulates sorting and processing of amyloid precursor protein through the endosomal system. *Nat. Commun.* **2013**, *4*, 2250. [CrossRef]
36. Watanabe, T.; Hikichi, Y.; Willuweit, A.; Shintani, Y.; Horiguchi, T. FBL2 regulates amyloid precursor protein (APP) metabolism by promoting ubiquitination-dependent APP degradation and inhibition of APP endocytosis. *J. Neurosci.* **2012**, *32*, 3352–3365. [CrossRef]
37. Zhang, Y.Q.; Sarge, K.D. Sumoylation of amyloid precursor protein negatively regulates Abeta aggregate levels. *Biochem. Biophys. Res. Commun.* **2008**, *374*, 673–678. [CrossRef]
38. Andrew, R.J.; Kellett, K.A.; Thinakaran, G.; Hooper, N.M. A Greek Tragedy: The Growing Complexity of Alzheimer Amyloid Precursor Protein Proteolysis. *J. Biol. Chem.* **2016**, *291*, 19235–19244. [CrossRef]
39. Edbauer, D.; Winkler, E.; Regula, J.T.; Pesold, B.; Steiner, H.; Haass, C. Reconstitution of gamma-secretase activity. *Nat. Cell Biol.* **2003**, *5*, 486–488. [CrossRef]
40. Kimura, A.; Hata, S.; Suzuki, T. Alternative Selection of β-Site APP-Cleaving Enzyme 1 (BACE1) Cleavage Sites in Amyloid β-Protein Precursor (APP) Harboring Protective and Pathogenic Mutations within the Aβ Sequence. *J. Biol. Chem.* **2016**, *291*, 24041–24053. [CrossRef]
41. Kim, D.; Tsai, L.H. Bridging physiology and pathology in AD. *Cell* **2009**, *137*, 997–1000. [CrossRef] [PubMed]
42. Nikolaev, A.; McLaughlin, T.; O'Leary, D.D.; Tessier-Lavigne, M. APP binds DR6 to trigger axon pruning and neuron death via distinct caspases. *Nature* **2009**, *457*, 981–989. [CrossRef] [PubMed]
43. Xu, K.; Olsen, O.; Tzvetkova-Robev, D.; Tessier-Lavigne, M.; Nikolov, D.B. The crystal structure of DR6 in complex with the amyloid precursor protein provides insight into death receptor activation. *Genes Dev.* **2015**, *29*, 785–790. [CrossRef] [PubMed]
44. Buoso, E.; Lanni, C.; Schettini, G.; Govoni, S.; Racchi, M. Beta-Amyloid precursor protein metabolism: Focus on the functions and degradation of its intracellular domain. *Pharmacol. Res.* **2010**, *62*, 308–317. [CrossRef]
45. Vingtdeux, V.; Hamdane, M.; Bégard, S.; Loyens, A.; Delacourte, A.; Beauvillain, J.C.; Buée, L.; Marambaud, P.; Sergeant, N. Intracellular pH regulates amyloid precursor protein intracellular domain accumulation. *Neurobiol. Dis.* **2007**, *25*, 686–696. [CrossRef]
46. Edbauer, D.; Willem, M.; Lammich, S.; Steiner, H.; Haass, C. Insulin-degrading enzyme rapidly removes the beta-amyloid precursor protein intracellular domain (AICD). *J. Biol. Chem.* **2002**, *277*, 13389–13393. [CrossRef]
47. Farris, W.; Mansourian, S.; Chang, Y.; Lindsley, L.; Eckman, E.A.; Frosch, M.P.; Eckman, C.B.; Tanzi, R.E.; Selkoe, D.J.; Guenette, S. Insulin-degrading enzyme regulates the levels of insulin, amyloid beta-protein, and the beta-amyloid precursor protein intracellular domain in vivo. *Proc. Natl. Acad. Sci. USA* **2003**, *100*, 4162–4167. [CrossRef]
48. Cao, X.; Südhof, T.C. A transcriptionally [correction of transcriptively] active complex of APP with Fe65 and histone acetyltrans-ferase Tip60. *Science* **2001**, *293*, 115–120. [CrossRef]
49. Grimm, M.O.; Mett, J.; Stahlmann, C.P.; Grösgen, S.; Haupenthal, V.J.; Blümel, T.; Hundsdörfer, B.; Zimmer, V.C.; Mylonas, N.T.; Tanila, H.; et al. APP intracellular domain derived from amyloidogenic β- and γ-secretase cleavage regulates neprilysin expression. *Front. Aging Neurosci.* **2015**, *7*, 77. [CrossRef]
50. Konietzko, U. AICD nuclear signaling and its possible contribution to Alzheimer's disease. *Curr. Alzheimer Res.* **2012**, *9*, 200–216. [CrossRef]

51. Von Rotz, R.C.; Kohli, B.M.; Bosset, J.; Meier, M.; Suzuki, T.; Nitsch, R.M.; Konietzko, U. The APP intracellular domain forms nuclear multiprotein complexes and regulates the transcription of its own precursor. *J. Cell Sci.* **2004**, *117*, 4435–4448. [CrossRef] [PubMed]
52. Scheinfeld, M.H.; Ghersi, E.; Laky, K.; Fowlkes, B.J.; D'Adamio, L. Processing of beta-amyloid precursor-like protein-1 and -2 by gamma-secretase regulates transcription. *J. Biol. Chem.* **2002**, *277*, 44195–44201. [CrossRef] [PubMed]
53. Cha, H.J.; Shen, J.; Kang, J. Regulation of gene expression by the APP family in the adult cerebral cortex. *Sci. Rep.* **2022**, *12*, 66. [CrossRef]
54. Xu, X. Gamma-secretase catalyzes sequential cleavages of the AbetaPP transmembrane domain. *J. Alzheimers Dis.* **2009**, *16*, 211–224. [CrossRef]
55. Takami, M.; Nagashima, Y.; Sano, Y.; Ishihara, S.; Morishima-Kawashima, M.; Funamoto, S.; Ihara, Y. gamma-Secretase: Successive tripeptide and tetrapeptide release from the transmembrane domain of beta-carboxyl terminal fragment. *J. Neurosci.* **2009**, *29*, 13042–13052. [CrossRef] [PubMed]
56. Hur, J.Y. γ-Secretase in Alzheimer's disease. *Exp. Mol. Med.* **2022**, *54*, 433–446. [CrossRef]
57. Long, J.M.; Holtzman, D.M. Alzheimer Disease: An Update on Pathobiology and Treatment Strategies. *Cell* **2019**, *179*, 312–339. [CrossRef]
58. Nhan, H.S.; Chiang, K.; Koo, E.H. The multifaceted nature of amyloid precursor protein and its proteolytic fragments: Friends and foes. *Acta Neuropathol.* **2015**, *129*, 1–19. [CrossRef]
59. Zhang, Z.; Song, M.; Liu, X.; Kang, S.S.; Kwon, I.S.; Duong, D.M.; Seyfried, N.T.; Hu, W.T.; Liu, Z.; Wang, J.Z.; et al. Cleavage of tau by asparagine endopeptidase mediates the neurofibrillary pathology in Alzheimer's disease. *Nat. Med.* **2014**, *20*, 1254–1262. [CrossRef]
60. Zhang, Z.; Song, M.; Liu, X.; Su Kang, S.; Duong, D.M.; Seyfried, N.T.; Cao, X.; Cheng, L.; Sun, Y.E.; Ping, Y.S.; et al. Delta-secretase cleaves amyloid precursor protein and regulates the pathogenesis in Alzheimer's disease. *Nat. Commun.* **2015**, *6*, 8762. [CrossRef]
61. Yao, Y.; Kang, S.S.; Xia, Y.; Wang, Z.H.; Liu, X.; Muller, T.; Sun, Y.E.; Ye, K. A delta-secretase-truncated APP fragment activates CEBPB, mediating Alzheimer's disease pathologies. *Brain* **2021**, *144*, 1833–1852. [CrossRef] [PubMed]
62. Baranger, K.; Khrestchatisky, M.; Rivera, S. MT5-MMP, just a new APP processing proteinase in Alzheimer's disease? *J. Neuroinflammation* **2016**, *13*, 167. [CrossRef] [PubMed]
63. Baranger, K.; Marchalant, Y.; Bonnet, A.E.; Crouzin, N.; Carrete, A.; Paumier, J.M.; Py, N.A.; Bernard, A.; Bauer, C.; Charrat, E.; et al. MT5-MMP is a new pro-amyloidogenic proteinase that promotes amyloid pathology and cognitive decline in a transgenic mouse model of Alzheimer's disease. *Cell Mol. Life Sci.* **2016**, *73*, 217–236. [CrossRef] [PubMed]
64. Willem, M.; Tahirovic, S.; Busche, M.A.; Ovsepian, S.V.; Chafai, M.; Kootar, S.; Hornburg, D.; Evans, L.D.; Moore, S.; Daria, A.; et al. η-Secretase processing of APP inhibits neuronal activity in the hippocampus. *Nature* **2015**, *526*, 443–447. [CrossRef] [PubMed]
65. Hernandez-Guillamon, M.; Mawhirt, S.; Blais, S.; Montaner, J.; Neubert, T.A.; Rostagno, A.; Ghiso, J. Sequential Amyloid-β Degradation by the Matrix Metalloproteases MMP-2 and MMP-9. *J. Biol. Chem.* **2015**, *290*, 15078–15091. [CrossRef]
66. Fragkouli, A.; Tsilibary, E.C.; Tzinia, A.K. Neuroprotective role of MMP-9 overexpression in the brain of Alzheimer's 5xFAD mice. *Neurobiol. Dis.* **2014**, *70*, 179–189. [CrossRef]
67. Schönherr, C.; Bien, J.; Isbert, S.; Wichert, R.; Prox, J.; Altmeppen, H.; Kumar, S.; Walter, J.; Lichtenthaler, S.F.; Weggen, S.; et al. Generation of aggregation prone N-terminally truncated amyloid β peptides by meprin β depends on the sequence specificity at the cleavage site. *Mol. Neurodegener.* **2016**, *11*, 19. [CrossRef]
68. Bien, J.; Jefferson, T.; Causević, M.; Jumpertz, T.; Munter, L.; Multhaup, G.; Weggen, S.; Becker-Pauly, C.; Pietrzik, C.U. The metalloprotease meprin β generates amino terminal-truncated amyloid β peptide species. *J. Biol. Chem.* **2012**, *287*, 33304–33313. [CrossRef]
69. Jefferson, T.; Čaušević, M.; auf dem Keller, U.; Schilling, O.; Isbert, S.; Geyer, R.; Maier, W.; Tschickardt, S.; Jumpertz, T.; Weggen, S.; et al. Metalloprotease meprin beta generates nontoxic N-terminal amyloid precursor protein fragments in vivo. *J. Biol. Chem.* **2011**, *286*, 27741–27750. [CrossRef]
70. Jäckle, F.; Schmidt, F.; Wichert, R.; Arnold, P.; Prox, J.; Mangold, M.; Ohler, A.; Pietrzik, C.U.; Koudelka, T.; Tholey, A.; et al. Metalloprotease meprin β is activated by transmembrane serine protease matriptase-2 at the cell surface thereby enhancing APP shedding. *Biochem. J.* **2015**, *470*, 91–103. [CrossRef]
71. Sun, X.; He, G.; Song, W. BACE2, as a novel APP theta-secretase, is not responsible for the pathogenesis of Alzheimer's disease in Down syndrome. *FASEB J.* **2006**, *20*, 1369–1376. [CrossRef]
72. Wang, Z.; Xu, Q.; Cai, F.; Liu, X.; Wu, Y.; Song, W. BACE2, a conditional β-secretase, contributes to Alzheimer's disease pathogenesis. *JCI Insight* **2019**, *4*, e123431. [CrossRef]
73. Qiu, K.; Liang, W.; Wang, S.; Kong, T.; Wang, X.; Li, C.; Wang, Z.; Wu, Y. BACE2 degradation is mediated by both the proteasome and lysosome pathways. *BMC Mol. Cell Biol.* **2020**, *21*, 13. [CrossRef] [PubMed]
74. Portelius, E.; Mattsson, N.; Andreasson, U.; Blennow, K.; Zetterberg, H. Novel Aβ isoforms in Alzheimer's disease-their role in diagnosis and treatment. *Curr. Pharm. Des.* **2011**, *17*, 2594–2602. [CrossRef] [PubMed]
75. Welzel, A.T.; Maggio, J.E.; Shankar, G.M.; Walker, D.E.; Ostaszewski, B.L.; Li, S.; Klyubin, I.; Rowan, M.J.; Seubert, P.; Walsh, D.M.; et al. Secreted amyloid β-proteins in a cell culture model include N-terminally extended peptides that impair synaptic plasticity. *Biochemistry* **2014**, *53*, 3908–3921. [CrossRef] [PubMed]

76. Portelius, E.; Brinkmalm, G.; Tran, A.; Andreasson, U.; Zetterberg, H.; Westman-Brinkmalm, A.; Blennow, K.; Ohrfelt, A. Identification of novel N-terminal fragments of amyloid precursor protein in cerebrospinal fluid. *Exp. Neurol.* **2010**, *223*, 351–358. [CrossRef] [PubMed]
77. Dawkins, E.; Gasperini, R.; Hu, Y.; Cui, H.; Vincent, A.J.; Bolós, M.; Young, K.M.; Foa, L.; Small, D.H. The N-terminal fragment of the β-amyloid precursor protein of Alzheimer's disease (N-APP) binds to phosphoinositide-rich domains on the surface of hippocampal neurons. *J. Neurosci. Res.* **2014**, *92*, 1478–1489. [CrossRef]
78. Fanutza, T.; Del Prete, D.; Ford, M.J.; Castillo, P.E.; D'Adamio, L. APP and APLP2 interact with the synaptic release machinery and facilitate transmitter release at hippocampal synapses. *eLife* **2015**, *4*, e09784. [CrossRef]
79. García-González, L.; Pilat, D.; Baranger, K.; Rivera, S. Emerging Alternative Proteinases in APP Metabolism and Alzheimer's Disease Pathogenesis: A Focus on MT1-MMP and MT5-MMP. *Front. Aging Neurosci.* **2019**, *11*, 244. [CrossRef]
80. Sun, B.; Zhou, Y.; Halabisky, B.; Lo, I.; Cho, S.H.; Mueller-Steiner, S.; Devidze, N.; Wang, X.; Grubb, A.; Gan, L. Cystatin C-cathepsin B axis regulates amyloid beta levels and associated neuronal deficits in an animal model of Alzheimer's disease. *Neuron* **2008**, *60*, 247–257. [CrossRef]
81. Hook, V.Y.; Kindy, M.; Hook, G. Inhibitors of cathepsin B improve memory and reduce beta-amyloid in transgenic Alzheimer disease mice expressing the wild-type, but not the Swedish mutant, beta-secretase site of the amyloid precursor protein. *J. Biol. Chem.* **2008**, *283*, 7745–7753. [CrossRef] [PubMed]
82. Gowrishankar, S.; Yuan, P.; Wu, Y.; Schrag, M.; Paradise, S.; Grutzendler, J.; De Camilli, P.; Ferguson, S.M. Massive accumulation of luminal protease-deficient axonal lysosomes at Alzheimer's disease amyloid plaques. *Proc. Natl. Acad. Sci. USA* **2015**, *112*, E3699–E3708. [CrossRef] [PubMed]
83. Hook, G.; Yu, J.; Toneff, T.; Kindy, M.; Hook, V. Brain pyroglutamate amyloid-β is produced by cathepsin B and is reduced by the cysteine protease inhibitor E64d, representing a potential Alzheimer's disease therapeutic. *J Alzheimer's Dis.* **2014**, *41*, 129–149. [CrossRef] [PubMed]
84. Mohamed, A.Z.; Nestor, P.J.; Cumming, P.; Nasrallah, F.A.; Alzheimer's Disease Neuroimaging Initiative. Traumatic brain injury fast-forwards Alzheimer's pathology: Evidence from amyloid positron emission tomorgraphy imaging. *J. Neurol.* **2022**, *269*, 873–884. [CrossRef]
85. Goetzl, E.J.; Peltz, C.B.; Mustapic, M.; Kapogiannis, D.; Yaffe, K. Neuron-Derived Plasma Exosome Proteins after Remote Traumatic Brain Injury. *J. Neurotrauma* **2020**, *37*, 382–388. [CrossRef] [PubMed]
86. Bogoslovsky, T.; Wilson, D.; Chen, Y.; Hanlon, D.; Gill, J.; Jeromin, A.; Song, L.; Moore, C.; Gong, Y.; Kenney, K.; et al. Increases of Plasma Levels of Glial Fibrillary Acidic Protein, Tau, and Amyloid β up to 90 Days after Traumatic Brain Injury. *J. Neurotrauma* **2017**, *34*, 66–73. [CrossRef]
87. Hu, W.; Tung, Y.C.; Zhang, Y.; Liu, F.; Iqbal, K. Involvement of Activation of Asparaginyl Endopeptidase in Tau Hyperphosphorylation in Repetitive Mild Traumatic Brain Injury. *J. Alzheimer's Dis.* **2018**, *64*, 709–722. [CrossRef]
88. Wu, Z.; Wang, Z.H.; Liu, X.; Zhang, Z.; Gu, X.; Yu, S.P.; Keene, C.D.; Cheng, L.; Ye, K. Traumatic brain injury triggers APP and Tau cleavage by delta-secretase, mediating Alzheimer's disease pathology. *Prog. Neurobiol.* **2020**, *185*, 101730. [CrossRef]
89. Wu, Z.; Chen, C.; Kang, S.S.; Liu, X.; Gu, X.; Yu, S.P.; Keene, C.D.; Cheng, L.; Ye, K. Neurotrophic signaling deficiency exacerbates environmental risks for Alzheimer's disease pathogenesis. *Proc. Natl. Acad. Sci. USA* **2021**, *118*, e2100986118. [CrossRef]
90. Hook, G.; Reinheckel, T.; Ni, J.; Wu, Z.; Kindy, M.; Peters, C.; Hook, V. Cathepsin B Gene Knockout Improves Behavioral Deficits and Reduces Pathology in Models of Neurologic Disorders. *Pharmacol. Rev.* **2022**, *74*, 600–629. [CrossRef]
91. Stone, J.R.; Okonkwo, D.O.; Singleton, R.H.; Mutlu, L.K.; Helm, G.A.; Povlishock, J.T. Caspase-3-mediated cleavage of amyloid precursor protein and formation of amyloid Beta peptide in traumatic axonal injury. *J. Neurotrauma* **2002**, *19*, 601–614. [CrossRef]
92. Abu Hamdeh, S.; Ciuculete, D.M.; Sarkisyan, D.; Bakalkin, G.; Ingelsson, M.; Schiöth, H.B.; Marklund, N. Differential DNA Methylation of the Genes for Amyloid Precursor Protein, Tau, and Neurofilaments in Human Traumatic Brain Injury. *J. Neurotrauma* **2021**, *38*, 1679–1688. [CrossRef] [PubMed]
93. Al-Sarraj, S.; Troakes, C.; Rutty, G.N. Axonal injury is detected by βAPP immunohistochemistry in rapid death from head injury following road traffic collision. *Int. J. Leg. Med.* **2022**, *136*, 1321–1339. [CrossRef] [PubMed]
94. Chaves, R.S.; Tran, M.; Holder, A.R.; Balcer, A.M.; Dickey, A.M.; Roberts, E.A.; Bober, B.G.; Gutierrez, E.; Head, B.P.; Groisman, A.; et al. Amyloidogenic Processing of Amyloid Precursor Protein Drives Stretch-Induced Disruption of Axonal Transport in hiPSC-Derived Neurons. *J. Neurosci.* **2021**, *41*, 10034–10053. [CrossRef] [PubMed]
95. Freude, K.K.; Penjwini, M.; Davis, J.L.; LaFerla, F.M.; Blurton-Jones, M. Soluble amyloid precursor protein induces rapid neural differentiation of human embryonic stem cells. *J. Biol. Chem.* **2011**, *286*, 24264–24274. [CrossRef]
96. Furukawa, K.; Sopher, B.L.; Rydel, R.E.; Begley, J.G.; Pham, D.G.; Martin, G.M.; Fox, M.; Mattson, M.P. Increased activity-regulating and neuroprotective efficacy of alpha-secretase-derived secreted amyloid precursor protein conferred by a C-terminal heparin-binding domain. *J. Neurochem.* **1996**, *67*, 1882–1896. [CrossRef] [PubMed]
97. Taylor, C.J.; Ireland, D.R.; Ballagh, I.; Bourne, K.; Marechal, N.M.; Turner, P.R.; Bilkey, D.K.; Tate, W.P.; Abraham, W.C. Endogenous secreted amyloid precursor protein-alpha regulates hippocampal NMDA receptor function, long-term potentiation and spatial memory. *Neurobiol. Dis.* **2008**, *31*, 250–260. [CrossRef]
98. Austin, S.A.; Combs, C.K. Mechanisms of microglial activation by amyloid precursor protein and its proteolytic fragments. In *Central Nervous System Diseases and Inflammation*, 2008th ed.; Lane, T.E., Carson, M., Bergmann, C., Wyss-Coray, T., Eds.; Springer: New York, NY, USA, 2008; pp. 13–32.

99. Barger, S.W.; Harmon, A.D. Microglial activation by Alzheimer amyloid precursor protein and modulation by apolipoprotein E. *Nature* **1997**, *388*, 878–881. [CrossRef]
100. Tamayev, R.; Matsuda, S.; Arancio, O.; D'Adamio, L. β- but not γ-secretase proteolysis of APP causes synaptic and memory deficits in a mouse model of dementia. *EMBO Mol. Med.* **2012**, *4*, 171–179. [CrossRef]
101. Bittner, T.; Fuhrmann, M.; Burgold, S.; Jung, C.K.; Volbracht, C.; Steiner, H.; Mitteregger, G.; Kretzschmar, H.A.; Haass, C.; Herms, J. Gamma-secretase inhibition reduces spine density in vivo via an amyloid precursor protein-dependent pathway. *J. Neurosci.* **2009**, *29*, 10405–10409. [CrossRef]
102. Lauritzen, I.; Pardossi-Piquard, R.; Bauer, C.; Brigham, E.; Abraham, J.D.; Ranaldi, S.; Fraser, P.; St-George-Hyslop, P.; Le Thuc, O.; Espin, V.; et al. The β-secretase-derived C-terminal fragment of βAPP, C99, but not Aβ, is a key contributor to early intraneuronal lesions in triple-transgenic mouse hippocampus. *J. Neurosci.* **2012**, *32*, 16243–16255. [CrossRef] [PubMed]
103. Mitani, Y.; Yarimizu, J.; Saita, K.; Uchino, H.; Akashiba, H.; Shitaka, Y.; Ni, K.; Matsuoka, N. Differential effects between β-secretase inhibitors and modulators on cognitive function in amyloid precursor protein-transgenic and nontransgenic mice. *J. Neurosci.* **2012**, *32*, 2037–2050. [CrossRef] [PubMed]
104. Yankner, B.A.; Dawes, L.R.; Fisher, S.; Villa-Komaroff, L.; Oster-Granite, M.L.; Neve, R.L. Neurotoxicity of a fragment of the amyloid precursor associated with Alzheimer's disease. *Science* **1989**, *245*, 417–420. [CrossRef]
105. Neve, R.L.; Kammesheidt, A.; Hohmann, C.F. Brain transplants of cells expressing the carboxyl-terminal fragment of the Alzheimer amyloid protein precursor cause specific neuropathology in vivo. *Proc. Natl. Acad. Sci. USA* **1992**, *89*, 3448–3452. [CrossRef] [PubMed]
106. Song, D.K.; Won, M.H.; Jung, J.S.; Lee, J.C.; Kang, T.C.; Suh, H.W.; Huh, S.O.; Paek, S.H.; Kim, Y.H.; Kim, S.H.; et al. Behavioral and neuropathologic changes induced by central injection of carboxyl-terminal fragment of beta-amyloid precursor protein in mice. *J. Neurochem.* **1998**, *71*, 875–878. [CrossRef]
107. Fukuchi, K.I.; Kunkel, D.D.; Schwartzkroin, P.A.; Kamino, K.; Ogburn, C.E.; Furlong, C.E.; Martin, G.M. Overexpression of a C-terminal portion of the beta-amyloid precursor protein in mouse brains by transplantation of transformed neuronal cells. *Exp. Neurol.* **1994**, *127*, 253–264. [CrossRef]
108. Multhaup, G.; Huber, O.; Buée, L.; Galas, M.C. Amyloid Precursor Protein (APP) Metabolites APP Intracellular Fragment (AICD), Aβ42, and Tau in Nuclear Roles. *J. Biol. Chem.* **2015**, *290*, 23515–23522. [CrossRef]
109. Beckett, C.; Nalivaeva, N.N.; Belyaev, N.D.; Turner, A.J. Nuclear signalling by membrane protein intracellular domains: The AICD enigma. *Cell Signal.* **2012**, *24*, 402–409. [CrossRef]
110. Kim, H.S.; Kim, E.M.; Lee, J.P.; Park, C.H.; Kim, S.; Seo, J.H.; Chang, K.A.; Yu, E.; Jeong, S.J.; Chong, Y.H.; et al. C-terminal fragments of amyloid precursor protein exert neurotoxicity by inducing glycogen synthase kinase-3beta expression. *FASEB J.* **2003**, *17*, 1951–1953. [CrossRef]
111. Ozaki, T.; Li, Y.; Kikuchi, H.; Tomita, T.; Iwatsubo, T.; Nakagawara, A. The intracellular domain of the amyloid precursor protein (AICD) enhances the p53-mediated apoptosis. *Biochem. Biophys. Res. Commun.* **2006**, *351*, 57–63. [CrossRef]
112. Passer, B.; Pellegrini, L.; Russo, C.; Siegel, R.M.; Lenardo, M.J.; Schettini, G.; Bachmann, M.; Tabaton, M.; D'Adamio, L. Generation of an apoptotic intracellular peptide by gamma-secretase cleavage of Alzheimer's amyloid beta protein precursor. *J. Alzheimers Dis.* **2000**, *2*, 289–301. [CrossRef]
113. Milosch, N.; Tanriöver, G.; Kundu, A.; Rami, A.; François, J.C.; Baumkötter, F.; Weyer, S.W.; Samanta, A.; Jäschke, A.; Brod, F.; et al. Holo-APP and G-protein-mediated signaling are required for sAPPα-induced activation of the Akt survival pathway. *Cell Death Dis.* **2014**, *5*, e1391. [CrossRef] [PubMed]
114. Chasseigneaux, S.; Allinquant, B. Functions of Aβ, sAPPα and sAPPβ: Similarities and differences. *J. Neurochem.* **2012**, *120* (Suppl. S1), 99–108. [CrossRef] [PubMed]
115. Small, D.H.; Nurcombe, V.; Reed, G.; Clarris, H.; Moir, R.; Beyreuther, K.; Masters, C.L. A heparin-binding domain in the amyloid protein precursor of Alzheimer's disease is involved in the regulation of neurite outgrowth. *J. Neurosci.* **1994**, *14*, 2117–2127. [CrossRef] [PubMed]
116. Corrigan, F.; Vink, R.; Blumbergs, P.C.; Masters, C.L.; Cappai, R.; van den Heuvel, C. sAPPα rescues deficits in amyloid precursor protein knockout mice following focal traumatic brain injury. *J. Neurochem.* **2012**, *122*, 208–220. [CrossRef] [PubMed]
117. Fol, R.; Braudeau, J.; Ludewig, S.; Abel, T.; Weyer, S.W.; Roederer, J.P.; Brod, F.; Audrain, M.; Bemelmans, A.P.; Buchholz, C.J.; et al. Viral gene transfer of APPsα rescues synaptic failure in an Alzheimer's disease mouse model. *Acta Neuropathol.* **2016**, *131*, 247–266. [CrossRef]
118. Hick, M.; Herrmann, U.; Weyer, S.W.; Mallm, J.P.; Tschäpe, J.A.; Borgers, M.; Mercken, M.; Roth, F.C.; Draguhn, A.; Slomianka, L.; et al. Acute function of secreted amyloid precursor protein fragment APPsα in synaptic plasticity. *Acta Neuropathol.* **2015**, *129*, 21–37. [CrossRef]
119. Jäger, S.; Leuchtenberger, S.; Martin, A.; Czirr, E.; Wesselowski, J.; Dieckmann, M.; Waldron, E.; Korth, C.; Koo, E.H.; Heneka, M.; et al. alpha-secretase mediated conversion of the amyloid precursor protein derived membrane stub C99 to C83 limits Abeta generation. *J. Neurochem.* **2009**, *111*, 1369–1382. [CrossRef]
120. Tian, Y.; Crump, C.J.; Li, Y.M. Dual role of alpha-secretase cleavage in the regulation of gamma-secretase activity for amyloid production. *J. Biol. Chem.* **2010**, *285*, 32549–32556. [CrossRef]

121. Jang, H.; Arce, F.T.; Ramachandran, S.; Capone, R.; Azimova, R.; Kagan, B.L.; Nussinov, R.; Lal, R. Truncated beta-amyloid peptide channels provide an alternative mechanism for Alzheimer's Disease and Down syndrome. *Proc. Natl. Acad. Sci. USA* **2010**, *107*, 6538–6543. [CrossRef]
122. Gowing, E.; Roher, A.E.; Woods, A.S.; Cotter, R.J.; Chaney, M.; Little, S.P.; Ball, M.J. Chemical characterization of A beta 17-42 peptide, a component of diffuse amyloid deposits of Alzheimer disease. *J. Biol. Chem.* **1994**, *269*, 10987–10990. [CrossRef] [PubMed]
123. Szczepanik, A.M.; Rampe, D.; Ringheim, G.E. Amyloid-beta peptide fragments p3 and p4 induce pro-inflammatory cytokine and chemokine production in vitro and in vivo. *J. Neurochem.* **2001**, *77*, 304–317. [CrossRef] [PubMed]
124. Rice, H.C.; de Malmazet, D.; Schreurs, A.; Frere, S.; Van Molle, I.; Volkov, A.N.; Creemers, E.; Vertkin, I.; Nys, J.; Ranaivoson, F.M.; et al. Secreted amyloid-β precursor protein functions as a GABABR1a ligand to modulate synaptic transmission. *Science* **2019**, *363*, eaao4827. [CrossRef] [PubMed]
125. Wang, H.; Sang, N.; Zhang, C.; Raghupathi, R.; Tanzi, R.E.; Saunders, A.; Cathepsin, L. Mediates the Degradation of Novel APP C-Terminal Fragments. *Biochemistry* **2015**, *54*, 2806–2816. [CrossRef]
126. Armbrust, F.; Bickenbach, K.; Marengo, L.; Pietrzik, C.; Becker-Pauly, C. The Swedish dilemma-the almost exclusive use of APPswe-based mouse models impedes adequate evaluation of alternative β-secretases. *Biochim. Biophys. Acta Mol. Cell Res.* **2022**, *1869*, 119164. [CrossRef]
127. Vella, L.J.; Cappai, R. Identification of a novel amyloid precursor protein processing pathway that generates secreted N-terminal fragments. *FASEB J.* **2012**, *26*, 2930–2940. [CrossRef]
128. Lu, D.C.; Rabizadeh, S.; Chandra, S.; Shayya, R.F.; Ellerby, L.M.; Ye, X.; Salvesen, G.S.; Koo, E.H.; Bredesen, D.E. A second cytotoxic proteolytic peptide derived from amyloid beta-protein precursor. *Nat. Med.* **2000**, *6*, 397–404. [CrossRef]
129. Bertrand, E.; Brouillet, E.; Caillé, I.; Bouillot, C.; Cole, G.M.; Prochiantz, A.; Allinquant, B. A short cytoplasmic domain of the amyloid precursor protein induces apoptosis in vitro and in vivo. *Mol. Cell Neurosci.* **2001**, *18*, 503–511. [CrossRef]
130. De Chiara, G.; Marcocci, M.E.; Civitelli, L.; Argnani, R.; Piacentini, R.; Ripoli, C.; Manservigi, R.; Grassi, C.; Garaci, E.; Palamara, A.T. APP processing induced by herpes simplex virus type 1 (HSV-1) yields several APP fragments in human and rat neuronal cells. *PLoS ONE* **2010**, *5*, e13989. [CrossRef]
131. Racchi, M.; Govoni, S. Rationalizing a pharmacological intervention on the amyloid precursor protein metabolism. *Trends Pharmacol. Sci.* **1999**, *20*, 418–423. [CrossRef]
132. Racchi, M.; Govoni, S. The pharmacology of amyloid precursor protein processing. *Exp. Gerontol.* **2003**, *38*, 145–157. [CrossRef] [PubMed]
133. Kögel, D.; Deller, T.; Behl, C. Roles of amyloid precursor protein family members in neuroprotection, stress signaling and aging. *Exp. Brain Res.* **2012**, *217*, 471–479. [CrossRef]
134. Westmark, C.J. What's hAPPening at synapses? The role of amyloid β-protein precursor and β-amyloid in neurological disorders. *Mol. Psychiatry* **2013**, *18*, 425–434. [CrossRef] [PubMed]
135. Ray, B.; Long, J.M.; Sokol, D.K.; Lahiri, D.K. Increased secreted amyloid precursor protein-α (sAPPα) in severe autism: Proposal of a specific, anabolic pathway and putative biomarker. *PLoS ONE* **2011**, *6*, e20405. [CrossRef]
136. Sokol, D.K.; Chen, D.; Farlow, M.R.; Dunn, D.W.; Maloney, B.; Zimmer, J.A.; Lahiri, D.K. High levels of Alzheimer beta-amyloid precursor protein (APP) in children with severely autistic behavior and aggression. *J. Child Neurol.* **2006**, *21*, 444–449. [CrossRef]
137. Palmert, M.R.; Usiak, M.; Mayeux, R.; Raskind, M.; Tourtellotte, W.W.; Younkin, S.G. Soluble derivatives of the beta amyloid protein precursor in cerebrospinal fluid: Alterations in normal aging and in Alzheimer's disease. *Neurology* **1990**, *40*, 1028–1034. [CrossRef] [PubMed]
138. Van Nostrand, W.E.; Wagner, S.L.; Shankle, W.R.; Farrow, J.S.; Dick, M.; Rozemuller, J.M.; Kuiper, M.A.; Wolters, E.C.; Zimmerman, J.; Cotman, C.W.; et al. Decreased levels of soluble amyloid beta-protein precursor in cerebrospinal fluid of live Alzheimer disease patients. *Proc. Natl. Acad. Sci. USA* **1992**, *89*, 2551–2555. [CrossRef]
139. Bergamaschi, S.; Binetti, G.; Govoni, S.; Wetsel, W.C.; Battaini, F.; Trabucchi, M.; Bianchetti, A.; Racchi, M. Defective phorbol ester-stimulated secretion of beta-amyloid precursor protein from Alzheimer's disease fibroblasts. *Neurosci. Lett.* **1995**, *201*, 1–5. [CrossRef]
140. Mattson, M.P. Cellular actions of beta-amyloid precursor protein and its soluble and fibrillogenic derivatives. *Physiol. Rev.* **1997**, *77*, 1081–1132. [CrossRef]
141. Buoso, E.; Biundo, F.; Lanni, C.; Aiello, S.; Grossi, S.; Schettini, G.; Govoni, S.; Racchi, M. Modulation of Rack-1/PKCβII signalling by soluble AβPPα in SH-SY5Y cells. *Curr. Alzheimer Res.* **2013**, *10*, 697–705. [CrossRef]
142. Thornton, E.; Vink, R.; Blumbergs, P.C.; Van Den Heuvel, C. Soluble amyloid precursor protein alpha reduces neuronal injury and improves functional outcome following diffuse traumatic brain injury in rats. *Brain Res.* **2006**, *1094*, 38–46. [CrossRef] [PubMed]
143. Kovalevich, J.; Santerre, M.; Langford, D. Considerations for the Use of SH-SY5Y Neuroblastoma Cells in Neurobiology. *Methods Mol. Biol.* **2021**, *2311*, 9–23. [CrossRef] [PubMed]
144. Skotak, M.; Wang, F.; Chandra, N. An in vitro injury model for SH-SY5Y neuroblastoma cells: Effect of strain and strain rate. *J. Neurosci. Methods* **2012**, *205*, 159–168. [CrossRef] [PubMed]
145. Gakhar-Koppole, N.; Hundeshagen, P.; Mandl, C.; Weyer, S.W.; Allinquant, B.; Müller, U.; Ciccolini, F. Activity requires soluble amyloid precursor protein alpha to promote neurite outgrowth in neural stem cell-derived neurons via activation of the MAPK pathway. *Eur. J. Neurosci.* **2008**, *28*, 871–882. [CrossRef]

146. Dong, Y.; Li, T.; Ma, Z.; Zhou, C.; Wang, X.; Li, J. HSPA1A, HSPA2, and HSPA8 Are Potential Molecular Biomarkers for Prognosis among HSP70 Family in Alzheimer's Disease. *Dis. Markers* **2022**, *2022*, 9480398. [CrossRef]
147. Hoffman, J.L.; Faccidomo, S.; Kim, M.; Taylor, S.M.; Agoglia, A.E.; May, A.M.; Smith, E.N.; Wong, L.C.; Hodge, C.W. Alcohol drinking exacerbates neural and behavioral pathology in the 3xTg-AD mouse model of Alzheimer's disease. *Int. Rev. Neurobiol.* **2019**, *148*, 169–230. [CrossRef]
148. Ramos, E.; Romero, A.; Marco-Contelles, J.; López-Muñoz, F.; Del Pino, J. Modulation of Heat Shock Response Proteins by ASS234, Targeted for Neurodegenerative Diseases Therapy. *Chem. Res. Toxicol.* **2018**, *31*, 839–842. [CrossRef]
149. Von Wittgenstein, J.; Zheng, F.; Wittmann, M.T.; Balta, E.A.; Ferrazzi, F.; Schäffner, I.; Häberle, B.M.; Valero-Aracama, M.J.; Koehl, M.; Miranda, C.J.; et al. Sox11 is an Activity-Regulated Gene with Dentate-Gyrus-Specific Expression Upon General Neural Activation. *Cereb. Cortex* **2020**, *30*, 3731–3743. [CrossRef]
150. Li, Y.; Struebing, F.L.; Wang, J.; King, R.; Geisert, E.E. Different Effect of Sox11 in Retinal Ganglion Cells Survival and Axon Regeneration. *Front. Genet.* **2018**, *9*, 633. [CrossRef]
151. Jankowski, M.P.; McIlwrath, S.L.; Jing, X.; Cornuet, P.K.; Salerno, K.M.; Koerber, H.R.; Albers, K.M. Sox11 transcription factor modulates peripheral nerve regeneration in adult mice. *Brain Res.* **2009**, *1256*, 43–54. [CrossRef]
152. Salerno, K.M.; Jing, X.; Diges, C.M.; Cornuet, P.K.; Glorioso, J.C.; Albers, K.M. Sox11 modulates brain-derived neurotrophic factor expression in an exon promoter-specific manner. *J. Neurosci. Res.* **2012**, *90*, 1011–1019. [CrossRef] [PubMed]
153. Guo, Y.; Liu, S.; Zhang, X.; Wang, L.; Zhang, X.; Hao, A.; Han, A.; Yang, J. Sox11 promotes endogenous neurogenesis and locomotor recovery in mice spinal cord injury. *Biochem. Biophys. Res. Commun.* **2014**, *446*, 830–835. [CrossRef] [PubMed]
154. Uemura, T.; Sato, T.; Aoki, T.; Yamamoto, A.; Okada, T.; Hirai, R.; Harada, R.; Mori, K.; Tagaya, M.; Harada, A. p31 deficiency influences endoplasmic reticulum tubular morphology and cell survival. *Mol. Cell Biol.* **2009**, *29*, 1869–1881. [CrossRef] [PubMed]
155. Parnell, E.; Shapiro, L.P.; Voorn, R.A.; Forrest, M.P.; Jalloul, H.A.; Loizzo, D.D.; Penzes, P. KALRN: A central regulator of synaptic function and synaptopathies. *Gene* **2021**, *768*, 145306. [CrossRef]
156. Russo-Savage, L.; Rao, V.K.S.; Eipper, B.A.; Mains, R.E. Role of Kalirin and mouse strain in retention of spatial memory training in an Alzheimer's disease model mouse line. *Neurobiol. Aging* **2020**, *95*, 69–80. [CrossRef]
157. Xie, Z.; Shapiro, L.P.; Cahill, M.E.; Russell, T.A.; Lacor, P.N.; Klein, W.L.; Penzes, P. Kalirin-7 prevents dendritic spine dysgenesis induced by amyloid beta-derived oligomers. *Eur. J. Neurosci.* **2019**, *49*, 1091–1101. [CrossRef]
158. Liu, M.; Zhong, W.; Li, C.; Su, W. Fluoxetine attenuates apoptosis in early brain injury after subarachnoid hemorrhage through Notch1/ASK1/p38 MAPK signaling pathway. *Bioengineered* **2022**, *13*, 8396–8411. [CrossRef]
159. Yeo, E.J.; Eum, W.S.; Yeo, H.J.; Choi, Y.J.; Sohn, E.J.; Kwon, H.J.; Kim, D.W.; Kim, D.S.; Cho, S.W.; Park, J.; et al. Protective Role of Transduced Tat-Thioredoxin1 (Trx1) against Oxidative Stress-Induced Neuronal Cell Death via ASK1-MAPK Signal Pathway. *Biomol. Ther.* **2021**, *29*, 321–330. [CrossRef]
160. Gómora-García, J.C.; Gerónimo-Olvera, C.; Pérez-Martínez, X.; Massieu, L. IRE1α RIDD activity induced under ER stress drives neuronal death by the degradation of 14-3-3 θ mRNA in cortical neurons during glucose deprivation. *Cell Death Discov.* **2021**, *7*, 131. [CrossRef]
161. Zou, D.; Li, R.; Huang, X.; Chen, G.; Liu, Y.; Meng, Y.; Wang, Y.; Wu, Y.; Mao, Y. Identification of molecular correlations of RBM8A with autophagy in Alzheimer's disease. *Aging* **2019**, *11*, 11673–11685. [CrossRef]
162. Maekawa, M.; Iwayama, Y.; Ohnishi, T.; Toyoshima, M.; Shimamoto, C.; Hisano, Y.; Toyota, T.; Balan, S.; Matsuzaki, H.; Iwata, Y.; et al. Investigation of the fatty acid transporter-encoding genes SLC27A3 and SLC27A4 in autism. *Sci. Rep.* **2015**, *5*, 16239. [CrossRef]
163. Fernandes, N.; Buchan, J.R. RPS28B mRNA acts as a scaffold promoting cis-translational interaction of proteins driving P-body assembly. *Nucleic Acids Res.* **2020**, *48*, 6265–6279. [CrossRef] [PubMed]
164. Riggs, C.L.; Kedersha, N.; Ivanov, P.; Anderson, P. Mammalian stress granules and P bodies at a glance. *J. Cell Sci.* **2020**, *133*, jcs242487. [CrossRef] [PubMed]
165. Singh, B.K.; Vatsa, N.; Kumar, V.; Shekhar, S.; Sharma, A.; Jana, N.R. Ube3a deficiency inhibits amyloid plaque formation in APPswe/PS1δE9 mouse model of Alzheimer's disease. *Hum. Mol. Genet.* **2017**, *26*, 4042–4054. [CrossRef]
166. Olabarria, M.; Pasini, S.; Corona, C.; Robador, P.; Song, C.; Patel, H.; Lefort, R. Dysfunction of the ubiquitin ligase E3A Ube3A/E6-AP contributes to synaptic pathology in Alzheimer's disease. *Commun. Biol.* **2019**, *2*, 111. [CrossRef]
167. Sacco, A.; Martelli, F.; Pal, A.; Saraceno, C.; Benussi, L.; Ghidoni, R.; Rongioletti, M.; Squitti, R. Regulatory miRNAs in Cardiovascular and Alzheimer's Disease: A Focus on Copper. *Int. J. Mol. Sci.* **2022**, *23*, 3327. [CrossRef] [PubMed]
168. Taylor, H.A.; Przemylska, L.; Clavane, E.M.; Meakin, P.J. BACE1, More than just a β-secretase. *Obes. Rev.* **2022**, *23*, e13430. [CrossRef]
169. Peters-Libeu, C.; Campagna, J.; Mitsumori, M.; Poksay, K.S.; Spilman, P.; Sabogal, A.; Bredesen, D.E.; John, V. sAβPPα is a Potent Endogenous Inhibitor of BACE1. *J. Alzheimers Dis.* **2015**, *47*, 545–555. [CrossRef]
170. Obregon, D.; Hou, H.; Deng, J.; Giunta, B.; Tian, J.; Darlington, D.; Shahaduzzaman, M.; Zhu, Y.; Mori, T.; Mattson, M.P.; et al. Soluble amyloid precursor protein-α modulates β-secretase activity and amyloid-β generation. *Nat. Commun.* **2012**, *3*, 777. [CrossRef]
171. Deng, J.; Habib, A.; Obregon, D.F.; Barger, S.W.; Giunta, B.; Wang, Y.J.; Hou, H.; Sawmiller, D.; Tan, J. Soluble amyloid precursor protein alpha inhibits tau phosphorylation through modulation of GSK3β signaling pathway. *J. Neurochem.* **2015**, *135*, 630–637. [CrossRef]

172. Tiwari-Woodruff, S.K.; Kaplan, R.; Kornblum, H.I.; Bronstein, J.M. Developmental expression of OAP-1/Tspan-3, a member of the tetraspanin superfamily. *J. Neurosci. Res.* **2004**, *77*, 166–173. [CrossRef] [PubMed]
173. Hemler, M.E. Tetraspanin functions and associated microdomains. *Nat. Rev. Mol. Cell Biol.* **2005**, *6*, 801–811. [CrossRef] [PubMed]
174. Boucheix, C.; Rubinstein, E. Tetraspanins. *Cell Mol. Life Sci.* **2001**, *58*, 1189–1205. [CrossRef]
175. Charrin, S.; le Naour, F.; Silvie, O.; Milhiet, P.E.; Boucheix, C.; Rubinstein, E. Lateral organization of membrane proteins: Tetraspanins spin their web. *Biochem. J.* **2009**, *420*, 133–154. [CrossRef]
176. Hemler, M.E. Tetraspanin proteins mediate cellular penetration, invasion, and fusion events and define a novel type of membrane microdomain. *Annu. Rev. Cell Dev. Biol.* **2003**, *19*, 397–422. [CrossRef]
177. Yáñez-Mó, M.; Barreiro, O.; Gordon-Alonso, M.; Sala-Valdés, M.; Sánchez-Madrid, F. Tetraspanin-enriched microdomains: A functional unit in cell plasma membranes. *Trends Cell Biol.* **2009**, *19*, 434–446. [CrossRef]
178. Charrin, S.; Jouannet, S.; Boucheix, C.; Rubinstein, E. Tetraspanins at a glance. *J. Cell Sci.* **2014**, *127*, 3641–3648. [CrossRef] [PubMed]
179. Bassani, S.; Cingolani, L.A.; Valnegri, P.; Folci, A.; Zapata, J.; Gianfelice, A.; Sala, C.; Goda, Y.; Passafaro, M. The X-linked intellectual disability protein TSPAN7 regulates excitatory synapse development and AMPAR trafficking. *Neuron* **2012**, *73*, 1143–1158. [CrossRef]
180. Murru, L.; Vezzoli, E.; Longatti, A.; Ponzoni, L.; Falqui, A.; Folci, A.; Moretto, E.; Bianchi, V.; Braida, D.; Sala, M.; et al. Pharmacological Modulation of AMPAR Rescues Intellectual Disability-Like Phenotype in Tm4sf2-/y Mice. *Cereb. Cortex* **2017**, *27*, 5369–5384. [CrossRef]
181. Murru, L.; Moretto, E.; Martano, G.; Passafaro, M. Tetraspanins shape the synapse. *Mol. Cell Neurosci.* **2018**, *91*, 76–81. [CrossRef]
182. Tiwari-Woodruff, S.K.; Buznikov, A.G.; Vu, T.Q.; Micevych, P.E.; Chen, K.; Kornblum, H.I.; Bronstein, J.M. OSP/claudin-11 forms a complex with a novel member of the tetraspanin super family and beta1 integrin and regulates proliferation and migration of oligodendrocytes. *J. Cell Biol.* **2001**, *153*, 295–305. [CrossRef] [PubMed]
183. Thiede-Stan, N.K.; Tews, B.; Albrecht, D.; Ristic, Z.; Ewers, H.; Schwab, M.E. Tetraspanin-3 is an organizer of the multi-subunit Nogo-A signaling complex. *J. Cell Sci.* **2015**, *128*, 3583–3596. [CrossRef] [PubMed]
184. Seipold, L.; Damme, M.; Prox, J.; Rabe, B.; Kasparek, P.; Sedlacek, R.; Altmeppen, H.; Willem, M.; Boland, B.; Glatzel, M.; et al. Tetraspanin 3, A central endocytic membrane component regulating the expression of ADAM10, presenilin and the amyloid precursor protein. *Biochim. Biophys. Acta Mol. Cell Res.* **2017**, *1864*, 217–230. [CrossRef] [PubMed]
185. Martinez, C.; González-Ramírez, J.; Marín, M.E.; Martínez-Coronilla, G.; Meza-Reyna, V.I.; Mora, R.; Díaz-Molina, R. Isthmin 2 is decreased in preeclampsia and highly expressed in choriocarcinoma. *Heliyon* **2020**, *6*, e05096. [CrossRef]
186. Hu, M.; Zhang, X.; Hu, C.; Teng, T.; Tang, Q.Z. A brief overview about the adipokine: Isthmin-1. *Front. Cardiovasc. Med.* **2022**, *9*, 939757. [CrossRef]
187. Yoshimoto, S.; Katayama, K.; Suzuki, T.; Dohmae, N.; Simizu, S. Regulation of N-glycosylation and secretion of Isthmin-1 by its C-mannosylation. *Biochim. Biophys. Acta Gen. Subj.* **2021**, *1865*, 129840. [CrossRef]
188. Xiang, W.; Ke, Z.; Zhang, Y.; Cheng, G.H.; Irwan, I.D.; Sulochana, K.N.; Potturi, P.; Wang, Z.; Yang, H.; Wang, J.; et al. Isthmin is a novel secreted angiogenesis inhibitor that inhibits tumour growth in mice. *J. Cell Mol. Med.* **2011**, *15*, 359–374. [CrossRef]
189. Zhang, Y.; Chen, M.; Venugopal, S.; Zhou, Y.; Xiang, W.; Li, Y.H.; Lin, Q.; Kini, R.M.; Chong, Y.S.; Ge, R. Isthmin exerts pro-survival and death-promoting effect on endothelial cells through alphavbeta5 integrin depending on its physical state. *Cell Death Dis.* **2011**, *2*, e153. [CrossRef]
190. Yuan, B.; Xian, R.; Ma, J.; Chen, Y.; Lin, C.; Song, Y. Isthmin inhibits glioma growth through antiangiogenesis in vivo. *J. Neurooncol.* **2012**, *109*, 245–252. [CrossRef]
191. Jiang, Z.; Zhao, M.; Voilquin, L.; Jung, Y.; Aikio, M.A.; Sahai, T.; Dou, F.Y.; Roche, A.M.; Carcamo-Orive, I.; Knowles, J.W.; et al. Isthmin-1 is an adipokine that promotes glucose uptake and improves glucose tolerance and hepatic steatosis. *Cell Metab.* **2021**, *33*, 1836–1852.e11. [CrossRef]
192. GeneCards. Available online: https://www.genecards.org/cgi-bin/carddisp.pl?gene=ISM2 (accessed on 10 October 2022).
193. Kundu, B.; Brock, A.A.; Englot, D.J.; Butson, C.R.; Rolston, J.D. Deep brain stimulation for the treatment of disorders of consciousness and cognition in traumatic brain injury patients: A review. *Neurosurg. Focus* **2018**, *45*, E14. [CrossRef]
194. Aronson, J.P.; Katnani, H.A.; Huguenard, A.; Mulvaney, G.; Bader, E.R.; Yang, J.C.; Eskandar, E.N. Phasic stimulation in the nucleus accumbens enhances learning after traumatic brain injury. *Cereb. Cortex Commun.* **2022**, *3*, tgac016. [CrossRef] [PubMed]
195. Osera, C.; Fassina, L.; Amadio, M.; Venturini, L.; Buoso, E.; Magenes, G.; Govoni, S.; Ricevuti, G.; Pascale, A. Cytoprotective response induced by electromagnetic stimulation on SH-SY5Y human neuroblastoma cell line. *Tissue Eng. Part A* **2011**, *17*, 2573–2582. [CrossRef] [PubMed]
196. Bolatai, A.; He, Y.; Wu, N. Vascular endothelial growth factor and its receptors regulation in gestational diabetes mellitus and eclampsia. *J. Transl. Med.* **2022**, *20*, 400. [CrossRef]
197. Apte, R.S.; Chen, D.S.; Ferrara, N. VEGF in Signaling and Disease: Beyond Discovery and Development. *Cell* **2019**, *176*, 1248–1264. [CrossRef]
198. Shi, Y.; Hu, Y.; Cui, B.; Zhuang, S.; Liu, N. Vascular endothelial growth factor-mediated peritoneal neoangiogenesis in peritoneal dialysis. *Perit. Dial. Int.* **2022**, *42*, 25–38. [CrossRef] [PubMed]
199. Theis, V.; Theiss, C. VEGF—A Stimulus for Neuronal Development and Regeneration in the CNS and PNS. *Curr. Protein. Pept. Sci.* **2018**, *19*, 589–597. [CrossRef]

200. Okabe, K.; Fukada, H.; Tai-Nagara, I.; Ando, T.; Honda, T.; Nakajima, K.; Takeda, N.; Fong, G.H.; Ema, M.; Kubota, Y. Neuron-derived VEGF contributes to cortical and hippocampal development independently of VEGFR1/2-mediated neurotrophism. *Dev. Biol.* **2020**, *459*, 65–71. [CrossRef]
201. Ureña-Guerrero, M.E.; Castañeda-Cabral, J.L.; Rivera-Cervantes, M.C.; Macias-Velez, R.J.; Jarero-Basulto, J.J.; Gudiño-Cabrera, G.; Beas-Zárate, C. Neuroprotective and Neurorestorative Effects of Epo and VEGF: Perspectives for New Therapeutic Approaches to Neurological Diseases. *Curr. Pharm. Des.* **2020**, *26*, 1263–1276. [CrossRef]
202. Carmeliet, P.; Ruiz de Almodovar, C. VEGF ligands and receptors: Implications in neurodevelopment and neurodegeneration. *Cell Mol. Life Sci.* **2013**, *70*, 1763–1778. [CrossRef]
203. Chiappelli, M.; Borroni, B.; Archetti, S.; Calabrese, E.; Corsi, M.M.; Franceschi, M.; Padovani, A.; Licastro, F. VEGF gene and phenotype relation with Alzheimer's disease and mild cognitive impairment. *Rejuvenation Res.* **2006**, *9*, 485–493. [CrossRef] [PubMed]
204. Xu, K.; Wu, C.L.; Wang, Z.X.; Wang, H.J.; Yin, F.J.; Li, W.D.; Liu, C.C.; Fan, H.N. VEGF Family Gene Expression as Prognostic Biomarkers for Alzheimer's Disease and Primary Liver Cancer. *Comput. Math Methods Med.* **2021**, *2021*, 3422393. [CrossRef] [PubMed]
205. Harper, S.J.; Bates, D.O. VEGF-A splicing: The key to anti-angiogenic therapeutics? *Nat. Rev. Cancer* **2008**, *8*, 880–887. [CrossRef]
206. Jackson, M.W.; Bentel, J.M.; Tilley, W.D. Vascular endothelial growth factor (VEGF) expression in prostate cancer and benign prostatic hyperplasia. *J. Urol.* **1997**, *157*, 2323–2328. [CrossRef]
207. Bucolo, C.; Barbieri, A.; Viganò, I.; Marchesi, N.; Bandello, F.; Drago, F.; Govoni, S.; Zerbini, G.; Pascale, A. Short-and Long-Term Expression of Vegf: A Temporal Regulation of a Key Factor in Diabetic Retinopathy. *Front. Pharmacol.* **2021**, *12*, 707909. [CrossRef] [PubMed]
208. Fahmideh, F.; Marchesi, N.; Campagnoli, L.I.M.; Landini, L.; Caramella, C.; Barbieri, A.; Govoni, S.; Pascale, A. Effect of troxerutin in counteracting hyperglycemia-induced VEGF upregulation in endothelial cells: A new option to target early stages of diabetic retinopathy? *Front. Pharmacol.* **2022**, *13*, 951833. [CrossRef] [PubMed]
209. Amadio, M.; Scapagnini, G.; Lupo, G.; Drago, F.; Govoni, S.; Pascale, A. PKCbetaII/HuR/VEGF: A new molecular cascade in retinal pericytes for the regulation of VEGF gene expression. *Pharmacol Res.* **2008**, *57*, 60–66. [CrossRef]
210. Pascale, A.; Govoni, S. The complex world of post-transcriptional mechanisms: Is their deregulation a common link for diseases? Focus on ELAV-like RNA-binding proteins. *Cell Mol. Life Sci.* **2012**, *69*, 501–517. [CrossRef]
211. Deschênes-Furry, J.; Perrone-Bizzozero, N.; Jasmin, B.J. The RNA-binding protein HuD: A regulator of neuronal differentiation, maintenance and plasticity. *Bioessays* **2006**, *28*, 822–833. [CrossRef]
212. Quattrone, A.; Pascale, A.; Nogues, X.; Zhao, W.; Gusev, P.; Pacini, A.; Alkon, D.L. Posttranscriptional regulation of gene expression in learning by the neuronal ELAV-like mRNA-stabilizing proteins. *Proc. Natl. Acad. Sci. USA* **2001**, *98*, 11668–11673. [CrossRef]
213. Pascale, A.; Gusev, P.A.; Amadio, M.; Dottorini, T.; Govoni, S.; Alkon, D.L.; Quattrone, A. Increase of the RNA-binding protein HuD and posttranscriptional up-regulation of the GAP-43 gene during spatial memory. *Proc. Natl. Acad. Sci. USA* **2004**, *101*, 1217–1222. [CrossRef] [PubMed]
214. Pascale, A.; Amadio, M.; Scapagnini, G.; Lanni, C.; Racchi, M.; Provenzani, A.; Govoni, S.; Alkon, D.L.; Quattrone, A. Neuronal ELAV proteins enhance mRNA stability by a PKCalpha-dependent pathway. *Proc. Natl. Acad. Sci. USA* **2005**, *102*, 12065–12070. [CrossRef] [PubMed]
215. Amadio, M.; Pascale, A.; Wang, J.; Ho, L.; Quattrone, A.; Gandy, S.; Haroutunian, V.; Racchi, M.; Pasinetti, G.M. nELAV proteins alteration in Alzheimer's disease brain: A novel putative target for amyloid-beta reverberating on AbetaPP processing. *J. Alzheimers Dis.* **2009**, *16*, 409–419. [CrossRef] [PubMed]
216. Marchesi, N.; Amadio, M.; Colombrita, C.; Govoni, S.; Ratti, A.; Pascale, A. PKC Activation Counteracts ADAM10 Deficit in HuD-Silenced Neuroblastoma Cells. *J. Alzheimers Dis.* **2016**, *54*, 535–547. [CrossRef] [PubMed]
217. Guo, H.; Xia, D.; Liao, S.; Niu, B.; Tang, J.; Hu, H.; Qian, H.; Cao, B. Vascular endothelial growth factor improves the cognitive decline of Alzheimer's disease via concurrently inducing the expression of ADAM10 and reducing the expression of β-site APP cleaving enzyme 1 in Tg2576 mice. *Neurosci. Res.* **2019**, *142*, 49–57. [CrossRef]
218. Baker, T.L.; Agoston, D.V.; Brady, R.D.; Major, B.; McDonald, S.J.; Mychasiuk, R.; Wright, D.K.; Yamakawa, G.R.; Sun, M.; Shultz, S.R. Targeting the Cerebrovascular System: Next-Generation Biomarkers and Treatment for Mild Traumatic Brain Injury. *Neuroscientist* **2021**, *28*, 594–612. [CrossRef]
219. Wang, K.; Jing, Y.; Xu, C.; Zhao, J.; Gong, Q.; Chen, S. HIF-1α and VEGF Are Involved in Deferoxamine-Ameliorated Traumatic Brain Injury. *J. Surg. Res.* **2020**, *246*, 419–426. [CrossRef]
220. Xu, Y.Q.; Sun, Z.Q.; Wang, Y.T.; Xiao, F.; Chen, M.W. Function of Nogo-A/Nogo-A receptor in Alzheimer's disease. *CNS Neurosci. Ther.* **2015**, *21*, 479–485. [CrossRef]
221. Corrigan, F.; Thornton, E.; Roisman, L.C.; Leonard, A.V.; Vink, R.; Blumbergs, P.C.; van den Heuvel, C.; Cappai, R. The neuroprotective activity of the amyloid precursor protein against traumatic brain injury is mediated via the heparin binding site in residues 96–110. *J. Neurochem.* **2014**, *128*, 196–204. [CrossRef]
222. Plummer, S.L.; Corrigan, F.; Thornton, E.; Woenig, J.A.; Vink, R.; Cappai, R.; Van Den Heuvel, C. The amyloid precursor protein derivative, APP96-110, is efficacious following intravenous administration after traumatic brain injury. *PLoS ONE* **2018**, *13*, e0190449. [CrossRef]

223. Hodgetts, S.I.; Lovett, S.J.; Baron-Heeris, D.; Fogliani, A.; Sturm, M.; Van den Heuvel, C.; Harvey, A.R. Effects of amyloid precursor protein peptide APP96-110, alone or with human mesenchymal stromal cells, on recovery after spinal cord injury. *Neural. Regen. Res.* **2022**, *17*, 1376–1386. [CrossRef] [PubMed]
224. Mockett, B.G.; Richter, M.; Abraham, W.C.; Müller, U.C. Therapeutic Potential of Secreted Amyloid Precursor Protein APPsα. *Front. Mol. Neurosci.* **2017**, *10*, 30. [CrossRef]
225. Mockett, B.G.; Ryan, M.M. The therapeutic potential of the neuroactive peptides of soluble amyloid precursor protein-alpha in Alzheimer's disease and related neurological disorders. *Semin. Cell Dev. Biol.* **2022**, *139*, 93–101. [CrossRef] [PubMed]
226. Buoso, E.; Lanni, C.; Molteni, E.; Rousset, F.; Corsini, E.; Racchi, M. Opposing effects of cortisol and dehydroepiandrosterone on the expression of the receptor for Activated C Kinase 1: Implications in immunosenescence. *Exp. Gerontol.* **2011**, *46*, 877–883. [CrossRef]
227. Buoso, E.; Galasso, M.; Ronfani, M.; Serafini, M.M.; Lanni, C.; Corsini, E.; Racchi, M. Role of spliceosome proteins in the regulation of glucocorticoid receptor isoforms by cortisol and dehydroepiandrosterone. *Pharmacol. Res.* **2017**, *120*, 180–187. [CrossRef]
228. Buoso, E.; Galasso, M.; Ronfani, M.; Papale, A.; Galbiati, V.; Eberini, I.; Marinovich, M.; Racchi, M.; Corsini, E. The scaffold protein RACK1 is a target of endocrine disrupting chemicals (EDCs) with important implication in immunity. *Toxicol. Appl. Pharmacol.* **2017**, *325*, 37–47. [CrossRef]
229. Racchi, M.; Buoso, E.; Ronfani, M.; Serafini, M.M.; Galasso, M.; Lanni, C.; Corsini, E. Role of Hormones in the Regulation of RACK1 Expression as a Signaling Checkpoint in Immunosenescence. *Int. J. Mol. Sci.* **2017**, *18*, 1453. [CrossRef]
230. Buoso, E.; Masi, M.; Galbiati, V.; Maddalon, A.; Iulini, M.; Kenda, M.; Sollner Dolenc, M.; Marinovich, M.; Racchi, M.; Corsini, E. Effect of estrogen-active compounds on the expression of RACK1 and immunological implications. *Arch. Toxicol.* **2020**, *94*, 2081–2095. [CrossRef]
231. Corsini, E.; Buoso, E.; Galbiati, V.; Racchi, M. Role of Protein Kinase C in Immune Cell Activation and Its Implication Chemical-Induced Immunotoxicity. *Adv. Exp. Med. Biol.* **2021**, *1275*, 151–163. [CrossRef] [PubMed]
232. Buoso, E.; Kenda, M.; Masi, M.; Linciano, P.; Galbiati, V.; Racchi, M.; Dolenc, M.S.; Corsini, E. Effects of Bisphenols on RACK1 Expression and Their Immunological Implications in THP-1 Cells. *Front. Pharmacol.* **2021**, *12*, 743991. [CrossRef]
233. Galbiati, V.; Buoso, E.; d'Emmanuele di Villa Bianca, R.; Paola, R.D.; Morroni, F.; Nocentini, G.; Racchi, M.; Viviani, B.; Corsini, E. Immune and Nervous Systems Interaction in Endocrine Disruptors Toxicity: The Case of Atrazine. *Front. Toxicol.* **2021**, *3*, 649024. [CrossRef] [PubMed]
234. Maddalon, A.; Masi, M.; Iulini, M.; Linciano, P.; Galbiati, V.; Marinovich, M.; Racchi, M.; Buoso, E.; Corsini, E. Effects of endocrine active contaminating pesticides on RACK1 expression and immunological consequences in THP-1 cells. *Environ. Toxicol. Pharmacol.* **2022**, *95*, 103971. [CrossRef] [PubMed]
235. Masi, M.; Maddalon, A.; Iulini, M.; Linciano, P.; Galbiati, V.; Marinovich, M.; Racchi, M.; Corsini, E.; Buoso, E. Effects of endocrine disrupting chemicals on the expression of RACK1 and LPS-induced THP-1 cell activation. *Toxicology* **2022**, *480*, 153321. [CrossRef] [PubMed]
236. Buoso, E.; Ronfani, M.; Galasso, M.; Ventura, D.; Corsini, E.; Racchi, M. Cortisol-induced SRSF3 expression promotes GR splicing, RACK1 expression and breast cancer cells migration. *Pharmacol. Res.* **2019**, *143*, 17–26. [CrossRef]
237. Buoso, E.; Masi, M.; Long, A.; Chiappini, C.; Travelli, C.; Govoni, S.; Racchi, M. Ribosomes as a nexus between translation and cancer progression: Focus on ribosomal Receptor for Activated C Kinase 1 (RACK1) in breast cancer. *Br. J. Pharmacol.* **2022**, *179*, 2813–2828. [CrossRef]
238. Buoso, E.; Masi, M.; Racchi, M.; Corsini, E. Endocrine-Disrupting Chemicals' (EDCs) Effects on Tumour Microenvironment and Cancer Progression: Emerging Contribution of RACK1. *Int. J. Mol. Sci.* **2020**, *21*, 9229. [CrossRef]
239. Masi, M.; Garattini, E.; Bolis, M.; Di Marino, D.; Maraccani, L.; Morelli, E.; Grolla, A.A.; Fagiani, F.; Corsini, E.; Travelli, C.; et al. OXER1 and RACK1-associated pathway: A promising drug target for breast cancer progression. *Oncogenesis* **2020**, *9*, 105. [CrossRef]
240. Masi, M.; Racchi, M.; Travelli, C.; Corsini, E.; Buoso, E. Molecular Characterization of Membrane Steroid Receptors in Hormone-Sensitive Cancers. *Cells* **2021**, *10*, 2999. [CrossRef]
241. Cheng, Z.F.; Cartwright, C.A. Rack1 maintains intestinal homeostasis by protecting the integrity of the epithelial barrier. *Am. J. Physiol. Gastrointest Liver Physiol.* **2018**, *314*, G263–G274. [CrossRef]
242. Cheng, Z.F.; Pai, R.K.; Cartwright, C.A. Rack1 function in intestinal epithelia: Regulating crypt cell proliferation and regeneration and promoting differentiation and apoptosis. *Am. J. Physiol. Gastrointest Liver Physiol.* **2018**, *314*, G1–G13. [CrossRef]
243. Kershner, L.; Welshhans, K. RACK1 regulates neural development. *Neural. Regen. Res.* **2017**, *12*, 1036–1039. [CrossRef] [PubMed]
244. Buoso, E.; Biundo, F.; Lanni, C.; Schettini, G.; Govoni, S.; Racchi, M. AβPP intracellular C-terminal domain function is related to its degradation processes. *J. Alzheimers Dis.* **2012**, *30*, 393–405. [CrossRef] [PubMed]
245. Battaini, F.; Pascale, A.; Paoletti, R.; Govoni, S. The role of anchoring protein RACK1 in PKC activation in the ageing rat brain. *Trends Neurosci.* **1997**, *20*, 410–415. [CrossRef]
246. Dwane, S.; Durack, E.; O'Connor, R.; Kiely, P.A. RACK1 promotes neurite outgrowth by scaffolding AGAP2 to FAK. *Cell Signal.* **2014**, *26*, 9–18. [CrossRef]
247. Kershner, L.; Welshhans, K. RACK1 is necessary for the formation of point contacts and regulates axon growth. *Dev. Neurobiol.* **2017**, *77*, 1038–1056. [CrossRef] [PubMed]

248. Romano, N.; Di Giacomo, B.; Nobile, V.; Borreca, A.; Willems, D.; Tilesi, F.; Catalani, E.; Agrawal, M.; Welshhans, K.; Ricciardi, S.; et al. Ribosomal RACK1 Regulates the Dendritic Arborization by Repressing FMRP Activity. *Int. J. Mol. Sci.* **2022**, *23*, 11857. [CrossRef] [PubMed]
249. Zhu, Q.; Chen, L.; Li, Y.; Huang, M.; Shao, J.; Li, S.; Cheng, J.; Yang, H.; Wu, Y.; Zhang, J.; et al. Rack1 is essential for corticogenesis by preventing p21-dependent senescence in neural stem cells. *Cell. Rep.* **2021**, *36*, 109639. [CrossRef]
250. Yaka, R.; Thornton, C.; Vagts, A.J.; Phamluong, K.; Bonci, A.; Ron, D. NMDA receptor function is regulated by the inhibitory scaffolding protein, RACK1. *Proc. Natl. Acad. Sci. USA* **2002**, *99*, 5710–5715. [CrossRef]
251. Ma, J.; Wu, R.; Zhang, Q.; Wu, J.B.; Lou, J.; Zheng, Z.; Ding, J.Q.; Yuan, Z. DJ-1 interacts with RACK1 and protects neurons from oxidative-stress-induced apoptosis. *Biochem. J.* **2014**, *462*, 489–497. [CrossRef]
252. He, D.Y.; Neasta, J.; Ron, D. Epigenetic regulation of BDNF expression via the scaffolding protein RACK1. *J. Biol. Chem.* **2010**, *285*, 19043–19050. [CrossRef]
253. Neasta, J.; Kiely, P.A.; He, D.Y.; Adams, D.R.; O'Connor, R.; Ron, D. Direct interaction between scaffolding proteins RACK1 and 14-3-3? regulates brain-derived neurotrophic factor (BDNF) transcription. *J. Biol. Chem.* **2012**, *287*, 322–336. [CrossRef]
254. Brivio, P.; Buoso, E.; Masi, M.; Gallo, M.T.; Gruca, P.; Lason, M.; Litwa, E.; Papp, M.; Fumagalli, F.; Racchi, M.; et al. The coupling of RACK1 with the beta isoform of the glucocorticoid receptor promotes resilience to chronic stress exposure. *Neurobiol. Stress* **2021**, *15*, 100372. [CrossRef] [PubMed]
255. Pascale, A.; Fortino, I.; Govoni, S.; Trabucchi, M.; Wetsel, W.C.; Battaini, F. Functional impairment in protein kinase C by RACK1 (receptor for activated C kinase 1) deficiency in aged rat brain cortex. *J. Neurochem.* **1996**, *67*, 2471–2477. [CrossRef] [PubMed]
256. Battaini, F.; Pascale, A.; Lucchi, L.; Pasinetti, G.M.; Govoni, S. Protein kinase C anchoring deficit in postmortem brains of Alzheimer's disease patients. *Exp. Neurol.* **1999**, *159*, 559–564. [CrossRef]
257. Battaini, F.; Pascale, A. Protein kinase C signal transduction regulation in physiological and pathological aging. *Ann. N. Y. Acad Sci.* **2005**, *1057*, 177–192. [CrossRef]
258. Liu, W.; Dou, F.; Feng, J.; Yan, Z. RACK1 is involved in β-amyloid impairment of muscarinic regulation of GABAergic transmission. *Neurobiol. Aging* **2011**, *32*, 1818–1826. [CrossRef] [PubMed]
259. Zhu, J.; Chen, X.; Song, Y.; Zhang, Y.; Zhou, L.; Wan, L. Deficit of RACK1 contributes to the spatial memory impairment via upregulating BECLIN1 to induce autophagy. *Life Sci.* **2016**, *151*, 115–121. [CrossRef]
260. Ni, H.; Rui, Q.; Xu, Y.; Zhu, J.; Gao, F.; Dang, B.; Li, D.; Gao, R.; Chen, G. RACK1 upregulation induces neuroprotection by activating the IRE1-XBP1 signaling pathway following traumatic brain injury in rats. *Exp. Neurol.* **2018**, *304*, 102–113. [CrossRef]
261. Amiri, S.; Azadmanesh, K.; Dehghan Shasaltaneh, M.; Mayahi, V.; Naghdi, N. The Implication of Androgens in the Presence of Protein Kinase C to Repair Alzheimer's Disease-Induced Cognitive Dysfunction. *Iran. Biomed. J.* **2020**, *24*, 64–80. [CrossRef]
262. He, W.; Tu, M.; Du, Y.; Li, J.; Pang, Y.; Dong, Z. Nicotine Promotes AβPP Nonamyloidogenic Processing via RACK1-Dependent Activation of PKC in SH-SY5Y-AβPP695 Cells. *J. Alzheimers Dis.* **2020**, *75*, 451–460. [CrossRef]
263. Liu, X.; Zhu, M.; Yang, X.; Wang, Y.; Qin, B.; Cui, C.; Chen, H.; Sang, A. Inhibition of RACK1 ameliorates choroidal neovascularization formation in vitro and in vivo. *Exp. Mol. Pathol.* **2016**, *100*, 451–459. [CrossRef] [PubMed]
264. Wang, F.; Yamauchi, M.; Muramatsu, M.; Osawa, T.; Tsuchida, R.; Shibuya, M. RACK1 regulates VEGF/Flt1-mediated cell migration via activation of a PI3K/Akt pathway. *J. Biol. Chem.* **2011**, *286*, 9097–9106. [CrossRef]
265. Almeida, J.; Costa, J.; Coelho, P.; Cea, V.; Galesio, M.; Noronha, J.P.; Diniz, M.S.; Prudêncio, C.; Soares, R.; Sala, C.; et al. Adipocyte proteome and secretome influence inflammatory and hormone pathways in glioma. *Metab. Brain Dis.* **2019**, *34*, 141–152. [CrossRef] [PubMed]
266. Zhang, X.; Liu, N.; Ma, D.; Liu, L.; Jiang, L.; Zhou, Y.; Zeng, X.; Li, J.; Chen, Q. Receptor for activated C kinase 1 (RACK1) promotes the progression of OSCC via the AKT/mTOR pathway. *Int. J. Oncol.* **2016**, *49*, 539–548. [CrossRef] [PubMed]
267. Marcelo, A.; Koppenol, R.; de Almeida, L.P.; Matos, C.A.; Nóbrega, C. Stress granules, RNA-binding proteins and polyglutamine diseases: Too much aggregation? *Cell Death Dis.* **2021**, *12*, 592. [CrossRef]
268. Jung, Y.D.; Kim, M.S.; Shin, B.A.; Chay, K.O.; Ahn, B.W.; Liu, W.; Bucana, C.D.; Gallick, G.E.; Ellis, L.M. EGCG, a major component of green tea, inhibits tumour growth by inhibiting VEGF induction in human colon carcinoma cells. *Br. J. Cancer* **2001**, *84*, 844–850. [CrossRef]
269. Sartippour, M.R.; Shao, Z.M.; Heber, D.; Beatty, P.; Zhang, L.; Liu, C.; Ellis, L.; Liu, W.; Go, V.L.; Brooks, M.N. Green tea inhibits vascular endothelial growth factor (VEGF) induction in human breast cancer cells. *J. Nutr.* **2002**, *132*, 2307–2311. [CrossRef]
270. Lanni, C.; Necchi, D.; Pinto, A.; Buoso, E.; Buizza, L.; Memo, M.; Uberti, D.; Govoni, S.; Racchi, M. Zyxin is a novel target for β-amyloid peptide: Characterization of its role in Alzheimer's pathogenesis. *J. Neurochem.* **2013**, *125*, 790–799. [CrossRef]

Disclaimer/Publisher's Note: The statements, opinions and data contained in all publications are solely those of the individual author(s) and contributor(s) and not of MDPI and/or the editor(s). MDPI and/or the editor(s) disclaim responsibility for any injury to people or property resulting from any ideas, methods, instructions or products referred to in the content.

MDPI
St. Alban-Anlage 66
4052 Basel
Switzerland
www.mdpi.com

International Journal of Molecular Sciences Editorial Office
E-mail: ijms@mdpi.com
www.mdpi.com/journal/ijms

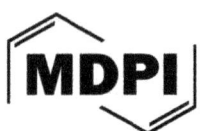

Disclaimer/Publisher's Note: The statements, opinions and data contained in all publications are solely those of the individual author(s) and contributor(s) and not of MDPI and/or the editor(s). MDPI and/or the editor(s) disclaim responsibility for any injury to people or property resulting from any ideas, methods, instructions or products referred to in the content.